CHIRAL CAPILLARY ELECTROPHORESIS IN CURRENT PHARMACEUTICAL AND BIOMEDICAL ANALYSIS

Authored by **Peter Mikuš**

Chiral Capillary Electrophoresis in Current Pharmaceutical and Biomedical Analysis
Authored by Peter Mikuš

Published by InTech
Janeza Trdine 9, 51000 Rijeka, Croatia

Publishing Process Manager Davor Vidic

Technical Editor Teodora Smiljanic

Cover Designer InTech Design Team

Additional hard copies can be obtained from orders@intechopen.com

Chiral Capillary Electrophoresis in Current Pharmaceutical and Biomedical Analysis,
Authored by Peter Mikuš
p. cm.
ISBN 978-953-51-0657-9

Meet the author

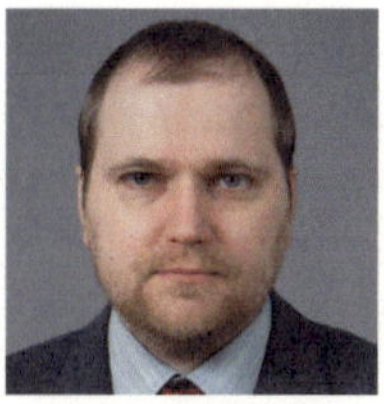

Dr Peter Mikuš (PM) received his M.Sc. in Analytical Chemistry in 1995 from the Faculty of Natural Sciences Comenius University in Bratislava, Slovak Republic. He received his Ph.D. in Analytical Chemistry from the same Faculty in 2002 under the supervision of Prof. Dr. Dusan Kaniansky, an excellent analyst and expert in the field of instrumental development of capillary electomigration techniques. During his Ph.D. study, in 1997, PM joined academic and research center, namely Consiglio Nazionale delle Ricerche, Istituto di Cromatografia in Rome, Italy. Here, he made research for a period of three months under the supervision of Prof. Dr. Salvatore Fanali, an expert in the field of advanced methodology and application of chiral capillary electomigration methods. From 2002 he worked at the Faculty of Pharmacy Comenius University as a teacher and research scientist. PM received his Assoc. Prof. qualification in Pharmaceutical Chemistry from the Faculty of Pharmacy Comenius University in 2007. Currently, he is Assistant Professor, the Head of the Department of Pharmaceutical Analysis and Nuclear Pharmacy, Vice-dean for Foreign Relations and Development of the Faculty, and Departmental Erasmus Coordinator at the Faculty of Pharmacy Comenius University.

Contents

Published by InTech with the financial support from
the Faculty of Pharmacy Comenius University.

Preface

Although the technologies on chiral/enantiomer separation and stereoselective analysis have matured in the past ca. 20 years, the development of new, even more advanced chiral separation materials, mechanisms and methods still belong to the more challenging tasks in separation science and analytical chemistry. An analysis of recent trends indicates that capillary electrophoresis (CE) can show real advantages over chromatographic methods in ultratrace chiral determination of biologically active ionogenic compounds in complex matrices, including mostly biological ones. This is due to the extremely high separation efficiency of CE, as well as numerous new chiral selectors providing a wide range of selectivities for CE. Along with these tools, there are many applicable in-capillary electromigration effects in CE (countercurrent migration, stacking effects, etc.) enhancing significantly separability and, moreover, enabling effective sample preparation (preconcentration, purification, analyte derivatization). Other possible on-line combinations of CE, such as column coupled CE-CE techniques and implementation of nonelectrophoretic techniques (extraction, membrane filtration, flow injection, etc.) into CE, offer additional approaches for highly effective sample preparation and separation. Chiral CE matured to a highly flexible and compatible technique enabling its hyphenation with powerful detection systems allows for extremely sensitive detection (e.g., laser induced fluorescence) and/or structural characterization of analytes (e.g., mass spectrometry). Within the last decade, more and less conventional analytical on-line approaches have been effectively utilized in this field, and their practical potentialities have been demonstrated in many application examples in the literature.

In the present scientific monograph, three main aspects of chiral analysis of biologically active compounds are highlighted and supported by a theoretical description. This comprehensive integrated view on the topic is composed from the sections dealing with (i) progressive enantioseparation approaches and new enantioselective agents, (ii) in-capillary sample preparation (preconcentration, purification, derivatization) and (iii) detection possibilities related to enhanced sensitivity of quantitative determination and/or structural characterization of analysed chiral molecules. The section dealing with the chiral separations is inserted prior to the section dealing with the sample preparation in this book. This is logical, because achieving chiral resolution is a prerequisite in chiral research and the optimization of chiral resolution is a starting point within the development of a new chiral method. Then, a sample preparation and detection can be optimized, method validated, and finally, applied.

Although this book deals with the advanced chiral CE, it should be realized that this methodology could be understood more generally as the advanced CE modified with a selector (chiral as well as achiral) providing a considerably higher application potential. This generalization is justified realizing the parallels between the chiral and achiral selector-mediated separation systems in terms of (i) the implementations of the selectors and separation mechanisms, (ii) compatibility of sample preparation, separation and detection steps in the presence of the selector, and (iii) the application of the CE method modified with the selector. Therefore, the reader can advantageously use this book as a guide when proposing the strategy for the advanced chiral analysis, as well as achiral one supported by the complexing equilibria.

The author wishes that the readers obtain an integral view on the topic, some new knowledge, a good source of the relevant thematic reviews, as well as original research works on the topic, and hopes the readers gain inspiration for solving their own problems when reading this book.

The author would like to thank the book reviewers, excellent chemists and analysts, Prof. Dr. Ladislav Novotný, Assoc. Prof. Dr. Jozef Polonský, Prof. Dr. Emil Havránek and Prof. Dr. Milan Remko, for their valuable advice and suggestions on the manuscript during its preparation and before its final editing and publication.

Peter Mikuš
Faculty of Pharmacy, Comenius University, Bratislava,
Slovak Republic

1

Introduction and Overview

1.1 Demands in chiral bioanalysis

It is well-established that in most cases of chiral drugs the pharmacological activity is restricted to one of the enantiomers (eutomer), whereas the other enantiomer (distomer) has either no effect or may show side effects - even being toxic [Ward T.J. & Ward K.D., 2010; Gilpin R.K. & Gilpin C.S., 2009; Bartos & Gorog, 2009; Gübitz & Schmid, 2008; Tzanavaras, 2010; Christodoulou, 2010; Zeng A.G. et al., 2010]. Information on the qualitative and quantitative composition of biologically active chiral compounds (enantiomers, diastereoisomers) in various real matrices, such as biological, pharmaceutical, environmental, food, beverage, etc., is required by control authorities and it is relevant in particular research areas, [see e.g., Hashim, 2010]. Enantioselective drug absorption, distribution, metabolism, elimination or liberation studies are included among the most advanced analytical problems being solved in pharmaceutical and biomedical research. This is due to (i) the multicomponent character of biological matrices (many potentially interfering compounds per sample), (ii) a very low concentration of the analyte(s) (pg-ng/mL) among the matrix constituents present in the sample in a wide concentration scale (pg-mg/mL), (iii) identical physicochemical properties of enantiomers in an achiral environment and in many cases (iv) limited/minute amounts of the sample [Maier et al., 2001; Camilleri, 1991; Bonato, 2003; Lin C.C. et al., 2003; Scriba, 2003, 2011; Van Eeckhaut & Michotte, 2006; Hernández et al., 2008, 2010; Caslavska & Thormann, 2011].

1.2 Possibilities of capillary electrophoresis in chiral bioanalysis

Among high performance separation techniques, high performance liquid chromatography (HPLC) is the most matured, universal, robust, sensitive, selective, and therefore, the most frequently used technique (also) for the analysis of biomarkers, drugs and their metabolites in biological samples, as it can be seen from many application examples, [see e.g., Maier et al., 2001; Camilleri, 1991; Bonato, 2003; Lin C.C. et al., 2003; Scriba, 2003; Van Eeckhaut & Michotte, 2006; Hernández et al., 2008; Konieczna et al., 2010; Gatti & Gioia, 2008; El-Enany et al., 2007]. On the other hand, among the benefits of capillary electrophoresis (CE), pronounced especially in the chiral field, we can count its high separation efficiency, versatility and simplicity in the creation of (chiral) separation systems, short analysis time, good compatibility with aqueous samples and low consumption of chiral selector (low cost of enantioselective analyses) [Chankvetadze, 2007; Altria K. et al., 2006; Ward T.J. & Baker, 2008; Suntornsuk, 2010; Preinerstorfer et al., 2009; Bartos & Gorog, 2009; Ward T.J. & Ward K.D., 2010; Frost et al., 2010; Scriba, 2011]. Moreover, an analysis of recent trends indicates that CE can show real advantages over chromatographic methods, especially when a high resolution power, high sensitivity and low limit of detection/quantitation is ensured. CE meeting these criteria is directly applicable in the area of (chiral) analysis of low molecular ionic (and in some cases also neutral) compounds, such as drugs, their metabolites, biomarkers, etc., present in complex matrices such as biological samples [Mikuš & Maráková, 2009; Bonato, 2003; Lin C.C. et al., 2003; Scriba, 2003, 2011; Van Eeckhaut & Michotte, 2006; Hernández et al., 2008, 2010; Kraly et al., 2006; Caslavska & Thormann, 2011; Kitagawa & Otsuka, 2011].

The high resolution power and low limit of detection/quantitation are provided in CE itself by (i) an extremely high peak efficiency and (ii) wide range of various applicable electromigration effects and electrophoretic experimental modes enhancing selectivity and/or decreasing limit of detection (LOD) [Mikuš & Maráková, 2009]. Among such effects/modes, the (countercurrent) movement of analytes/selectors via electroosmotic flow (EOF), countercurrent migration of charged analyte and oppositely charged selector, in-capillary stacking effects for the analyte preconcentration, removing of undesired compounds by electrokinetic injection of the sample and/or by electronic switching in on-line coupled electrophoretic systems are of the highest importance [Lin C.H. & Kaneta, 2004; Hernández et al., 2008, 2010; Chankvetadze, 1997; Chankvetadze et al., 2001; Scriba 2002; Simpson et al., 2008; Kaniansky & Marák, 1990; Danková et al., 1999; Fanali et al., 2000; Breadmore et al., 2009; Malá et al., 2009; Mikuš & Maráková, 2010].

CE matured to a highly flexible and compatible technique also enables (iii) on-line combinations of CE with nonelectrophoretic techniques (e.g., extraction, membrane filtration, microdialysis, flow injection, etc.) offering additional approaches for the highly effective sample preparation (especially sample clean-up, but also preconcentration) and separation [Breadmore et al., 2009; Chen Y. et al., 2008; Wu X.Z., 2003; Kataoka, 2003; Lü W.J. et al., 2009; de Jong et al., 2006; Mikuš & Maráková, 2010].

The utilization of unique methodological effects and modes mentioned in (ii) and (iii) can significantly enhance analytical potential and the practical use of conventional (single-column) CE, solving its weakest points, such as a poor sensitivity and high concentration LOD, high risk of capillary overloading by major sample matrix constituents and peak overlapping, by numerous matrix constituents. In this way, the need for off-line sample preparation (isolation and concentration of analytes), especially when complex matrices are used (such as proteinic blood derived samples, ionic urine samples, tissue homogenates etc.), can be overcome.

Possibilities to combine CE with various detection techniques are comparable with chromatographic techniques. The high flexibility and compatibility of CE can be demonstrated by on-column and end-column coupling (hyphenation) with powerful detection systems covering demands on extremely sensitive detection (e.g., laser induced fluorescence, LIF), as well as structural characterization of analytes (e.g., mass spectrometry, MS) [Hernández et al., 2008, 2010; Swinney & Bornhop, 2000; Hempel G., 2000; Kok et al., 1998]. Such hyphenation is an essential part of advanced CE methods applied in modern highly demanding analytical research [Mikuš & Maráková, 2009].

1.3 Aim and scope

This scientific monograph deals with the theory and practice of the advanced chiral analysis of biologically active substances, beginning with the chiral separation, continuing with sample preparation and finishing with detection. The knowledge and findings from the review and research papers (involving also the author's works) included here give an integral and comprehensive view on the progressive performance of the chiral separations, analyses in complex matrices, pharmacokinetic and metabolic studies of drugs and analysis of biomarkers in various models and real matrices. The cited papers cover mainly the period from the year 2000 until now, although several former illustrative works are also included [see extensive reviews, e.g., Mikuš & Maráková, 2009; Scriba, 2003, 2011; Bonato, 2003; Lin C.C. et al., 2003; Hernández et al., 2008, 2010; Ward T.J. & Hamburg, 2004; Natishan, 2005; Van Eeckhaut & Michotte, 2006; Ha P.T. et al., 2006; Gübitz & Schmid, 2006, 2007; Caslavska & Thormann, 2011]. Mikuš and Maráková [Mikuš & Maráková, 2009] recently provided a review on the advanced capillary electrophoresis for the chiral analysis of drugs, metabolites and biomarkers in biological samples discussing chiral, sample preparation and detection aspects supported by the application examples. Other extensive review papers by Bonato [Bonato, 2003], Caslavska and Thormann [Caslavska & Thormann, 2011] and Scriba [Scriba, 2011] cover recent advances in the determination of enantiomeric drugs and their metabolites in biological matrices (e.g., biological fluids, tissues, microsomal preparations), as well as pharmaceuticals by CE mediated microanalysis and provide, besides many examples, also a detailed background on this topic. Other beneficial review papers in this area include refs. by Lin et al. [Lin C.C. et al., 2003] discussing recent progress in pharmacokinetic applications of CE, Scriba [Scriba, 2003] giving a view on pharmaceutical and biomedical applications of chiral CE and capillary electrochromatography (CEC), Hernández et al. [Hernández et al., 2008, 2010] giving an update on sensitive chiral analysis by CE in a variety of real samples including complex biological matrices. Several other review papers dealing with pharmaceutical and biomedical applications of chiral electromigration methods have also appeared in recent years [Van Eeckhaut & Michotte, 2006; Ward T.J. & Hamburg, 2004; Natishan, 2005; Ha et al., 2006; Gübitz & Schmid, 2006, 2007].

The aim of this scientific monograph is to demonstrate comprehensively the current position of CE in the area of advanced chiral analysis of biologically active substances in samples with complex matrices (mainly biological). Therefore, the aim is not only to illustrate this by various practical applications, but, especially, to highlight and critically evaluate the progressive of the analytical approaches employed/applied in such examples. These, included in the present book, cover new findings in (i) chiral CE separation approaches (progressive arrangements of separation systems, new chiral selectors), (ii) preconcentration, purification and derivatization pretreatment of complex samples (on-line combinations of various sample preparation techniques with chiral CE) and (iii) detection monitoring of qualitative and quantitative composition of separated electrophoretic zones in complex samples (sensitive detection and/or structural evaluation of analytes). Such advanced approaches, playing a key role in the automatization and miniaturization of analytical procedures along with providing maximum analytical information, are comprehensively described in terms of basic theory, advantages and limitations, and documented by representative application examples.

2

Advanced Chiral Separation

2.1 Chiral electromigration modes and enantioselective agents - introduction

Chiral separations by CE can be performed either indirectly, using a chiral derivatization agent forming irreversible diastereomeric pairs which can be resolved under achiral conditions, or directly, using chiral selectors as additives to the electrolyte, where reversible diastereomeric associates, enantiomer-chiral selector, are created that can be subsequently transformed into mobility differences of the individual stereoisomers [Chankvetadze & Blaschke, 2001; Rizzi, 2001]. In capillary electrochromatography (CEC), a hybrid CE / HPLC technique (i.e., CE with stationary phase), chiral stationary phases or chiral mobile phase additives are applied in enantioseparations [Huo & Kok, 2008].

Several disadvantages of the indirect enantioseparation approach, such as (i) the need of a functional group which can be derivatized, (ii) the derivatization reagent has to be of high enantiomeric purity, (iii) the derivatization represents an additional time consuming step with a risk of racemization under the reaction conditions, result in it being rarely used. Therefore, it is not surprising that only a few new chiral derivatization procedures, employing new chiral derivatization reagents, have been developed recently [Cheng J. & Kang J., 2006; Zhao S. et al., 2006a, 2006b].

More attractive and therefore much more frequently used are direct enantioseparations representing elegant and simple solutions in the majority of problems in chiral analysis. See, for instance, recent (2000-2011) chiral separations of drugs, their metabolites and biomarkers in various (mostly biological) samples listed in Tables 2.1 and 3.1 of this book (these tables are divided according to the manner of a sample preparation step, i.e., off- or on-line). In this chapter and Table 2.1 a chiral separation step is accompanied by a conventional off-line sample pretreatment and the chiral separation mechanism itself is highlighted. The latest fundamental reviews on chiral separations are given by Ward T.J. and Ward K.D. [Ward T.J. & Ward K.D., 2010] and Scriba [Scriba, 2011]. The papers by Gübitz and Schmid [Gübitz & Schmid, 2000a, 2007, 2008], Eeckhaut and Michotte [Van Eeckhaut & Michotte, 2006] and Preinerstorfer et al. [Preinerstorfer et al., 2009] provide detailed overviews on the different classes of chiral selectors, including newly introduced ones, that are used in common CE techniques, but also in MEEKC and MCE.

The following subsections summarize (i) basic electromigration modes and their possibilities in chiral separations, as well as (ii) basic characteristics of different groups of chiral selectors - giving a view on their complexing abilities (types of useful analytes) and advantages and limitations when introduced into CE. Recent applications in the enantioseparation of drugs in biological samples are discussed in the text and tabulated.

2.2 Electromigration techniques in chiral separations

Effective chiral separations can be performed by a wide range of electromigration techniques that provide a great variety of applicable separation mechanisms and, by that, a high application potential both analytically and preparatively. For the basic instrumental scheme of CE see Figure 2.1.

The latest review on advances of enantioseparations in CE is given by Lu and Chen [Lu H.A. & Chen G.N., 2011] and Scriba [Scriba, 2011]. Gübitz and Schmid [Gübitz & Schmid, 2000a, 2007, 2008] show recent progress in chiral separation principles in various CE techniques, namely capillary zone electrophoresis (CZE), capillary gel electrophoresis (CGE), isotachophoresis (ITP), isoelectric focusing (IEF), capillary electrokinetic chromatography (EKC) and capillary electrochromatography (CEC). The authors included into their latest review [Gübitz & Schmid, 2008] microchip CE (MCE). Among the most recent reviews also belong refs. by Gebauer et al. [Gebauer et al., 2009, 2011], Silva [Silva, 2009] and Ryan et al. [Ryan et al., 2009] describing recent advances in the methodology, optimization and application of ITP, micellar EKC (MEKC) and microemulsion EKC (MEEKC), respectively. Preinerstorfer et al. [Preinerstorfer et al., 2009] included, besides common CE techniques, also MEEKC and MCE.

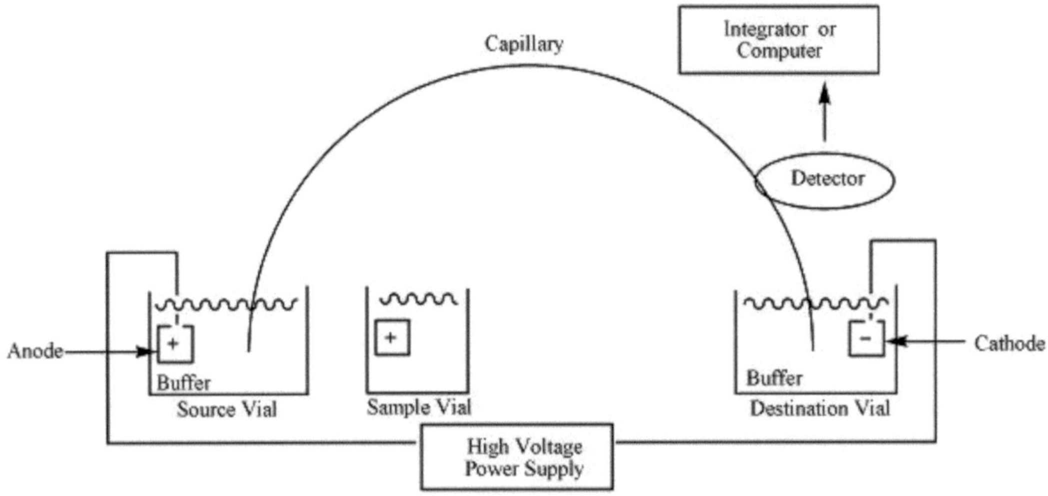

Figure 2.1. Instrumental scheme of capillary electrophoresis system.

Analyte	Separation method	Chiral selector[a]	pH	Biological sample	Sample preparation method[b]	Detection	LOQ	Application	Ref.
Amino acids, mexiletine	CEC	β-CD derivatives CSP	5.5-8.5	Human plasma	SPE	UV		Spiked samples	Li Y. et al., 2010
Catechin isomers	CDEKC	β-CD		Human plasma	PP	UV (high sensitivity detection cell)	4.1 and 1.5 ng/mL (LOD)	Real samples	El-Hady & El-Maali, 2008
Cetirizine and hydroxyzine	Polymeric EKC	maltodextrin	2.0	Human plasma	LLE	UV	10 ng/mL (LOD)	Spiked samples	Nojavan & Fakhari, 2011
Dioxopromethazine hydrochloride	CDEKC	β-CD	2.5	Human urine	LLE	ECL	4.0×10^{-6} M (LOD)	Spiked samples	Li X. et al., 2009
Ofloxacin	CDEKC	M-β-CD	2.8	Caco-cells	LLE, EK	UV	11.4-10.8 ng/mL	Spiked samples	Awadallah et al., 2003
Citalopram, desmethyl-citalopram	CDEKC	S-β-CD + acetonitrile	2.5	Plasma	LPME (19-31x)	UV	4.4-11.2 ng/mL	Clinical samples	Andersen et al., 2003
Primaquine, carboxyprimaquine	EKC	Maltodextrin	3.0	Mitochondrial fraction of liver of rats, plasma	LLE	DAD	40-100 ng/mL	Spiked samples	Bortocan & Bonato, 2004
Hydroxychloroquine and its metabolites	CDEKC	S-β-CD + HP-β-CD	9.0	Liver homogenate, plasma	LLE	DAD	129 ng/mL	Spiked samples	Cardoso et al., 2006
Propaphenone and its metabolites	CDEKC	S-β-CD + methanol	2.0	Serum	LLE	UV	10-12 ng/mL (LOD)	Spiked samples	Afshar & Thormann, 2006

Ketoprofen	CDEKC	HTM-β-CD	5.0	Serum	LLE	UV	500-1000 ng/mL	Pharmacokinetic study	Glowka & Karzniewicz, 2004a
Indobufen	CDEKC	HTM-β-CD	5.0	Serum	LLE	UV	200 ng/mL	Pharmacokinetic study	Glowka & Karzniewicz, 2004b
Apomorfine	CDEKC	HP-β-CD	3.0	Caco-cells	Direct injection	DAD	0.5×10^{-6} M	Spiked samples	Ha et al., 2004a
Lactic acid	CDEKC	HP-β-CD	7.0	Plasma	PP (10x)	DAD	$15\text{-}20 \times 10^{-6}$ M	Spiked samples	Tan et al., 2005
Serine	CDEKC	HP-γ-CD + D(+)-glucose	10.0	Neuronal cells (rat's brain)	Microdialysis, AD	LIF	0.3×10^{-6} M	Clinical samples	Quan et al., 2005
Methadone	CDEKC	S-β-CD	5.0	Serum	LLE, EK	UV	-	Clinical samples	Esteban et al., 2004
Mirtazapine and its metabolites	CDEKC	CM-β-CD	2.5	Plasma	SPE (37,5x)	DAD	5 ng/mL	Clinical samples	Mandrioli et al., 2004
Anisodamine	CDEKC	CM-γ-CD	2.5	Plasma (rabbits)	LLE, EK	UV	40-60 ng/mL	Pharmacokinetic study	Fan et al., 2004
Salbutamol	NACE (CDEKC)	HDAS-β-CD	6.0	Urine	SPE	DAD	375 ng/mL	Spiked samples	Servais et al., 2004
Metamphetamine and related compounds	CDEKC	HDAS-β-CD	1.7	Urine	LLE	MS	5 ng/mL	Spiked samples	Iio et al., 2005
t-tramadol, t-O-demethyltramadol	CDEKC	SBE-β-CD	2.5	Plasma, urine	LLE	UV	1.25 ng/mL	Pharmacokinetic study	Liu H.C. et al., 2004
Labetalol	CDEKC	ODAS-γ-CD, HDAS-β-CD	2.5	Plasma	SPE	DAD	-	Spiked samples	Goel et al., 2004
Deprenyl metabolites	CDEKC	DM-β-CD + CM-β-CD	2.7	Urine	SPE	UV	$0.1\text{-}0.5 \times 10^{-6}$ M	Metabolic study	Szökö et al., 2004
Mirtazapine and its metabolites	CDEKC	CE-β-CD	2.5	Urine	LPME, EH	DAD	62.5 ng/mL	Pharmacokinetic study	de Santana et al., 2008

Hydroxychloroquine and its metabotites	CDEKC	S-β-CD + HP-β-CD	9.0	Urine	LPME	DAD	10-21 ng/mL	Pharmacokinetic study	de Oliveira et al., 2007
Tioridazine 5-sulfoxide	CDEKC	HP-β-CD + S-β-CD	3.0	Plasma	LLE	DAD	250 ng/mL	Spiked samples	de Gaitani et al., 2003
Baclofen	CDEKC	S-β-CD	9.5	Plasma	PP, AD	LIF	$50x10^{-9}$ M (LOD)	Spiked samples	Kavran-Belin et al., 2005
Disopyramide	CDEKC	S-β-CD	4.5	Plasma	LLE	ECL	$8x10^{-8}$-1.10^{-7} M (LOD)	Spiked samples	Fang L. et al., 2006
Amlodipine	CDEKC	HP-β-CD	2.5	Serum	LLE	UV	700 ng/mL	Clinical samples	Wang R. et al., 2007
Ibuprofen and its metabolites	CDEKC	HTM-β-CD	5.0	Urine, plasma	SPE	UV	110 ng/mL (plasma), 1.0-$1.1x10^{3}$ ng/mL (urine)	Pharmacokinetic study	Glowka & Karazniewicz, 2007
Cetirizine	CDEKC	S-β-CD	8.7	Plasma	LLE	UV	500 ng/mL (LOD)	Spiked samples	Chou et al., 2008
Warfarin	MEKC	Polysodium-N-undecenoyl-L,L-leucyl-valinate	6.0	Plasma	SPE	MS	100 ng/mL (LOD)	Clinical samples	Hou, J. et al., 2007
Ketamine, norketamine	CDEKC	S-β-CD	2.5	Plasma (horse)	LLE	DAD	10 ng/mL (LOD)	Clinical samples	Theurillat et al., 2005
Amphetamine derivates	CDEKC	S-γ-CD	2.5	Plasma	LLE	MS	100-400 ng/mL (LOD)	Spiked samples	Rudaz et al., 2005
Salbutamol	NACE (CDEKC)	HDAS-β-CD		Urine	SPE	MS	18-20 ng/mL	Spiked samples	Servais et al., 2006

3,4-metylendioxy-metamphetamine and its metabolites	CDMEKC	β-CD + sodium cholate	2.3	Urine	LLE	LIF	-	Spiked samples	Huang Y.S. et al., 2003
Hydroxy-mebendazole, hydroxyamino-mebendazole, aminomebendazole	CDEKC	S-β-CD	4.2	Plasma	LLE	UV	10-40 ng/mL (LOD)	Clinical samples	Theurillat & Thormann, 2008
Cinchona alkaloids	CDEKC	HDM-β-CD	5.0	Urine	SPE (10x)	DAD	100 ng/mL	Clinical samples	Tsimachidis et al., 2008
Ketamine and its metabolites	CDEKC	S-β-CD (multiple isomer)	2.5	Plasma, urine	LLE	DAD	-	Metabolic study	Theurillat et al., 2007
Methadone	CDEKC	S-γ-CD	2.5	Plasma	LLE-EK, PP-HD	MS	0.5 ng/mL (LLE-EK), 250 ng/mL (PP-HD)	Clinical samples	Schappler et al., 2008
Methadone	CDEKC	HS-γ-CD	4.5	Oral fluids	LLE	DAD	7.6-8.1 ng/mL	Clinical samples	Martins et al., 2008
Mirtazapine and its metabolites	CEC	Vancomycin CSP	6.0	Urine	SPE	DAD	1000-2000 ng/mL	Spiked samples	Aturki et al., 2007
Albendazole sulfoxide	CDEKC	S-β-CD	7.0	Plasma, saliva	LLE	UV, LIF	100 ng/mL (LOD)	Clinical samples	Prost et al., 2002
Phenprocoumone	CDEKC	α-CD	5.4	Urine	Direct injection	LIF	200 ng/mL	Clinical samples	Chankvetadze et al., 2001b
Baclofen	CDEKC	α-CD	9.5	Plasma	PP, AD	LIF	10 ng/mL (LOD)	Spiked samples	Chiang et al., 2001
Clenbuterol	CDEKC	DM-β-CD	2.5	Plasma	SPE	MS	740 ng/mL	Spiked samples	Toussaint et al., 2001
Tramadol and its metabolites	CDEKC	SBE-β-CD	4.0	Plasma	LLE	MS	-	Metabolic study	Rudaz et al., 2000

Ofloxacin and its metabolites	CDEKC	SB-β-CD	2.0	Urine	Direct injection	LIF	100-250 ng/mL	Metabolic study	Horstkötter & Blaschke, 2001
Methadone and its metabolites	CDEKC	CM-β-CD	4.0	Serum	LLE (10x)	MS	-	Clinical samples	Cherkaoui et al., 2001
Benzoporfyrine derivate mono and diacid	MEKC	Sodium cholate	9.2	Serum, microsomes	PP, SPE	LIF	2180-3500 ng/mL	Metabolic study	Penget al., 2002
Tramadol	CDEKC	CM-β-CD + M-β-CD	10.0	Urine	Direct injection	LIF	100 ng/mL	Pharmacokinetic study	Soetebeer et al., 2001
Carvedilol	CDEKC	succinyl-β-CD + M-α-CD	3.0	Plasma	LLE	LIF	1.56 ng/mL	Pharmacokinetic study	Behn et al., 2001
Chloroquine, deethylchloroquine	CDEKC	HP-γ-CD, CM-γ-CD, S-γ-CD	9.65	Plasma	LLE	LIF	0.5 ng/mL (LOD)	Clinical samples	Müller & Blaschke, 2000

Table 2.1. Chiral CE determinations of biologically active compounds in various biological matrices employing conventional (off-line) sample preparation.

[a] Mixed selector systems are indicated by a plus sign. Charge of ionizable chiral selectors is obvious from pH (next column).

[b] Preconcentration factor is given in brackets.

ITP = isotachophoresis, EKC = electrokinetic chromatography, MEKC = micellar electrokinetic chromatography, CDEKC = cyclodextrin mediated electrokinetic chromatography, CDMEKC = cyclodextrin mediated micellar electrokinetic chromatography, NACE = non-aqueous capillary electrophoresis, MCE = electrophoresis on microchip, CEC = capillary electrochromatography, S-β-CD = sulphated-β–CD, S-γ–CD = sulphated-γ-CD, HS-γ-CD = highly sulphated-γ-CD, M-α-CD = methyl-α-CD, M-β-CD = methyl-β-CD, DM-β–CD = dimethyl-β–CD, CM-β–CD = carboxymethyl-β-CD, CM-γ-CD = carboxymethyl-γ-CD, CE-β-CD = carboxyethyl-β-CD, HP-β-CD = hydroxypropyl-β-CD, HP-γ-CD = hydroxypropyl-γ-CD, HTM-β-CD = heptakistrimethyl-β-CD, SBE-β-CD = sulfobuthylether-β-CD, SB-β-CD = sulfobuthyl-β-CD, HDAS-β-CD = heptakisdiacethylsulfo-β-CD, ODAS-γ-CD = oktakisdiacethylsulfo-γ-CD, AD = analyte derivatization, EH = enzymatic hydrolysis, HD = hydrodynamic injection, EK = electrokinetic injection, FESS = field-enhanced sample stacking, LVSS = large volume sample stacking, SPE = solid-phase extraction, LLE = liquid-liquid extraction, LPME = liquid-phase microextraction, PP = protein precipitation, DAD = diode array detection, UV-ultraviolet (absorbance detection), ECL = electrochemiluminiscent detection, LIF = laser induced fluorescent detection, MS = mass spectrometry, LOQ = limit of quantification, LOD = limit of detection.

2.2.1 Capillary electrophoresis

The unique properties of CE in terms of enantioresolution, due to a combination of extremely high separation efficiency (N) and various electomigration effects, are comprehensively summarized by Chankvetadze [Chankvetadze, 2007] and generally described by the Equation 2.1 [Giddings, 1969]:

$$R_S = \frac{1}{4}\sqrt{N}\frac{\Delta\mu}{\mu_{av}} \qquad 2.1$$

where μ_{av} is the effective averaged mobility $\{\mu_{av}=1/2(\mu_1+\mu_2)\}$ and $\Delta\mu$ is the mobility difference ($\Delta\mu=\mu_1-\mu_2$).

For enantioresolutions by CE the effective mobilities of the enantiomers have to be different ($\mu_1\neq\mu_2$). This occurs due to (i) a difference in the complex formation constants of the enantiomer-chiral selector complexes ($K_1\neq K_2$) and (ii) a difference in the mobility of the enantiomer-chiral selector complexes ($\mu_{c1}\neq\mu_{c2}$), as well as the mobility of the free enantiomer and the enantiomer-selector complex ($\mu_f\neq\mu_{c1}$, $\mu_f\neq\mu_{c2}$), as it can be seen from the mobility difference ($\Delta\mu$) model (Equation 2.2) developed for two enantiomers (*1, 2*) and the concentration of selector (C) by Wren and Rowe [Wren & Rowe, 1992, 1993]:

$$\Delta\mu = \mu_1 - \mu_2 = \frac{\mu_f + \mu_{c1}K_1[C]}{1+K_1[C]} - \frac{\mu_f + \mu_{c2}K_2[C]}{1+K_2[C]} \qquad 2.2$$

It is apparent from this equation that CE offers many possibilities to manipulate enantioresolution via electromigration and complexing effects. This is also discussed in detail in the following subsections.

Besides electromigration and complexing effects, flow counterbalancing [Chankvetadze et al., 1999], as a combination of the bulk flow moving with the opposite migration of both a chiral selector and a chiral analyte, is another interesting possibility to effectively manipulate enantioresolution that will be briefly mentioned later.

The great advantages of CE in terms of the arrangement of the chiral separation system flexibly and simply are: (i) creation of continuous (CZE) and discontinuous / gradient (ITP, IEF) electrolyte systems providing a high variety of separation mechanisms. For basic CE modes see Figure 2.2. Here, interesting separation, as well as preseparation, possibilities are given by the differences in arrangement and diffusion properties of electrophoretic zones. (ii) Implementation of chiral selector(s) or, in other words, chiral pseudostationary phase(s), merely by their dissolving in such separation systems, creating a proper chiral separation environment. An extremely high resolution power of chiral CE can be amplified further by a large excess of a chiral selector dissolved in the electrolyte solution compared to the separation techniques with immobilized chiral selectors (CEC, HPLC) [Chankvetadze & Blaschke, 2001].

In fact, enantiomeric separations performed by CE may be included in an EKC mode because the discrimination of the enantiomers of a chiral compound is due to their different interactions with a chiral selector, that is, enantiomers are distributed in a different way between the bulk solution and the chiral selector according to a chromatographic (interaction) mechanism. So the electrophoretic and chromatographic principles are acting simultaneously in EKC (notice that is principally true not only for chiral but also achiral separations modified by a selector). Therefore, in this monograph we consider all the enantiomeric separations performed in the zone electrophoretic mode to be EKC separations with the exception of chiral ITP and chiral IEF separations (no alternative terms are introduced in the literature).

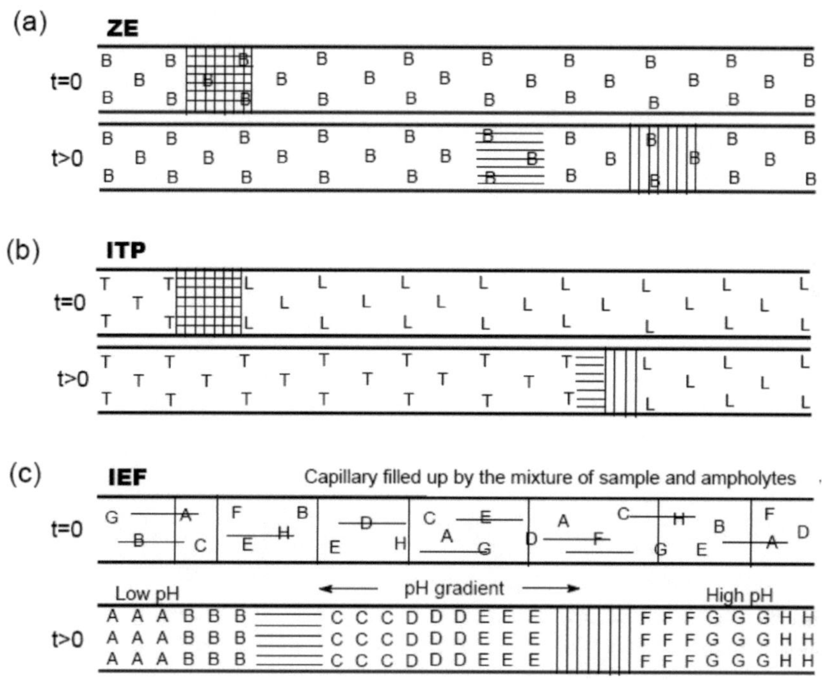

Figure 2.2. Separation principles in capillary electrophoresis: (a) zone electrophoresis (ZE), where B is background electrolyte, (b) isotachophoresis (ITP), where L is leading electrolyte and T is terminating electrolyte, with different electrophoretic mobilities of these electrolytes, (c) isoelectric focusing (IEF), where A-H are ampholytic electrolytes, with different pI values of these electrolytes. Reprinted from ref. [Boček, 1987].

2.2.1.1 Interactions in enantioseparations and their manipulation

Thanks to a great variety of applicable chiral selectors with different physico chemical properties and complexing abilities (see section 2.3), chiral CE separation systems with high performance variability can be created. Here, several basic enantioresolution mechanisms can be recognized that are based on:

- Inclusion (host-guest) complexation {cyclodextrins (CDs), crown ethers (CWEs)},
- Ligand-exchange (metal complexes),

- Affinity interactions (proteinic biopolymers, macrocyclic antibiotics),
- Polymeric complexation (saccharidic biopolymers),
- Micelle / microemulsion solubilization (micelles, micelle polymers, oils),
- Ion-pairing (ionic compounds in non-aqueous media).

Thus, the separations of enantiomeric couples with a wide range of polarities, charges and sizes can be easily accomplished [Gübitz & Schmid, 2000a, 2007, 2008; Preinerstorfer et al., 2009; Gebauer et al., 2009, 2011; Silva, 2009; Ryan et al., 2009], see examples in section 2.4, Table 2.1 and Table 3.1.

On the other hand, very subtle differences/modifications of the structure within the same group of chiral selectors also can provide significant differences in (enantio)selectivity, see Table 2.2 (notice differences in CE enantioresolutions under the same conditions, but different chiral selector – differing in one methyl group in their molecules). This demonstrates another powerful tool to manipulate (enantio)selectivity from the complex forming point of view in CE enantioseparations.

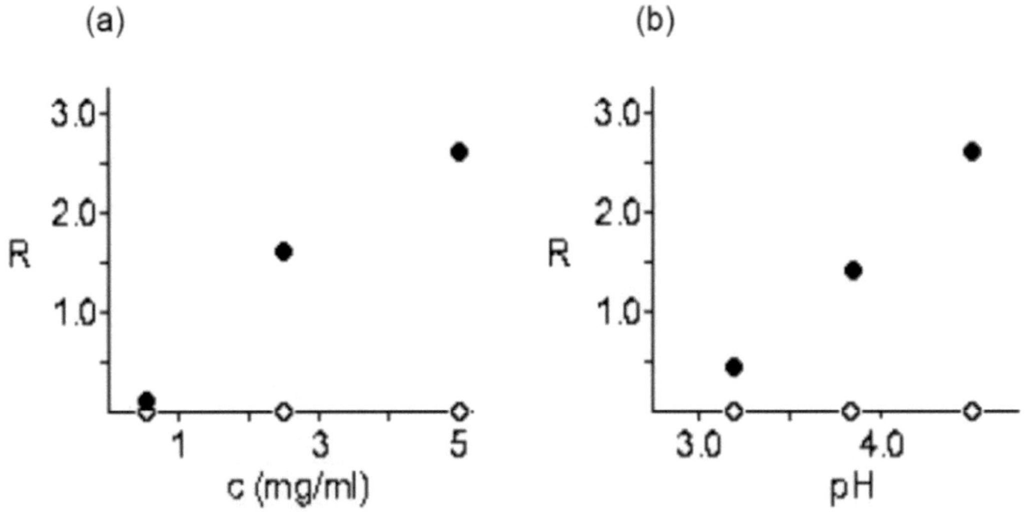

Figure 2.3. Influence of pH and concentration of chiral selector on the resolution of pheniramine enantiomers demonstrating the effectivity of charged chiral selector and countercurrent separation mechanism in EKC enantioseparation. (a) The concentration dependences at 0.5, 2.5 and 5.0 mg/mL concentrations of CE-β-CD (•) and native β-CD (○) were obtained at pH 4.5 (20 mM ε-aminocaproic acid - acetic acid BGE); (b) the pH dependences were obtained at 5 mg/mL concentrations of the CDs and the glycine- or ε-aminocaproic acid – acetic acid BGEs with pH 3.2-3.8 or 4.5, respectively. 0.2% (w/v) methyl-hydroxyethylcellulose served as an EOF suppressor in BGE. The driving current was stabilized at 100-120 μA. CE-β-CD = carboxyethyl-β-cyclodextrin. Reprinted from ref. [Mikuš et al., 2005a].

Analyte	Electrolyte system				
DNP-D,L-amino acid	R [ES2]	R [ES3]	R [ES4]	R [ES6]	R [ES7]
DNP-D,L-glutamic acid	2.6	1.0	1.6	0.4	1.7
DNP-D,L-methioninesulfone	0.9	0.0	1.6	0.0	1.3
DNP-D,L-methionine sulfoxide	0.9	0.3	1.1	0.0	0.9
DNP-D,L-α-amino-n-butyric acid	2.4	0.0	1.4	0.5	1.2
DNP-D,L-norvaline	2.7	1.7	2.4	0.8	2.2
DNP-D,L-citrulline	1.3	0.0	1.3	0.0	1.0
DNP-D,L-methionine	2.1	3.2	4.3	0.9	3.3
DNP-D,L-norleucine	5.1	6.5	6.0	1.3	4.5
DNP-D,L-ethionine	3.1	5.2	5.9	0.8	4.2
DNP-D,L-isoleucine	7.2	6.0	8.6	1.7	5.3
DNP-D,L-leucine	11.8	9.9	12.1	2.2	7.6

Table 2.2. Enantioresolutions of 2,4-dinitrophenyl (DNP) labelled amino acids under different complexing and acid-base conditions[a]

[a]Electrolyte systems (ESs) were prepared at two different pH values: (i) 100 mM morpholinoethanesulfonic acid + 10 mM histidine + 0.2% methylhydroxyethylcellulose (w/v) + 20 mM cyclodextrin derivative, pH 5.2, (ii) 50 mM H_3BO_3 + 100 mM 1,3-bis(tris(hydroxymethyl)-methylamino)propane + 0.2% methylhydroxyethylcellulose (w/v) + 20 mM cyclodextrin (CD) derivative, pH 9.6. ES1: 6^I-deoxy-6^I-monomethylamino-β-CD positively charged at pH 5.2, ES2: 6^I-deoxy-6^I-dimethylamino-β-CD positively charged at pH 5.2, ES3: 6^I-deoxy-6^I-trimethylammonium-β-CD positively charged at pH 5.2, ES4: 6^I-deoxy-6^I-monomethylamino-β-CD uncharged at pH 9.6, ES5: 6^I-deoxy-6^I-trimethylammonium-β-CD positively charged at pH 9.6.

R – enantioresolution (for a given ES).

Reprinted from ref. [Mikuš & Kaniansky, 2007].

Aqueous media. In CE, the improved separation enantioselectivity of charged solutes can be observed, in many cases, with oppositely charged chiral selectors compared to neutral ones (**Figure 2.3**). Higher stability of the formed complexes is one of the factors responsible for this enhanced enantioselectivity, as it was demonstrated by CE [Vespalec & Boček, 2000; Wenz et al., 2008] as well as nuclear magnetic resonance (NMR) measurements [Kitae et al., 1998], and as it is described in terms of complex formation mechanisms with particular chiral selectors in section 2.3. In aqueous media the complexing ability of ionizable compounds can be tuned by the pH of the buffer (changing the size of the effective charge) in this way creating optimal CE separating conditions (**Figure 2.3b**). Due to an enhanced enantioresolution power of such systems, very low amounts of charged chiral selectors are often sufficient for the successful CE enantioseparations (**Figure 2.3a**), and in some cases even micromolar concentrations are sufficient [Gübitz & Schmid, 2000a; Blanco & Valverde, 2003].

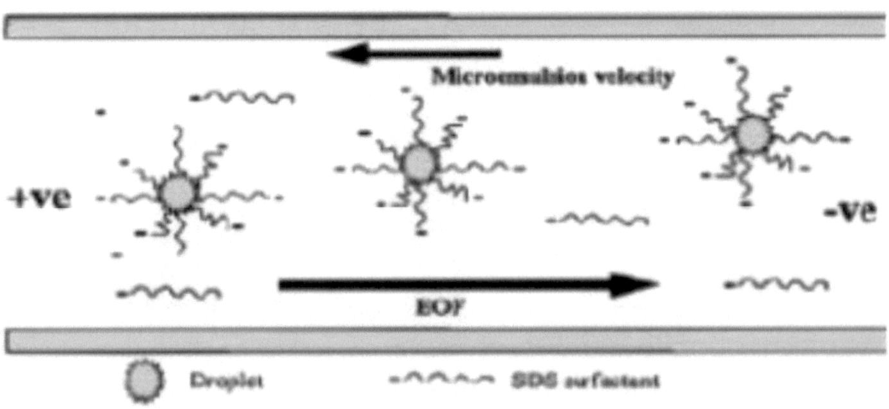

Figure 2.4. Schematic representation of MEEKC separation. MEKC separation has principally the same experimental arrangement but no oil droplets are present in micelle cores. Hydrophobic analytes are distributed preferably into droplet (MEEKC) or micelle core (MEKC). Reproduced from [Altria K.D. et al., 2003].

Amphiphilic media. CE is usually carried out in aqueous background electrolytes (BGEs) and therefore it is useful for the separation of hydrophilic solutes and samples of aqueous nature. On the other hand, the formation of stable complexes (associates) of hydrophobic analytes (that are many of natural biologically active compounds) can be accomplished in aqueous solutions using amphiphilic pseudostationary phases with proper hydrophobic bounding sites. Thus, typically, chiral micelles or chiral mixed micelles (in MEKC) and microemulsions (in MEEKC) help solving additional problems in chiral CE, such as enantioseparation of hydrophobic analytes in aqueous buffers [Preinerstorfer et al., 2009; Silva, 2009; Ryan et al., 2009; Kahle & Foley, 2007a], see **Figure 2.4**. In this field, chiral micelle polymers appeared recently as a very attractive alternative to the conventional micelle systems offering significant benefits not only in separation (fast complexing kinetics), but also detection (especially MS) schemes (see 2.3.8). Such amphiphilic systems are beneficial for the analyses of water-based samples, such as body fluids, creating a powerful alternative to HPLC-MS.

Non-aqueous media. The elimination of the aqueous media in non-aqueous CE (NACE) can provide additional selectivity with respect to that obtained in aqueous CE, and favours the analysis of solutes with poor water solubility [Karbaum & Jira, 1999; Valkó et al., 1996; Wang F. & Khaledi, 1996]. In the same manner, non-aqueous solvents show several advantages regarding solubility of chiral selectors and reduce unwanted interactions with the capillary wall. Different forms of chemical equilibria in aqueous and non-aqueous systems can lead to different selectivities as a result of the fact that weak interactions which are disrupted by water can become effective in non-aqueous systems (see e.g., ion-pair formation, 2.3.7). Moreover, in non-aqueous solvents, less Joule heating is produced and since higher voltage can be applied, retention times are shorter.

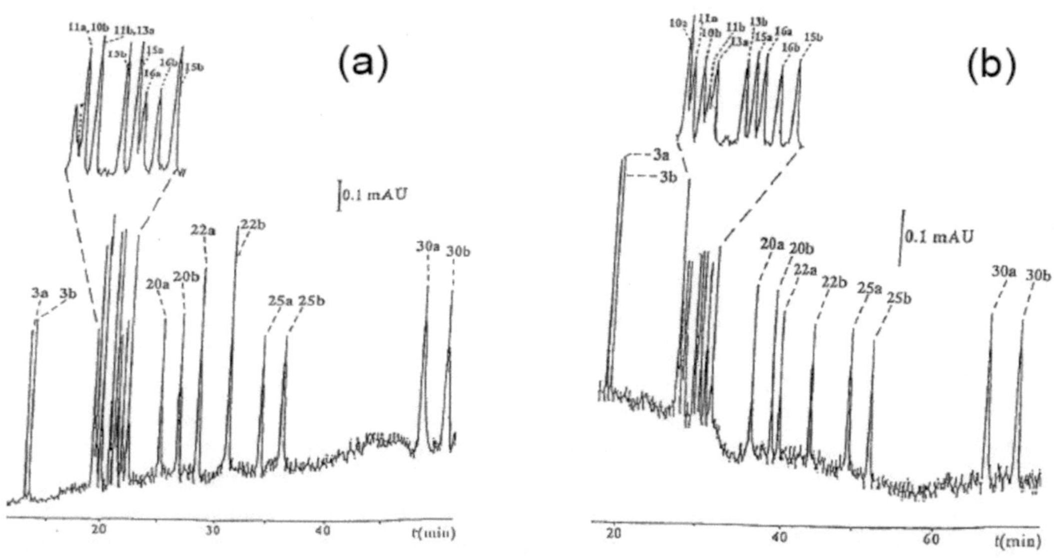

Figure 2.5. Influence of complementary complexing agents on the CE separation of a mixture of DNP-amino acid racemates. Electrolyte system with pH 5.2 and 20 mM 6^{I}-deoxy-6^{I}-monomethylamino-β-CD (as in Table 2.2) without any other coselector (a), with addition of 2 mM γ-CD (b). Peak labelling: 3 = DNP-DL-glutamic acid, 10 = DNP-DL-methioninesulfone, 11 = DNP-DL-methionine sulfoxide, 13 = DNP-DL-α-amino-n-butyric acid, 15 = DNP-DL-norvaline, 16 = DNP-DL-citruline, 20 = DNP-DL-methionine, 22 = DNP-DL-norleucine, 25 = DNP-DL-ethionine, 30 = DNP-DL-α-amino-caprylic acid. Reproduced from [Mikuš et al., 2001].

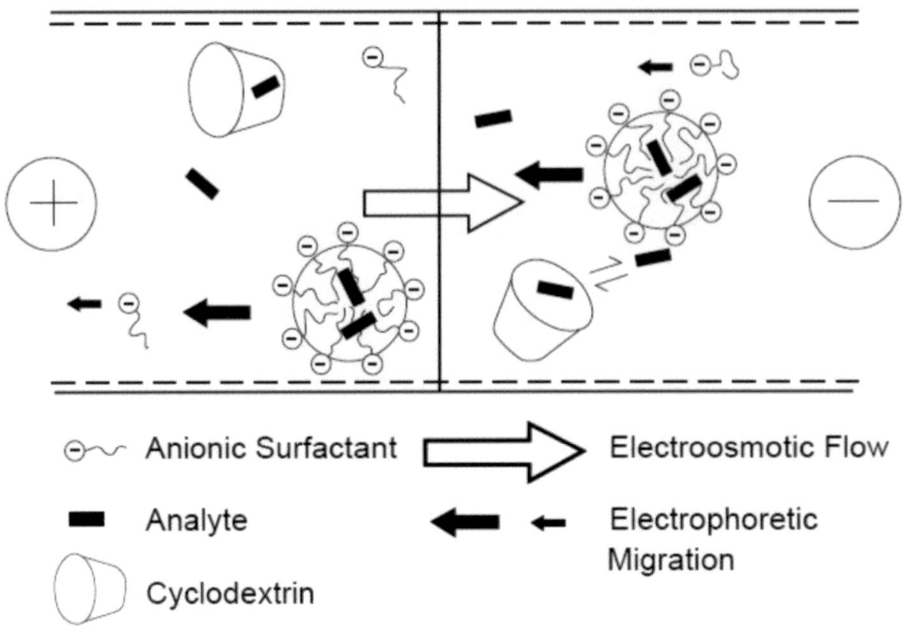

Figure 2.6. Schematic of the separation principle of CDMEKC showing multiple complexing equilibria. The detector window is assumed to be positioned near the negative electrode. Reproduced from [Terabe, 1992].

Combinations of selectors. The possibility of various chiral selectors being easily combined with one another, as well as with achiral additive(s) (introducing multiple complexing equilibria), increases the chance of successfully separating not only particular enantiomeric pairs (via enhanced chiral recognition), but also multicomponent mixtures of enantiomeric pairs (via enhanced molecular recognition) [Mikuš & Kaniansky, 2007; Mikuš et al., 2001; Carlavilla et al., 2006], see Figure 2.5. MEKC systems based on mixed micelles (micelle plus another selector, e.g., CD), introduced by Terabe et al. [Nishi, H. et al., 1991], can provide new and interesting possibilities in (enantio)recognition in comparison with single type micelle systems. For the scheme of the separation principle of CDMEKC showing multiple complexing equilibria see Figure 2.6. Rundlett and Armstrong [Rundlett & Armstrong, 1995] proposed another chiral system based on mixed micelles with vancomycin where the authors illustrated the presence of the mixed micelle as a qualitatively new chiral selector (Figure 2.7). As a special case, dual selector systems can be presented, composed from two different chiral selectors being inactive in enantiorecognition when used alone, acting via synergistic effect and providing unique enantioseparation possibilities in CE [Gübitz & Schmid, 2008; Lurie, 1997; Fillet et al., 2000].

The possibility of combining different chiral systems in on-line coupled CE techniques (i.e., different chiral selectors in different CE techniques) can be utilized for a further significant enhancing of enantioresolution in comparison to single column application [Fanali et al., 2000].

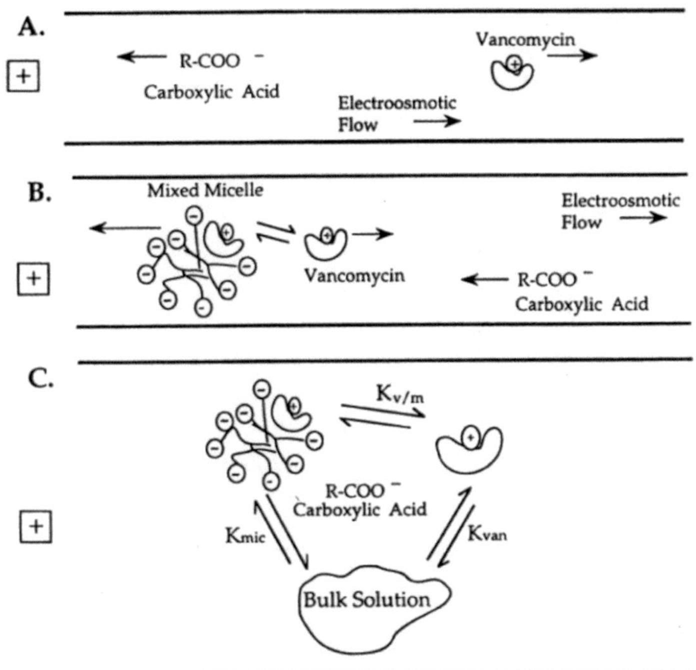

Figure 2.7. Representation of the electrophoretic mobilities of the analytes, chiral selector and mixed micelles in (A) buffer containing vancomycin (relative migration times: $t_{vancomycin}<t_{eof}<t_{acid}$) and (B) buffer containing vancomycin and SDS (relative migration times: $t_{eof}<t_{acid}<t_{vancomycin}<t_{SDS}$). (C) Shows the equilibria of acid analytes (between the bulk solution and the free vancomycin or mixed micelle). Reproduced from ref. [Rundlett & Armstrong, 1995].

2.2.1.2 Electromigration effects in enantioseparations and their manipulation

In chromatographic techniques the selectivity of enantioseparations is entirely defined by the chiral recognition, i.e., by the difference between the affinities of the enantiomers towards the chiral selector. Therefore, the selectivity of enantioseparations in common chromatographic techniques may, in the best case, approach the thermodynamic selectivity of the chiral recognition, but will never exceed it. One major consequence of the mobility contribution in separations in CE is that the apparent separation selectivity may exceed the thermodynamic selectivity of the recognition [Chankvetadze, 2007]. This belongs among unique features of electromigration methods, being not present in chromatographic methods, which can be advantageously utilized in enantiomeric separations. See the reviews on fundamental aspects of chiral electromigration techniques discussing the general aspects of migration models and the enantiomer migration order [Scriba, 2003; Chankvetadze, 1997; Chankvetadze & Blaschke, 2001]. A high enantioresolution power of CE, given by an extremely high separation (peak) efficiency, can be therefore further enhanced by electromigration effects based on increasing mobility difference between free and complexed forms of the enantiomer, as proposed by Wren and Rowe [Wren & Rowe, 1992, 1993], see Equation 2.2 in section 2.2.1. A contribution of intrinsic mobility of the chiral selector to changes of effective mobility of the charged as well as electroneutral compounds in CE is illustrated in simplified form in Figure 2.8. Moreover, the EOF mobility can additionally influence overall mobility of analytes according to the principles of additivity of particular mobility terms. From these facts the enormous potential of CE to manipulate the separability is apparent, including chiral compounds.

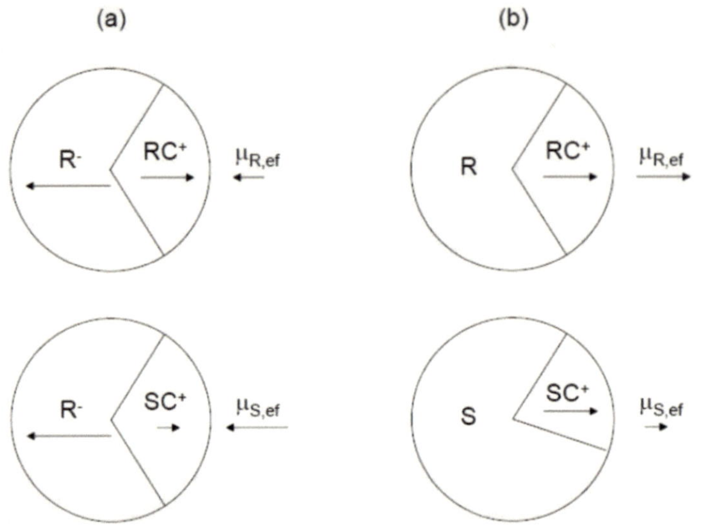

Figure 2.8. Influencing of the effective mobility of: (a) ionic enantiomers R, S, (b) neutral enantiomers R, S, by a charged chiral selector C^+. Inside the diagrams, the arrows indicate mobility contributions while the cut-outs indicate complex stability contributions. As some of the possible examples, diagrams (a) illustrate the main role of mobility differences between complexes while diagrams (b) illustrate the main role of complex stability differences between complexes for obtaining differences in effective mobilities of R and S enantiomers, $\mu_{R,ef}$, $\mu_{S,ef}$.

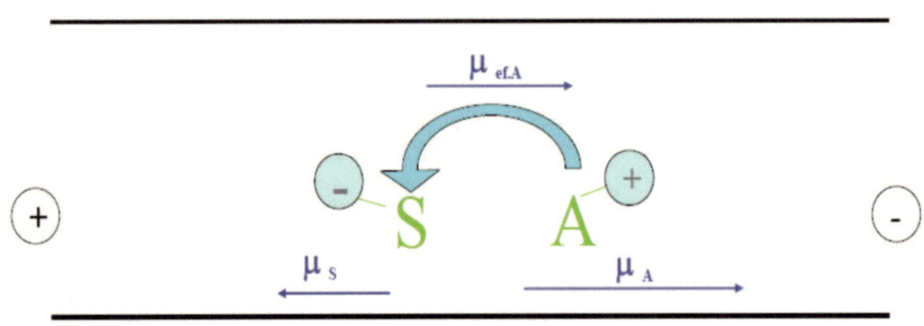

Figure 2.9. Scheme of a countercurrent migration CE system. A = analyte, S = selector.

Countercurrent migration systems. The electromigration effects enhancing enantioresolution can be implemented into CE via countercurrent migration of charged chiral selector and oppositely charged analyte enantiomers, see Figure 2.8a and Figure 2.9. Electrophoretic mobility of ionizable chiral selectors can be effectively tuned by the pH of the buffer creating very efficient chiral countercurrent migration CE systems, see the results from the relevant CE measurements in Figure 2.3b and Table 2.2. Enhanced effectivity of such systems is reflected in considerably decreased amounts of charged chiral selectors necessary for the successful CE enantioseparations (Figure 2.3a). Thanks to the many new charged chiral selectors (especially CDs and micelles) the possibilities to create new, effective countercurrent separation systems increase, see examples in section 2.4, Table 2.1 and Table 3.1. Besides enhanced enantioresolution, this migration mode is extremely useful also for hyphenated detection systems, eliminating detection interferences of chiral selectors due to their migration from the detector site (see chapter 4).

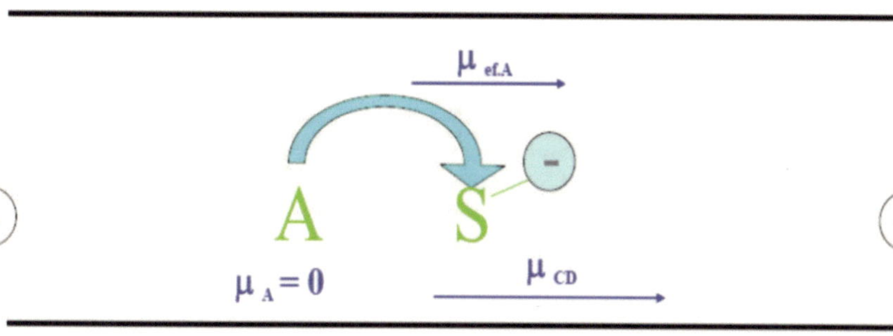

Figure 2.10. Scheme of a carrier molecule-based CE system. A = analyte, S = selector.

Carrier molecule-based migration systems. In addition, charged chiral selectors (or charged chiral pseudostationary phases) spread the application range of CE separating uncharged enantiomers according to their distribution between moving selector and solution phase, making CE (e.g., MEKC, CD-EKC) a universal separation technique like HPLC [Mikuš et al., 2005b; Zandkarimi et al., 2009], see Figure 2.8b and Figure 2.10 and examples in section 2.4.

EOF supported migration systems. Great variability of direct, countercurrent and carrier migration modes in CE, producing electrophoretic systems of different separation selectivities, is given not only by possible combinations of one or more charged and uncharged, as well as chiral and achiral additives, but also by the EOF modifying velocity and direction of movement of the species (analytes, selectors) present in the separation system, and by combinations of both electrophoretic and electroosmotic migration effects (Figures 2.4, 2.6, 2.7). These effects can also be utilized, besides enhancing enantioresolution and/or speeding analysis, for the manipulation of the enantiomer migration order [Scriba, 2003].

The benefits of the advanced migration modes can be pronounced not only in chiral resolution, but they can also simultaneously take effect in achiral resolution [Mikuš et al., 2001, 2006a; Marák et al., 2007; Mikuš & Kaniansky, 2007]. In biomedical analyses, they can be useful in simultaneous separation of structurally related analytes, e.g., chiral drugs and their metabolites, chiral drugs in multicomponent matrices, etc., see examples in section 2.4, Table 2.1 and Table 3.1. In this way, enhanced achiral resolution can also minimize requirements on sample preparation (purification) isolating the enantiomers of the interest from the matrix constituents during electrophoretic run [Mikuš et al., 2006a].

2.2.1.3 Counter-flow in enantioseparations and its manipulation

Another promising mode of chiral CE separations is flow counterbalanced capillary electrophoresis (FCCE). The difference between countercurrent [Chankvetadze et al., 1994] and flow counterbalancing CE [Chankvetadze et al., 1999] techniques is that in the latter case a chiral selector and a chiral analyte do not migrate in the opposite directions to each other, but the bulk flow moves with a defined velocity in the opposite direction to the effective mobility of the analyte zone. The principle of this technique is schematically shown in Figure 2.11 [Chankvetadze et al., 1999].

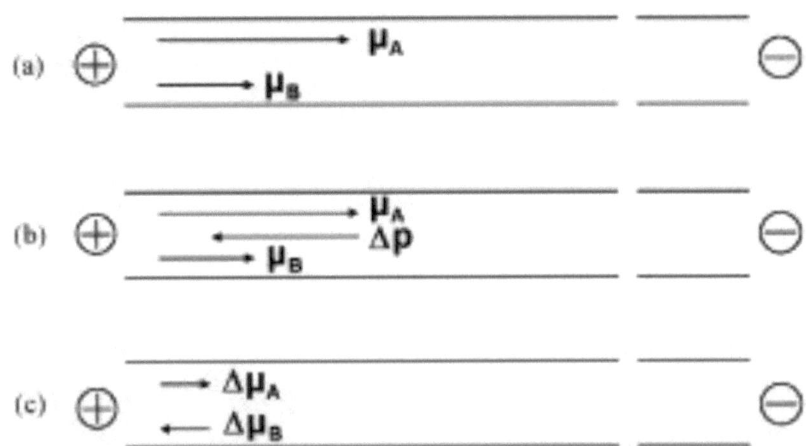

Figure 2.11. A schematic representation of the flow counterbalanced separation principle in CE: (a) without counterbalanced flow; (b) with counterbalanced flow; (c) resulting mobilities. Reproduced from ref. [Chankvetadze et al., 1999].

In FCCE, the sample is driven forward by electromigration and then backward by a pressure-induced flow. The pressure/vacuum, the EOF, hydrodynamic pressure (levelling of the inlet and outlet vials), etc., may be used as a driving force for countermobilities in this technique [Chankvetadze et al., 1999]. The samples travel back and forth in the capillary until sufficient separation is obtained [Zhao J. et al., 1999]. In the mode of FCCE as proposed by Culbertson and Jorgenson [Culbertson & Jorgenson, 1994], the electric field and the pressure are applied alternatively, but not simultaneously as the driving forces. In another mode of FCCE, the counterbalancing driving force, such as pressure, may be applied to the separation chamber continuously during the entire time of electrokinetic separation [Chankvetadze et al., 1999]. An enormous increase of apparent separation factor in chiral and achiral CE separations may be achieved using this technique.

The potential advantage of FCCE can be seen from the Equation 2.3 [Zhao J. et al., 1999]:

$$R_S = (\mu_1 - \mu_2)\frac{E\sqrt{t}}{4\sqrt{2D}} \qquad 2.3$$

where E is the electric field strength, D is the average effective diffusion coefficient of two analytes (*1, 2*), and t is the electrophoretic migration time. The advantages of the flow counterbalancing technique include the following: (i) enormous, in principle unlimited, enhancement of the apparent separation factor may be achieved in zonal discontinuous separations as shown in section 2.4. (ii) This technique allows easy discontinuous zonal separation of a binary mixture into a continuous separation with stepwise migration of the sample components from the inlet towards the outlet vial. (iii) FCCE may be used for micropreparative purposes and offers significantly higher sample capacity compared to discontinuous separations. Other potential advantages of mobility counterbalancing techniques are discussed in ref. [Chankvetadze et al., 1999].

The mobility counterbalancing technique is certainly not limited to binary mixtures and it can easily be applied in a stepwise mode for the separation of multicomponent samples. Counterbalancing of analyte electrophoretic mobility by pressure has been tried by Culbertson and Jorgenson [Culbertson & Jorgenson, 1994] for the enhancement of the detection sensitivity in achiral CE. Later, the same technique was used for the separation of isotopomers of phenylalanine [Culbertson & Jorgenson, 1999]. Several FCCE modes have been developed and applied for enantioseparations so far, see examples in section 2.4.

2.2.2 Capillary electrochromatography

Capillary electrochromatography (CEC) combines electrophoretic and chromatographic separation mechanisms that can be beneficial in highly effective enantioresolutions, for the recent advances in this field see the review by Lu and Chen [Lu H.A. & Chen G.N., 2011]. For the CEC separation principle see Figure 2.12. Chiral stationary phases (CSPs) known from HPLC may be used in CEC. CSPs are based on immobilization of chiral selector onto/into appropriate polymeric matrix (e.g., polysiloxanes, modified silica structures, methacrylates). CDs, proteins, polysaccharides, macrocyclic antibiotics are the most often used chiral molecules for the chiral stationary phases, offering in this rigid state modified enantioselectivity in comparison with their free (mobile) forms. In addition to those, new CSPs, such as ionic liquids functionalized β-cyclodextrin-and carbosilane dendrimer-bonded chiral stationary phases, are synthesized for producing modified enantioselectivity, [see e.g., Zhou Z. et al., 2010; Shou et al., 2008]. Moreover, the polymeric structure of these stationary phases can additionally influence CEC enantioresolution. An overview of previous developments in chiral CEC is given in former review articles [Gübitz & Schmid, 2000b; 2008; Lämmerhofer et al., 2000; Fanali et al., 2001; Kang et al., 2002].

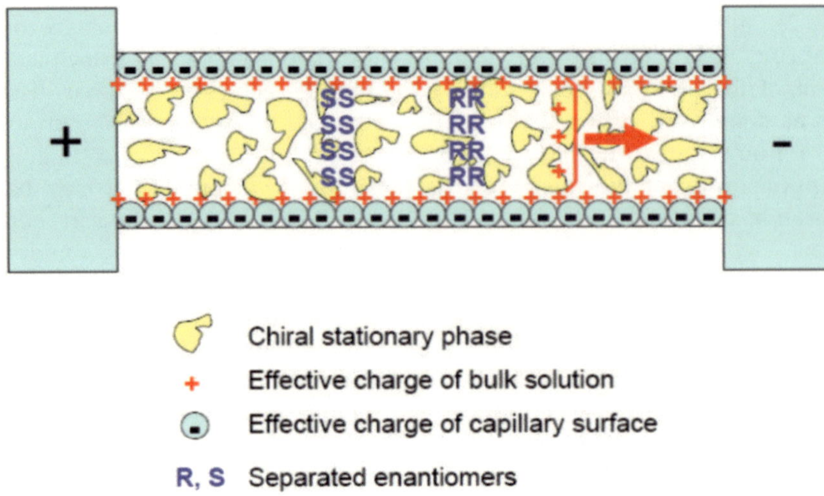

Figure 2.12. Separation principle of capillary electrochromatography.

Chiral CEC stationary phases included in capillary wall coatings, particle packings or monolytes (as an example see Figure 2.13) are beneficial in situations with special requirements on separation buffer (aqueous, non-aqueous), stability and solubility of compounds (analytes, selectors, additives, etc.) in separation system, and some on-line detection modes (e.g., avoiding a contamination of detector by selector, often in the case of UV absorbance and mass spectrometry) [Huo Y. & Kok, 2008]. Depending on a chiral selector embedded into the monolith, the resulting chiral monolith can provide significant differences in the chiral selectivity, as illustrated in Figure 2.14. Imprinted chiral phases can offer an enhanced specificity of chiral CEC analyses [Nilsson et al., 2004; Turiel & Martin-Esteban, 2004].

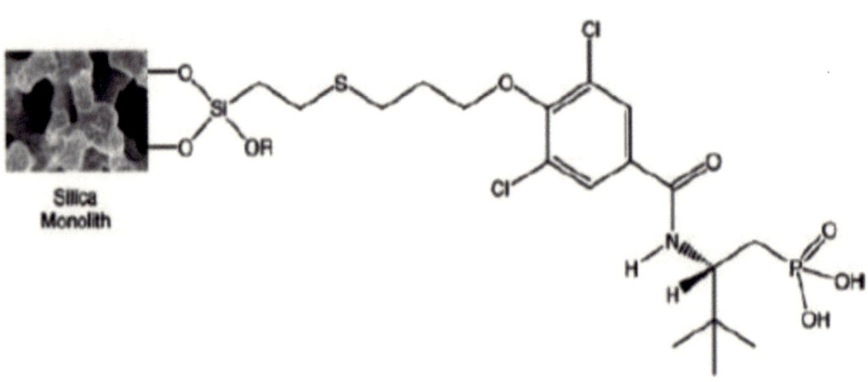

Figure 2.13. Surface-structure of enantioselective silica-based monolithic cation-exchange capillary column with aminophosphonic acid-derived chiral selector. Reproduced from ref. [Preinerstorfer et al., 2006].

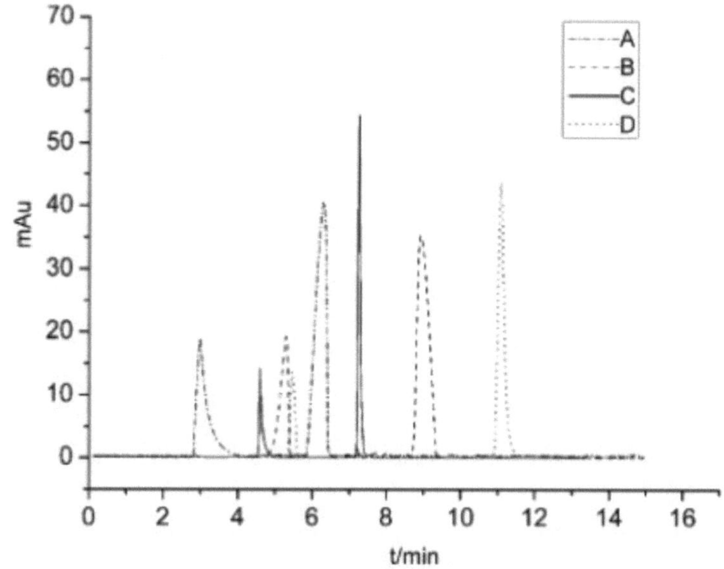

Figure 2.14. Separation of D,L-phenylalanine by four chiral monolithic CSPs. (A) Fabricated with NH_2-β-CD; (B) fabricated with β-CD; (C) fabricated with Asp-β-CD; (D) fabricated with HP-β-CD. Temperature: 20°C; voltage: −10 kV; injection:−2 kV, 2 s; mobile phase: phosphate, 5mM, pH= 6.5. Reprinted from ref. [Li Y. et al., 2010].

Compared to HPLC, where a conical flow profile caused by hydrodynamic flow leads to band broadening, in CEC a rather plug-like profile generated by the EOF (see Figure 2.12) results in higher peak efficiency. However, there are also several disadvantages in CEC such as the complicated packing procedures, formation of air bubbles in the case of packed capillaries due to Joule heating, lower reproducibility of migration times due to fluctuation of EOF with different packings and sample matrices [Gübitz & Schmid, 2000, 2008; Lämmerhofer et al., 2000; Fanali et al., 2001; Kang et al., 2002]. Pretreatment of samples with complex matrices is necessary before CEC analysis to maintain separation reproducibility (cleaning of CEC columns is much more difficult and less efficient than CE columns), see examples in section 2.4 and Table 2.1.

2.2.3 Microchip capillary electrophoresis

Microfluidic devices, such as microchips (Figure 2.15), can provide several additional advantages over electromigration techniques performed in capillary format [Li O.L. et al., 2008]. The heat dissipation is much better in chip format compared with that in a capillary and therefore, higher electric fields can be applied across microchip channels. This fact enables, along with a considerably reduced length of channels, significant shortening of separation time, see an example in Figure 2.16. Sample and reagent consumption is markedly reduced in microchannels, hence, the chiral MCE can provide the unique possibility of ultraspeed enantiomeric separations of microscale sample amounts. Both electrophoretic [Gong & Hauser, 2006; Piehl et al., 2004; Belder et al., 2006; Belder, 2006] and electrochromatographic modes are applicable [Weng X. et al., 2006].

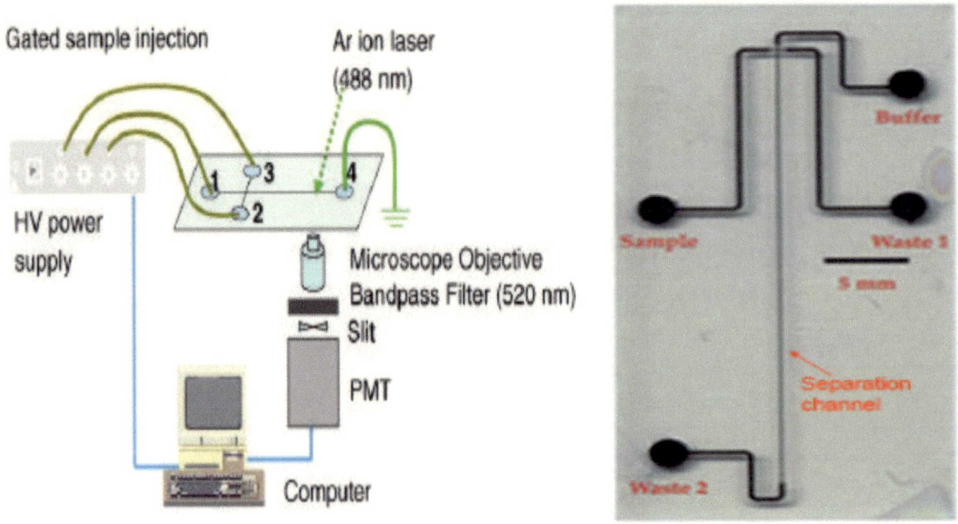

Figure 2.15. MCE. Experimental arrangement of microchip electrophoresis (left). Arrangement in the left single-channel chip: (1) sample, (2) run buffer, (3) sample waste and (4) buffer waste. The electrophoretic microchip – real detail (right). Arrangement in the right single-channel chip: reservoirs (sample, buffer, waste) and separation channel. For a chiral MCE, separation channel can be filled with chiral electrolyte (CE mode), or chiral/achiral electrolyte with chiral/achiral stationary phase (CEC mode). Reproduced (left) from [Kim M.S. et al., 2005].

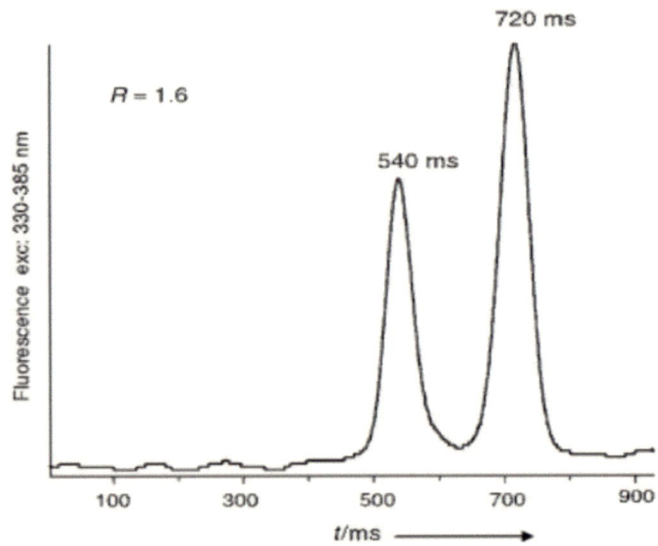

Figure 2.16. Subsecond chiral separation of DNS-tryptophan. Electrolyte: 2% HS-γ–CD, 25 mM triethylammonium phosphate buffer pH 2.5. A high field strength up to 2600 V/cm and short separation length of several millimetres were employed. Reproduced from ref. [Belder, 2006].

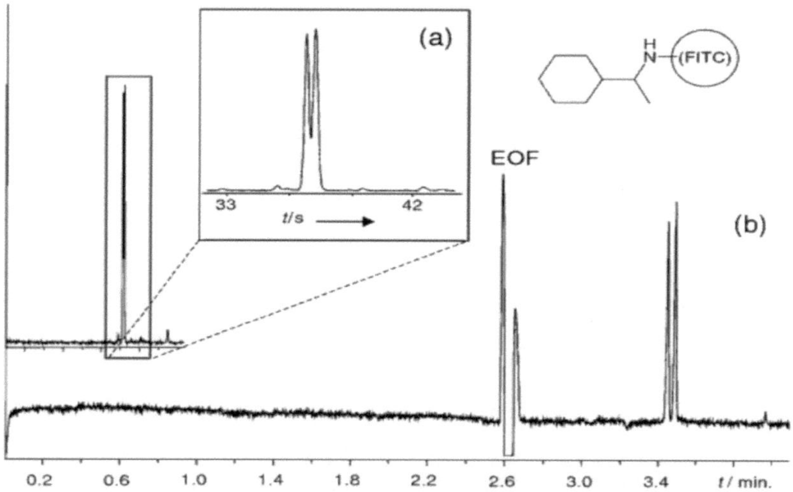

Figure 2.17. Comparison of chiral separations obtained in microchip electrophoresis (MCE) (a) and in classical capillary electrophoresis (CE) (b). For both the experiments the same electrolyte was used, while the column length was limited to 7 cm in MCE, a column of 40 cm effective length was used in CE. Reproduced from ref. [Belder, 2006].

In practice, however, the resolution achievable in MCE devices is often lower compared to that obtainable in classical CE utilizing considerably longer separation capillaries. This is shown in Figure 2.17, where the chiral separation of an FITC-labelled amine obtained at typical conditions in MCE and in classical CE is compared. In order to obtain sufficient resolution in chiral MCE, different strategies have been used [Belder, 2006], such as (i) enhancing the enantioselectivity of the system as much as possible (changing the type and amount of chiral selector, adding coselector, etc.), (ii) using folded separation channels, the column length can be extended without enlarging the compact footprint of the device, as shown in Figure 2.18, (iii) using coated channels, internal coatings improve separation performance by the suppression of both analyte wall interaction and electroosmosis; the impact of channel coating with poly(vinyl alcohol) on a chiral separation in MCE is shown in Figure 2.19 for the separation of an FITC-labelled amine. The use/combination of the above-mentioned tools applicable in MCE gives a good chance for real-time process control and for multidimensional separations, and makes MCE a powerful tool in real chiral applications (pharmaceutical, biomedical, etc.).

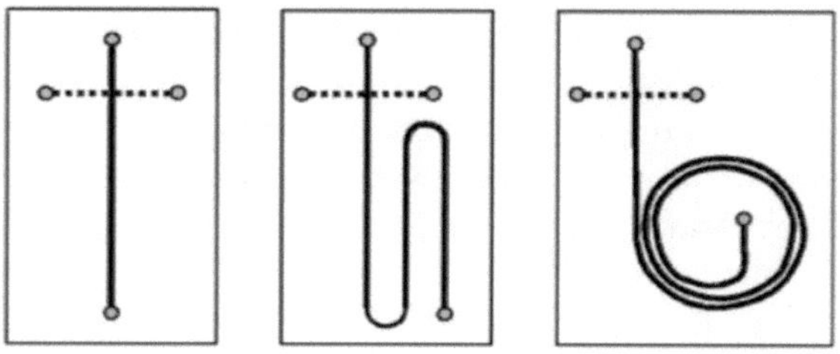

Figure 2.18. Channel layouts enabling long separation channels on a small device. Reproduced from ref. [Belder, 2006].

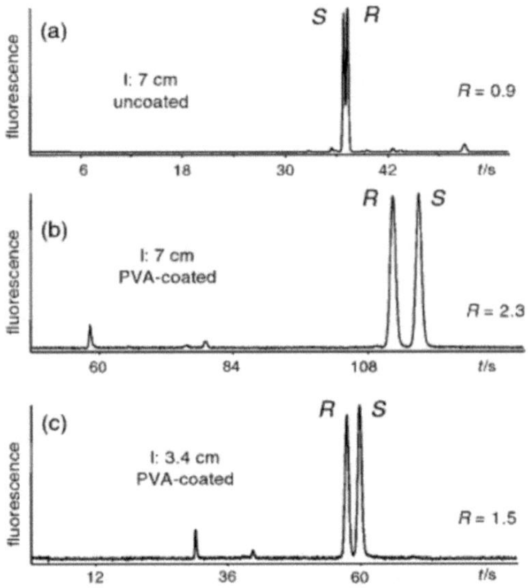

Figure 2.19. Influence of PVA-channel coating on chiral resolution of FITC-labelled (R)- (-) and (S)-(+)-1-cyclohexylethylamine in MCE. The effective separation lengths were 7 cm for the uncoated channel (a) and 7 cm (b) and 3.4 cm (c) for the PVA-coated microchip. Buffer: 40 mM CHES, 6.25 mM HP-γ-CD, pH 9.2. Reproduced from ref. [Belder, 2006].

For examples of practical applications of the chiral MCE, see section 2.4 and Table 3.1. A brief comparison of CE and MCE, and clinical applications of MCE are reviewed in ref. [Li, S.F.Y. & Kricka L.J., 2006]. Chiral separations in microfluidic devices are nicely reviewed by Belder [2006].

2.3 Chiral selectors as complexing agents, advantages and limitations

Conventional as well as new chiral selectors suitable for CE are described in the following subsections. From this description, showing complexing properties (i.e., mechanism of chiral discrimination), advantages and limitations of various classes of chiral selectors, the high flexibility of chiral CE for the separation of a wide range of structurally different compounds is apparent.

2.3.1 Cyclodextrins

Cyclodextrins (CDs), cyclic oligosaccharides with (typically) 6-8 D-glucose units in the macrocycle (α-, β-, γ-CDs, see Figure 2.20, although recently δ-CD was also introduced into CE [Wistuba et al., 2006]), are the most often employed chiral additives for the CE enantiomeric separations of low molecular organic compounds due to their outstanding broad selectivity spectra and other beneficial properties, such as UV transparency, availability, wide application range (polar, nonpolar, charged, uncharged analytes), and reasonable solubility in water [Chankvetadze, 2008; Scriba, 2008; Juvancz et al., 2008; Cserhati, 2008; Fanali, 2009]. Moreover, a fast complex forming kinetics with CDs is beneficial for highly efficient CE enantioseparations. From these reasons (and other facts discussed below) it is not surprising that CDs are dominating chiral selectors also in enantioselective analysis of many drugs in biological samples, as it is apparent from Table 2.1 and Table 3.1.

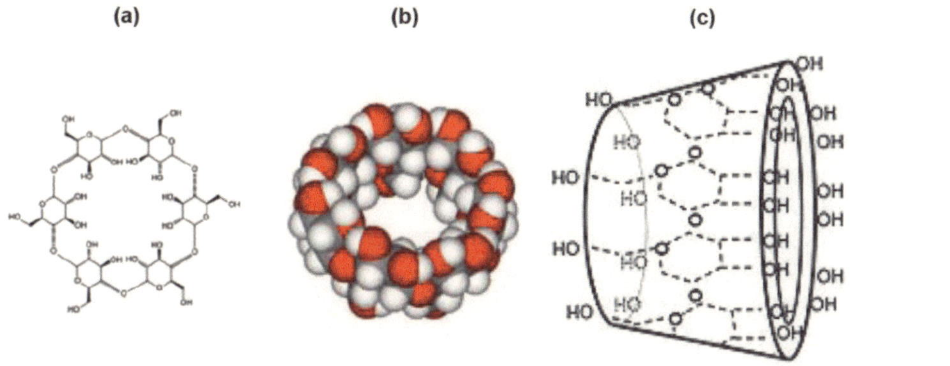

Figure 2.20. Cyclodextrins. (a) Chemical structure of α-CD. (b) Space filling model of β-CD. (c) γ-CD toroid structure showing spatial arrangement.

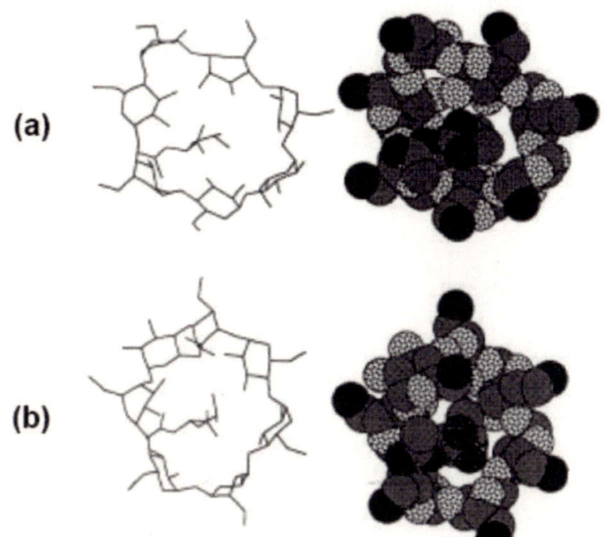

Figure 2.21. Structures of inclusion CD complexes. (a) per-NH_3^+-β-CD-(S)-AcLeu complex, (b) per-NH_3^+-β-CD-(R)-AcLeu complex. The complexes were derived from the molecular mechanics - molecular dynamics (MM-MD) calculations. Reproduced from ref. [Kitae et al., 1998].

The basic mechanism of chiral discrimination using CDs is based on the inclusion of the analyte (guest), or at least its hydrophobic part, into the relatively hydrophobic cavity of CD (host), see an example in Figure 2.21. Here different sterical arrangements of chiral compounds in chiral CD cavity results in differences in stability of the formed complexes.

Compounds containing an aromatic system in their molecules, including many drugs, are usually well-suited for inclusion into the CD cavity and hence, a good enantiorecognition between enantiomers is often easily achieved [Vespalec & Boček, 2000; Mikuš et al., 2002; Thiele et al., 2009; Denmark, 2011; Palcut & Rabara, 2009].

The hydroxyl groups present on the rim of the CD can be easily modified by chemical reactions with various functional groups creating a great amount of derivatized CDs with the desired properties, especially (i) complex forming ability, (ii) solubility, (iii) migration and (iv) detection capabilities. Therefore, it is not surprising that even in the field of newly developed chiral selectors the novel CD derivatives prevail significantly [Preinerstorfer et al., 2009]. The preparation of selectively substituted derivatives [Gübitz & Schmid, 2000a; Nzeadibe & Vigh, 2007; Cucinotta et al., 2010] is preferred as this eliminates the creation of mixtures of CDs having different substitution patterns, and, by that, different complexing / electromigration properties, see Figure 2.22, that can cause difficulties with separation reproducibility in CE [Vespalec & Boček, 1999; Mikuš et al., 1999; Mikuš & Kaniansky, 2007]. Several different groups of CD derivatives can be distinguished, namely (i) neutral CDs, (ii) negatively and positively charged CDs, (iii) amphoteric CDs and (iv) polymerized CDs.

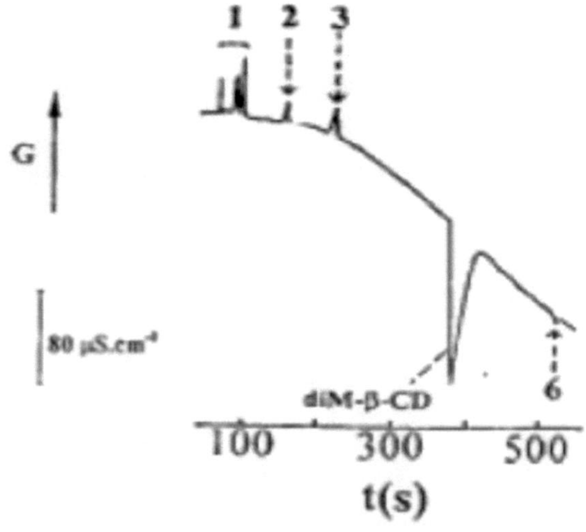

Figure 2.22. Electropherograms showing different electromigration properties of the β-CD aminoderivates. The sample constituents were separated according to differences in their actual ionic mobilities. There are clearly visible differences in migration velocities of the CD derivatives with different substitution degree (peaks 2, 3, and diM-β-CD) in the electropherogram. The concentration of the monoaminoderivative, 6^{I}-deoxy-6^{I}-dimethylamino-β-CD, the major constituent in the analysed preparative, was ca. 1.7 mM. Tentative peak assignments: 1 = a migration region of the alkali and alkaline earth metal cations and alkyl- and arylamines; 2 = triamino-β-CD derivatives; 3 = diamino-β-CD derivatives; diM-β-CD = 6^{I}-deoxy-6^{I}-dimethylamino-β-CD; 6 = unidentified constituents. Contactless conductivity detection was used in this CE experiment to monitor the non-absorbing analytes. Reproduced from ref. [Mikuš et al., 1999].

Neutral CDs (e.g., replacing hydroxyl groups with alkyl or hydroxyalkyl groups) can offer modified depth and flexibility of the cavity, as well as the free cross-section of its smaller opening, leading to better accommodation of the guest and increased stability of the resulting inclusion complex [Vespalec & Boček, 2000; Blanco & Valverde, 2003], as an example see Figure 2.23. This can improve solubility of CDs and their complexes, as well as enantiomeric recognition in comparison with their native forms as illustrated on many biological samples (urine, plasma, rat brain), such as 2-hydroxypropyl-β-CD vs. lorazepam and its chiral 3O-glucuronides, methyl-O-β-CD vs. isoproterenol [Hadviger et al., 1996], hydroxypropyl-β-CD vs. amlodipine [Mikuš et al., 2008a], 2-hydroxypropyl-β-CD and 2-hydroxypropyl-γ-CD vs. 4-fluoro-7-nitro-2,1,3-benzoxadiazole (NBD-F) or cyanobenz[*f*]isoindole (CBI) derivatives of serine [Quan et al., 2005; Zhao S. L. et al., 2005a], for details see Table 2.1 and Table 3.1.

(a)

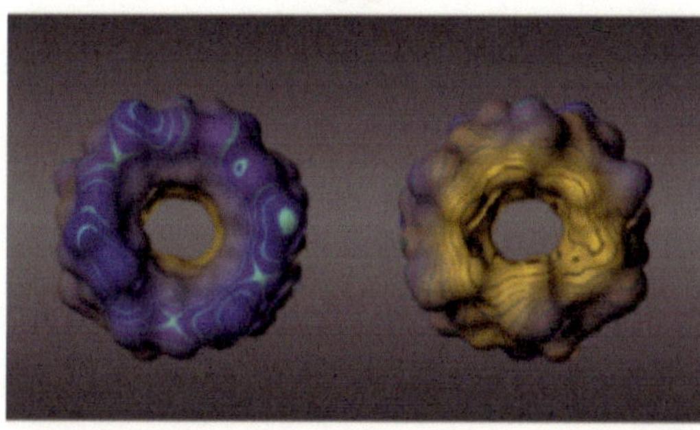

(b)

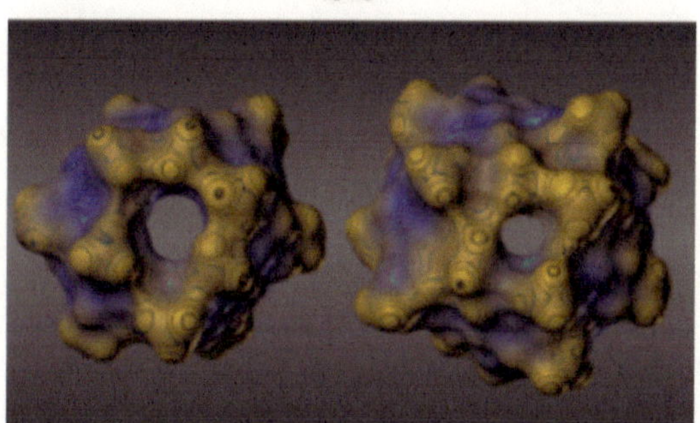

Figure 2.23. Modification of the structure and character of α-CD after its derivatization. (a) native α-CD, (b) per-O-methyl-α-CD. In the MOLCAD (molecular computer-aided design) structures the hydrophilic parts are coloured with blue while the hydrophobic parts are coloured with yellow. Reprinted from [csi.chemie.tu-darmstadt.de].

The improved chiral recognition was observed many times with charged CDs compared to neutral ones, see Figure 2.24 {compare NMR traces (b) and (d)}, as a result of the enhanced stability of host-guest complexes due to the additional strong electrostatic (Coulombic) interactions of oppositely charged functional groups of complexing partners [Vespalec & Boček, 2000; Wenz et al., 2008; Kitae et al., 1998]. For an example of the CD complex stabilized by the Coulombic interaction see Figure 2.25. The complex stability depends on the size of charge that is important especially for the effective use of ionizable CD derivatives in CE (having carboxyl or amino groups in macrocycle), as it was demonstrated (mainly from the electromigration point of view) in section 2.2. Substitution pattern is another tool for a quite significant tuning of the enantiorecognition ability of charged CDs [Mikuš & Kaniansky, 2007; Kitae et al., 1998], as illustrated in Figure 2.24 {compare NMR traces (b) and (c)}. The ionic character of CD derivatives is also responsible for their excellent water solubility. Enhanced enantiomeric recognition as well as solubility of these CDs and their complexes in comparison with their native forms was illustrated on many biological samples (urine, squirrel brain, human plasma), including carboxyethyl-β-CD vs. H_1-antihistaminic drugs (dioxopromethazine, dimethindene, pheniramine) [Mikuš et al., 2006a, 2008b; Marák et al., 2007], a highly sulfated-β-CD vs. CBI derivatives of serine, glutamate and aspartate [Kirschner et al., 2007], a highly sulfated-β-CD vs. CBI derivatized baclofen [Kavran-Belin et al., 2005], a highly sulfated-β-CD vs. a racemic antiarrhythmic drug (disopyramide) [Fang, L. et al., 2006], for details see Table 2.1 and Table 3.1.

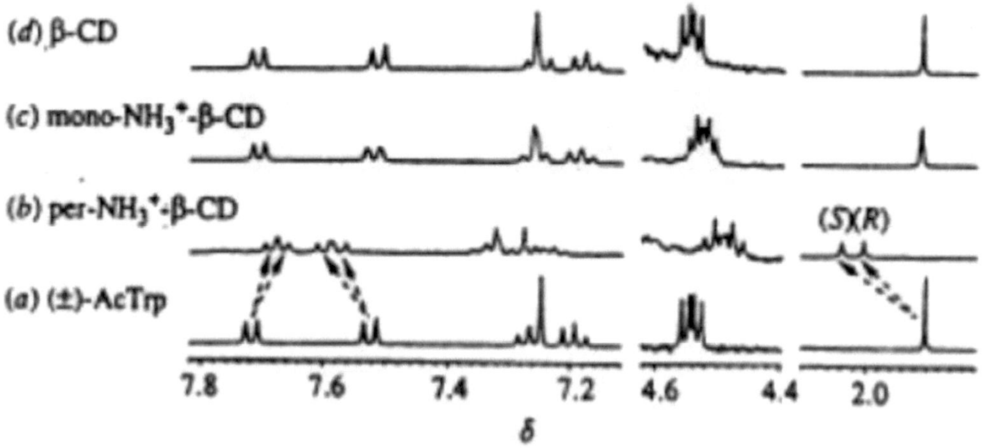

Figure 2.24. ¹H NMR spectra of (±)-AcTrp (2x10^{-3} M) in D_2O at pD 6.0 in the absence and the presence of native β-CD, and selectively substituted β-CD derivatives (8x10^{-3} M). Here, only per-NH_3^+-β-CD exhibited enantiorecognition capability for (±)-AcTrp (split NMR signals). Reproduced from ref. [Kitae et al., 1998].

Polymerized CDs are mostly prepared by cross-linking the CDs with bifunctional reagents like diepoxydes and diisocyanates [Fenyvesi, 1988]. Associated analytes have more reduced mobility (close to zero) that can lead, for some analytes, to their better CE enantioseparation in comparison with the use of the native monomeric CDs. Moreover, improved solubility and rigid structure of CD cavites in polymer can additionally influence (enantio)recognition and utilization [Fenyvesi, 1988; Ingelse et al., 1995; Ševčík et al., 1996]. For example, polymeric β-CD exhibited excellent molecular recognition for multicomponent mixtures of amino acid enantiomers [Mikuš et al., 2001].

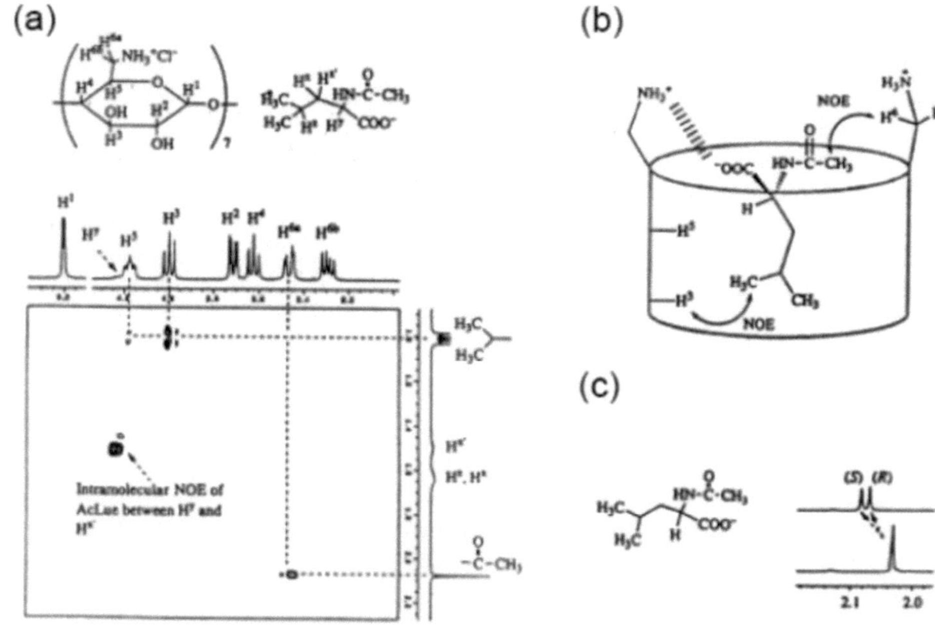

Figure 2.25. Illustration of the enhanced chiral recognition due to Coulomb interaction as an attractive force. (a) ROESY spectrum of the per-NH_3^+-β-CD-(S)-AcLeu system in D_2O at pD 6.0 and 25°C. The spectrum was measured for the solution of a mixture of per-NH_3^+-β-CD ($8x10^{-3}$ M) and (S)-AcLeu ($4x10^{-3}$ M) in N_2-saturated D_2O. The mixing time for the ROESY measurement was 250 ms. (b) A plausible structure of the per-NH_3^+-β-CD-(S)-AcLeu complex deduced from ^1H NMR spectroscopy. (c) ^1H NMR signals of the CH_3 protons at the acetyl group of *N*-acetylated leucine, AcLeu, ($2x10^{-3}$ M) in the absence (lower) and the presence of protonated heptakis(6-amino-6-deoxy)-β-cyclodextrin, per-NH_3^+-β-CD, ($8x10^{-3}$ M) (upper) in D_2O at pD 6.0 and 25°C. Reproduced from ref. [Kitae et al., 1998].

2.3.2 Crown ethers

Chiral crown ethers (CWEs) are cyclic polyethers that form stereoselectively inclusion complexes with primary amines (**Figure 2.26**). The CWE complexation differs from CD complexation by the inclusion of the hydrophilic part of the analyte (e.g., protonated amino group) in the cavity [Kuhn, 1999].

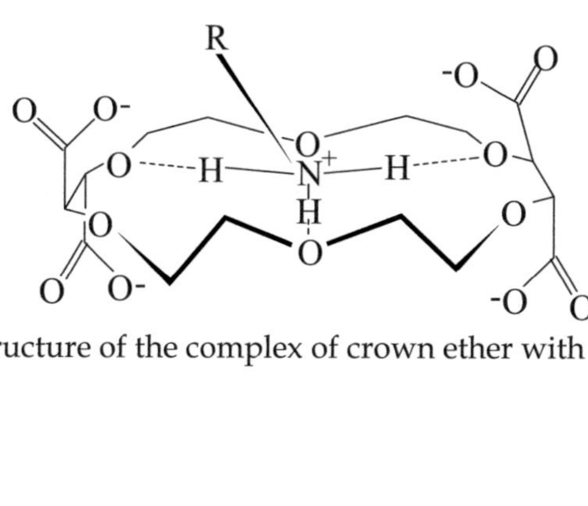

Figure 2.26. Chemical structure of the complex of crown ether with primary amine.

18-Crown-6-tetracarboxylic acid ($18C_6H_{14}$) found widespread application as a chiral selector in CE for the chiral separation of amino acids, dipeptides, sympathomimetics and various drugs containing primary amino groups [Kuhn, 1999]. Wang et al. [Wang C.Y. et al., 2003] demonstrated applicability of a new CWE, (S,S)-1,7-bis(4-benzyl-5-hydroxy-2-oxo-3-azapentyl)-1,7-diaza-12-crown-4, for the chiral CE separations. However, there are several limitations with CWEs. The separation electrolyte may not contain cations, such as potassium or ammonium ions, because they compete with the enantiomers for the CWE cavity. This increases claims on the purity and composition of electrolyte systems, and limits some applications. Therefore, according to our best knowledge, there is only one application of CWE to the chiral analysis of biological sample from 2000 [Cho et al., 2004]. $18C_6H_{14}$ was applied for enantioseparation of gemifloxacin in urine (for detail see Table 3.1).

2.3.3 Polysaccharides/oligosacharides

A variety of linear neutral and charged carbohydrates were found to be applicable as selectors for chiral CE separations. The low UV absorption and often high attainable separation efficiency make these selectors attractive for CE [Riekkola et al., 1997]. The enantiorecognition capability of various neutral oligo- polysacharides (maltodextrins, dextrins, dextrans) is significantly influenced by their higher molecular structures, like helical hydrophobic cavities or pores of polymeric networks [Nishi, H. et al., 1996a]. Two applications to biological samples from 2000 [Bortocan & Bonato, 2004; Nojavan & Fakhari, 2011] show enantioselective separation and determination of primaquine and its metabolite, carboxyprimaquine, in rat liver mitochondrial fraction and plasma samples, and cetirizine and hydroxyzine in human plasma, by maltodextrin as chiral selector (for detail see Table 2.1).

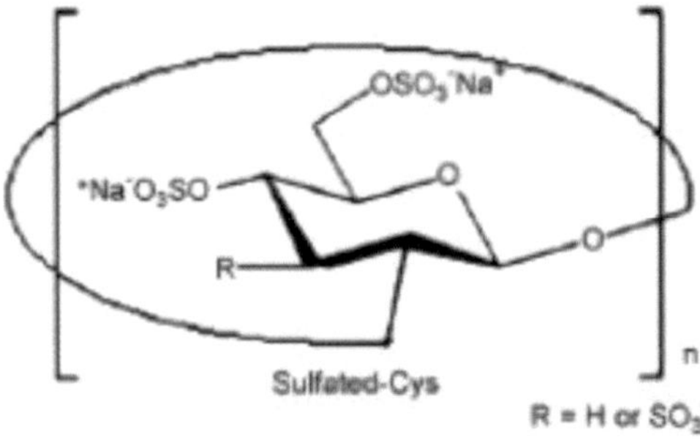

Figure 2.27. Chemical structure of HS-Cys. Reprinted from ref. [Park et al., 2004].

Electrostatic interactions provide additional stereoselectivity effects in the case of ionic polysacharides [Nishi H., 1997] (heparin, dextran sulphate, chondroitin sulphate, hyaluronate, chitosans, aminoglycosides, colominic acid, highly sulfated cyclosophoraoses) suitable for a variety of basic drugs such as β-blockers and sympathomimetics [Nishi H., 1997; Nishi, H.S. et al., 1996b; Du et al., 2002; Park et al., 2004]. For example, recently Park et al. [Park et al., 2004] synthesized highly sulfated cyclosophoraoses (HS-Cys) (Figure 2.27) from a family of neutral cyclosophoraoses isolated from *Rhizobium leguminosarum* and applied them as chiral selectors for the resolution of β-blocker and sympathomimetic enantiomers. Contrary to the sulfated compounds, the neutral cyclosophoraoses themselves showed no chiral recognition ability for these drugs investigated.

2.3.4 Proteins

Proteins provide strong and highly selective interactions, so called affinity interactions, with the analytes. Stereoselectivity is further influenced by the tertiary structure of proteins. Different analytes can selectively bind to different binding sites of proteins. Proteins can be used, depending on their ionization state, for neutral, basic or acidic analytes. However, there are several limitations associated with the use of proteins in CE enantioseparations, mainly low obtainable separation efficiency, adsorption of proteins to the capillary wall and high UV absorption. To eliminate these disturbing effects, capillary coating and/or partial filling techniques and/or indirect detection have to be used [Vespalec & Boček, 2000; Tanaka & Terabe, 1995; Armstrong et al., 1994a].

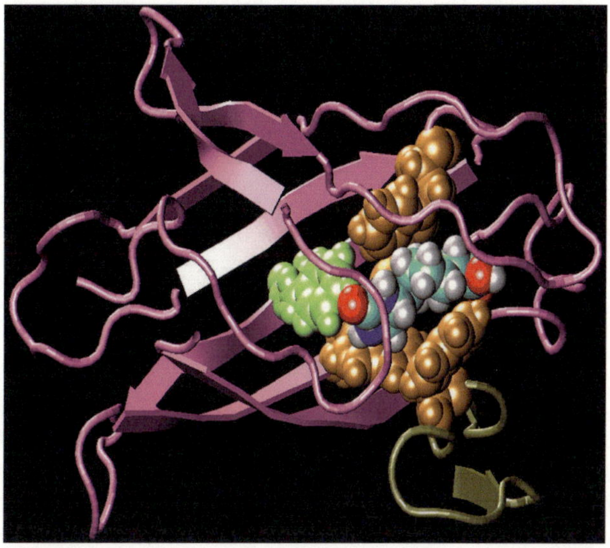

Figure 2.28. 3D structure of avidin. A typical arrangement of avidin complex (avidin-biotin). Reprinted from [ks.uiuc.edu].

Various proteins, e.g., bovine serum albumin, α1-acid glycoprotein, ovomucoid, avidin (Figure 2.28), transferring, pepsin, penicillin G acylase, have been successfully employed in CE enantioseparations of amino acids and drugs. [Haginaka, 2000; Hödl et al., 2006; Gotti et al., 2006; Martínez-Gómez et al., 2007]. Although this group of selectors is frequently used in model CE enantioseparations, it is less often applied in pharmaceutical analysis, see e.g., ref. by Martinez-Gomez et al. [Martínez-Gómez et al., 2007] devoted to the enantiomeric quality control of antihistamines in pharmaceuticals by affinity electrokinetic chromatography with human serum albumin as chiral selector. However, no chiral application to biological samples has been referred from 2000, probably because of achieving the goal with less problematic selectors such as CDs and their derivatives.

2.3.5 Macrocyclic antibiotics

Macrocyclic antibiotics, introduced by Armstrong et al. [Armstrong et al., 1994b], possess several asymmetric centres and many functional groups and structures (like hydrophobic pocket) allowing multiple interactions (affinity, inclusion, etc.) with the analytes and providing extremely high enantiorecognition capability. Since these compounds have strong UV absorption, partial filling methods [Desiderio et al., 1997] and countercurrent approaches [Oswald & Ward, 1999] have been applied to overcome detection problems. Moreover, capillaries have to be coated for the elimination of adsorption of antibiotics at the capillary wall [Wang Z. et al., 2007].

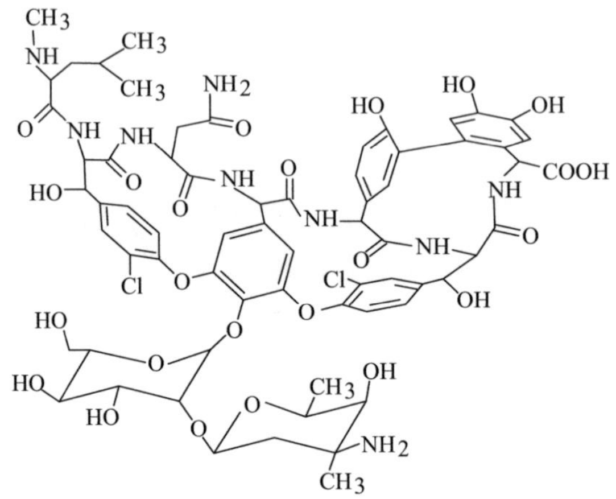

Figure 2.29. Chemical structure of vancomycin.

Several classes of antibiotics have been introduced as chiral selectors showing different enantiorecognition capabilities towards amino acids, drugs, etc.: ansamycins (rifamycin B, rifamycin SV), glycopeptides (vancomycin, ristocetin, teicoplanin, avoparcin), aminoglycosides (streptomycin sulfate, kanamycin sulfate, fradiomycin sulfate), macrolides (erythromycin), polypeptides, [see e.g., Wang Z. et al., 2007; Hou J.G. et al., 2003; Ha P.T.T. et al., 2004b]. For the chemical structure of vancomycin see Figure 2.29.

Lack of recent CE applications to biological samples can be explained by the same arguments used for proteins. On the other hand, applications in this field were accomplished by antibiotics immobilized in CEC stationary phases (see section 2.2.2 and Table 2.1).

2.3.6 Ligand-exchange selectors

Ligand-exchange selectors {usually chelate complexes (hemicomplexes) of amino acids with metal cations, e.g., histidine-copper(II)} can form ternary complexes with appropriate analytes (compounds containing aminocarboxyl or hydroxycarboxyl groups like amino acids and hydroxyl acids) having different stability for the two enantiomers [Gassmann et al., 1985]. Rizkov et al. [Rizkov et al., 2010] demonstrated beta-Amino alcohol selectors for enantioselective separation of amino acids by ligand-exchange capillary zone electrophoresis in a low molecular weight organogel. An approach related to the ligand-exchange of metal complexes is the formation of mixed borate–diol ternary complexes [Kodama et al., 2006]. For example, recently the use of (5S)-pinandiol (SPD) as the chiral selector in the presence of borate as a central ion and SDS has been described (**Figure 2.30**) [Kodama et al., 2005]. Three diols (1-phenyl-1,2-ethanediol, 3-phenoxy-1,2-propanediol and 3-benzyloxy-1,2-propanediol) were successfully resolved by this technique. Di-n-amyl L-tartrate-boric acid complex chiral selector in situ synthesis and its application in chiral non-aqueous capillary electrophoresis is presented by Wang et al. [Wang L.J. et al., 2011].

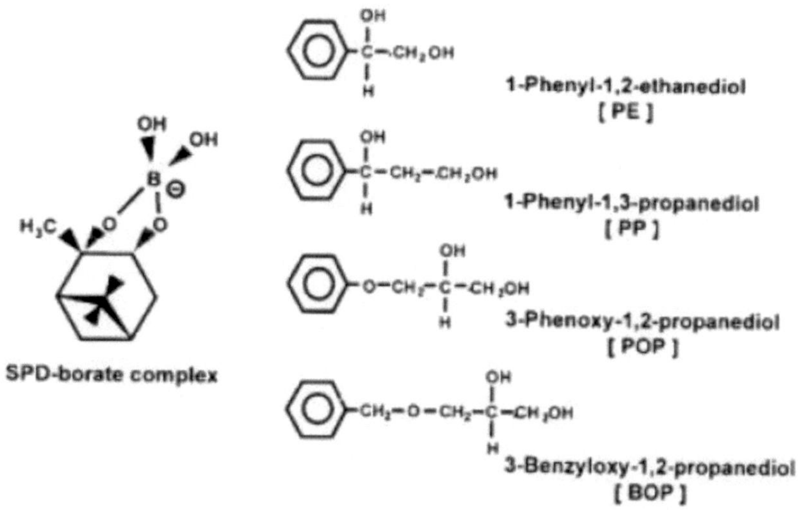

Figure 2.30. Chemical structures of SPD–borate complex and analytes. Reprinted from ref. from [Kodama et al., 2005].

The limited stability of these selectors, their UV absorption (detection difficulties) and rather slow ligand-exchange kinetics (poor enantioresolution) [Blanco & Valverde, 2003] could be the main reasons for a rare utilization of these selectors in chiral CE. Recently, tartaric acid–Cu(II) complex has been used as a selector for the chiral separation of drugs with amino alcohol structure [Hödl et al., 2007], however, it has not been employed in real bioanalyses so far.

2.3.7 Ion-pairing reagents

Ion-pairing reagents {e.g., (+)-*S*-Camphor-10-sulfonic acid; 2*R*,3*S*,4*R*,5*S* (−) 2,3,4,6-di-*O*-isopropylidene-2-keto-l-gulonic acid; 1*S*,4*R*(+) ketopinic acid, see examples in Figure 2.31}, are applicable in CE usually in non-aqueous medium as the essential interactions (hydrogen bondings and dipole–dipole interactions) are less effective in aqueous medium [Bjornsdottir et al., 1996; Carlsson et al., 2001; Hedeland et al., 2007]. Exceptions are the use of chiral counterions as supporting agents for separations with coselectors (e.g., CDs) in aqueous organic mixtures [Kodama et al., 2003].

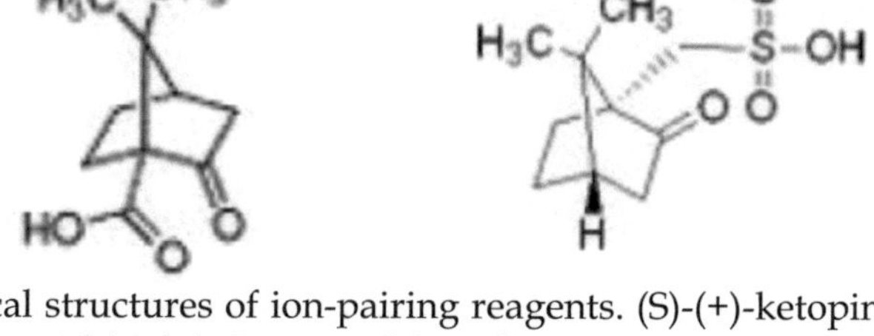

Figure 2.31. Chemical structures of ion-pairing reagents. (S)-(+)-ketopinic acid (left), (+)-(S)-camphor-10-sulfonic acid (right). Reprinted from [sigmaaldrich.com].

The ion-pairing mechanism under non-aqueous conditions took part in the enantioseparation of many drugs such as β-blockers [Bjornsdottir et al., 1996; Carlsson et al., 2001; Hedeland et al., 2007]. It cooperated also in bioanalytical applications separating enantiomers of salbutamol with heptakis-(2,3-di-O-acetyl-6-O-sulfo)-β-CD in urine samples under non-aqueous EKC conditions [Servais et al., 2004, 2006] (for detail see Table 2.1).

2.3.8 Amphiphilic molecules, micelles, micelle polymers and microemulsions

Amphiphilic molecules, composed of a polar head group and a hydrophobic tail, can form micelles above their critical micelle concentration (Figure 2.32). Micelles are aggregates (usually spherical) with a surface created by heads and core by tails. A typical recognition of analytes is based on the formation of associates with the micelles (less polar parts of analytes tend to enter the micelle core) having different stability for the two analytes of different hydrophobicity, or in other words, differences in their partition coefficients between the micelle phase and the electrolyte bulk phase. Chiral recognition is given by modifying partition coefficients of chiral analytes due to different steric effects between chiral analytes and chiral core or chiral surface of micelles. Micelle pseudostationary phases were introduced into CE by Terabe et al. [Terabe et al., 1984]. Different classes of charged as well as neutral amphiphilic molecules, namely bile salts, saponines, long-chain *N*-alkyl-lamino acids, *N*-alkanoyl-L-amino acids, *N*-dodecoxycarbonyl amino acids, alkylglycosides, alkylglucosides, were applied as chiral selectors in aqueous solutions for a wide range of substances of a hydrophilic or hydrophobic nature, see the specialized review article [Palmer & McCarney, 2004a]. For example, sodium cholate was used for the enantiomeric separation of mono and diacid benzoporfyrine derivates in serum and microsome samples [Peng et al., 2002] (for details see Table 2.1).

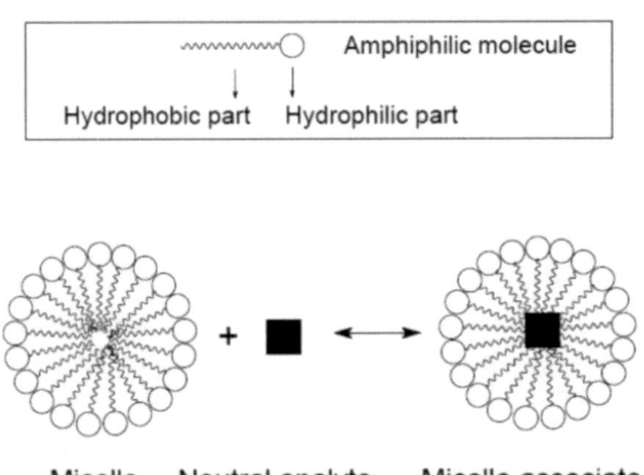

Figure 2.32. Mechanism of formation of micelle associate with neutral molecule. Reprinted from ref. [Terabe et al., 1984].

Micelle polymers {e.g., poly- sodium *N*-undecenoxy carbonyl-L-leucinate/isoleucinate (Figure 2.33), 3-[(3-dehydroabietamidopropyl)dimethyl-ammonio]-1-propane-sulfonate, undecyl-L-valine} can offer additional benefits in comparison to conventional micelles, such as elimination of intrinsic micelle equilibrium (enhanced chiral recognition), wide concentration range applicable (no critical micelle concentration) and therefore, higher obtainable signal to noise ratio (S/N). Further, the covalent bonds between surfactant monomers are stable (less background noise from ionized surfactant monomers of low molecular weights in mass spectrometer) and there are no disruptions in micelle formation (wider range of buffer additives applicable, e.g., organic modifiers). Micelle polymers have lower surface activity, association kinetics is fast due to a shallower and faster penetration of the solute into the compact polymeric structure (enhanced efficiency) [Riekkola et al., 1997; Palmer & McCarney, 2004b; Palmer, 2007; Zhao, S. et al., 2007; Akbay et al., 2005; Hou, J. G. et al., 2006; Rizvi et al., 2007]. Many of these properties are beneficial for enhancing chiral, as well as achiral, recognition {a broad range of structurally diverse racemic compounds such as phenylethylamines, β-blockers, 2-(2-chlorophenoxy) propionic acid, benzoin derivatives, derivatized amino acids and benzodiazepines} and for improving detection (very pronounced in MS) when compared with traditional micelle systems [Rizvi et al., 2007]. Therefore, the utilization of these selectors tends to rise up as it is apparent from the following recent applications in biological samples (human urine, plasma), such as poly(sodium *N*-undecenoxy carbonyl-L-leucine) sulfate vs. pseudoephedrine [Rizvi et al., 2007], polysodium-*N*-undecenoyl-L,L-leucyl-valinate vs. warfarin [Hou, J. et al., 2007], for details see Table 2.1.

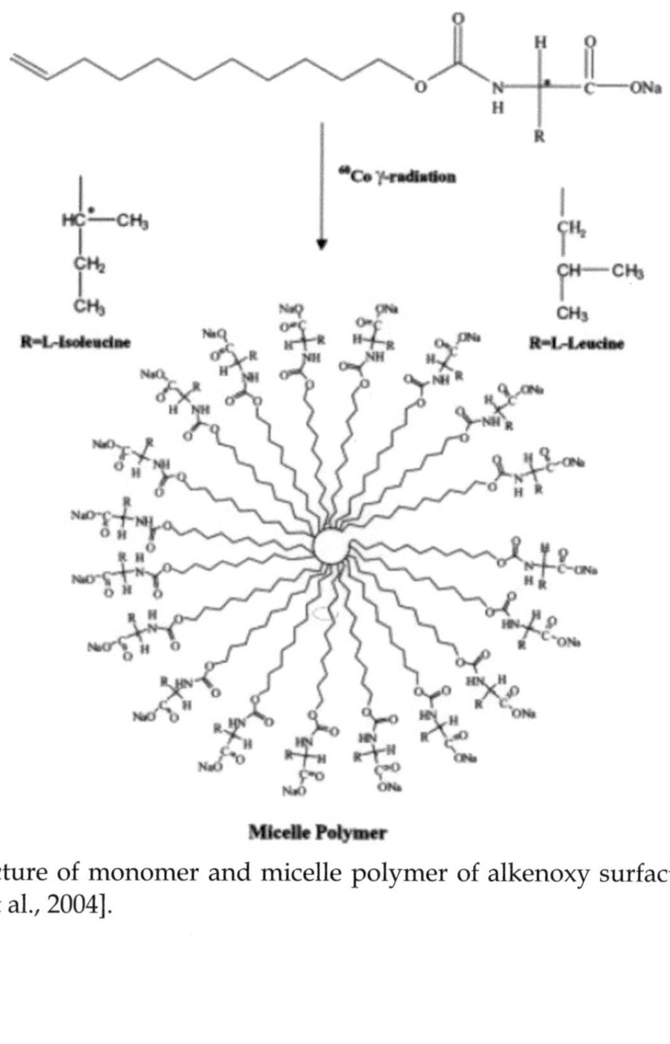

Figure 2.33. Structure of monomer and micelle polymer of alkenoxy surfactants. Reprinted from ref. [Rizvi et al., 2004].

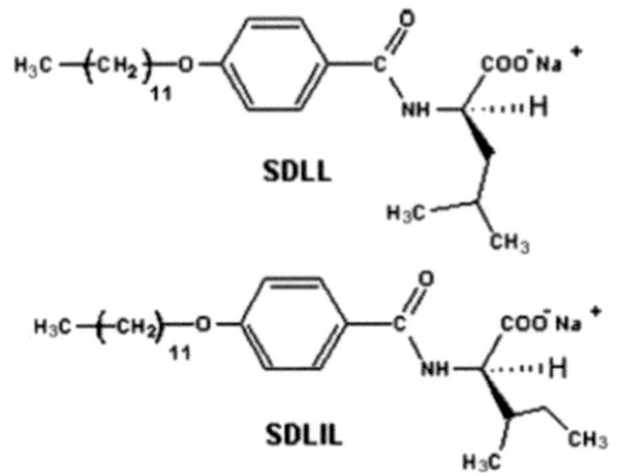

Figure 2.34. Molecular structures of the vesicle-forming amphiphilic molecules. Sodium *N*-[4-*n*-dodecyloxybenzoyl]-L-leucinate (SDLL) and sodium *N*-[4-*n*-dodecyloxybenzoyl]-L-isoleucinate (SDLIL). Reprinted from ref. [Mohanty & Dey, 2006].

The use of vesicle-forming amphiphilic molecules (e.g., sodium N-[4-n-dodecyloxybenzoyl]-L-leucinate) [Mohanty & Dey, 2006] and ionic liquids (i.e., salts in the liquid state, organic salts with low melting points soluble in both polar and nonpolar solvents, e.g., undecenoxycarbonyl-L-pyrrolidinol bromide) [Rizvi & Shamsi, 2006] can be counted among the recent trends in chiral CE with new potentialities for biologically active chiral compounds. For example, two vesicle-forming single-tailed amino acid derivatized surfactants sodium *N*-[4-*n*-dodecyloxybenzoyl]-L-leucinate (SDLL) and sodium *N*-[4-*n*-dodecyloxybenzoyl]-L-isoleucinate (SDLIL) (Figure 2.34) have been synthesized and used as a pseudo-stationary phase in MEKC for various model chiral analytes, namely atropisomers (±)-1,1′-bi-2-naphthol, (±)-1,1′-binaphthyl-2,2′-diamine, (±)-1,1′-binaphthyl-2,2′-diylhydrogen phosphate and Tröger's base and chiral compound benzoin [Mohanty & Dey, 2006]. Results of these studies have suggested formation of vesicles in aqueous solutions. Microenvironment of the vesicle determined the depth of penetration of the analytes into vesicle, and, in this way, it influenced the separation selectivity. The application of novel ionic liquid-like surfactants and their polymers for chiral separation of acidic analytes in MEKC was reported first by Rizvi and Shamsi in 2006 [Rizvi & Shamsi, 2006]. The two model acidic analytes, (*rac*)-α-bromophenylacetic acid and (*rac*)-2-(2-chlorophenoxy)propanoic acid, were successfully separated with the amino alcohol-derived chiral ionic liquids (given in Figure 2.35) and their polymers at 25 mM surfactant concentration.

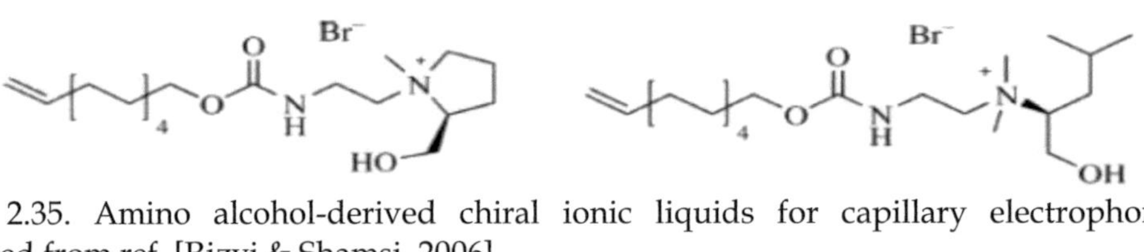

Figure 2.35. Amino alcohol-derived chiral ionic liquids for capillary electrophoresis. Reprinted from ref. [Rizvi & Shamsi, 2006].

Microemulsions, spherical aggregates of nanometre size consisting of an oil core covered/stabilized by amphiphilic molecules in water solution (Figure 2.36), are optically transparent and thermodynamically stable phases that offer a new alternative to micelles for chiral separations aimed at hydrophobic molecules. Chiral microemulsions can utilize one chiral entity (either surfactant, cosurfactant or oil are chiral) or more than one chiral entity (e.g., both surfactant and cosurfactant are chiral) [Ryan et al., 2009; Kahle & Foley, 2006]. Only a few applications to chiral separations have been described (none yet in biological samples), including chiral oils, chiral amphiphilic molecules, as well as CDs as chiral additives [Marsh et al., 2004; McEvoy et al., 2007]. Kahle and Foley [Kahle & Foley, 2007a; 2007b, 2007c] investigated one-, two- and three-chiral-component microemulsions, composed of the chiral surfactant dodecoxycarbonylvaline, the cosurfactant 2-hexanol and one of the chiral oils dibutyl or diethyl tartrate for MEEKC. Six basic drugs, viz. four ephedrine derivatives and two β-blockers, were used as test solutes. For most analytes, enantioselectivity, as well as resolution, were higher with the best dual-chirality system compared with the best one-chiral-component microemulsion due to synergistic effects.

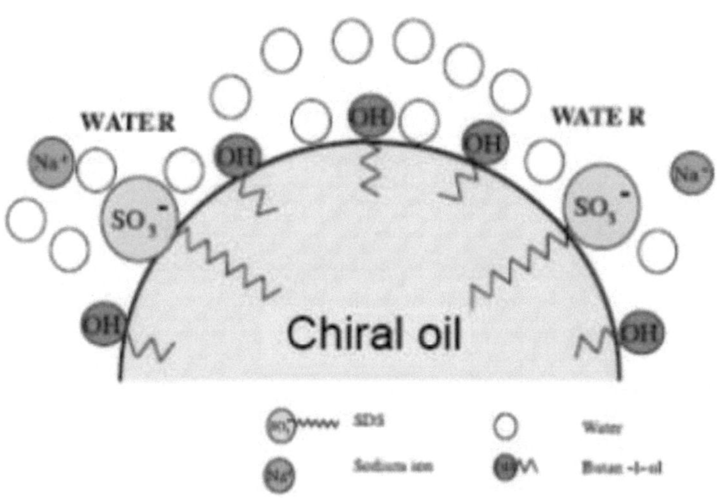

Figure 2.36. Schematic representation of an oil-in-water microemulsion droplet. Adapted from ref. [Ryan et al., 2009].

2.3.9 Alternative chiral selectors

Several alternative chiral selectors, compared to those described in sections 2.3.1-2.3.8, have been employed in chiral CE, including calixarenes (macrocyclic compounds consisting of benzene rings linked by methylene groups and chiral substituent, see Figure 2.37), cyclosphoraoses (unbranched cyclic β-D-glucans), hemispherodextrins (capped CDs), tergurides (ergot alkaloids), amphiphilic aminosaccharides, cyclopeptides, guanosine gels, aptamers (single-stranded RNA or DNA oligonucleotides 15 to 60 base in length that bind with high affinity to specific molecular targets), e.g., anti-arginine 1-RNA aptamer, dendrimers (repetitively branched cascade molecules, see Figure 2.38), etc. [Van Eeckhaut & Michotte, 2006; Gübitz & Schmid, 2004, 2008; Riekkola et al., 1997; Mokhtari et al., 2011, Chen Y.M. et al. 1998]. These selectors can solve particular/specific problems in chiral separations, however, their use is less universal in most cases as they can be expensive and their availability is limited. This could also be the reason why no application in chiral bioanalysis has been demonstrated so far.

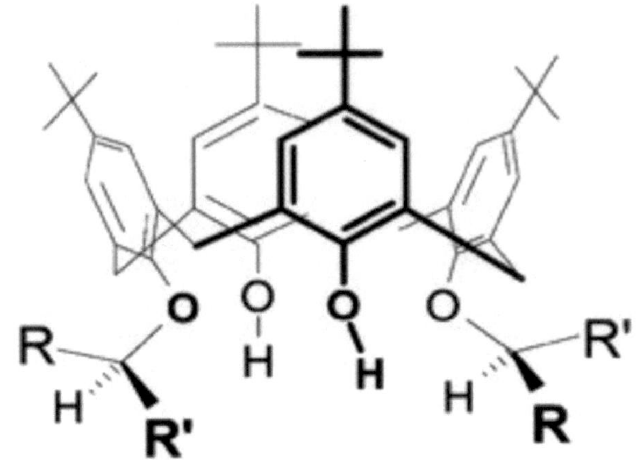

Figure 2.37. Chiral calixarene. Reprinted from [rsc.org].

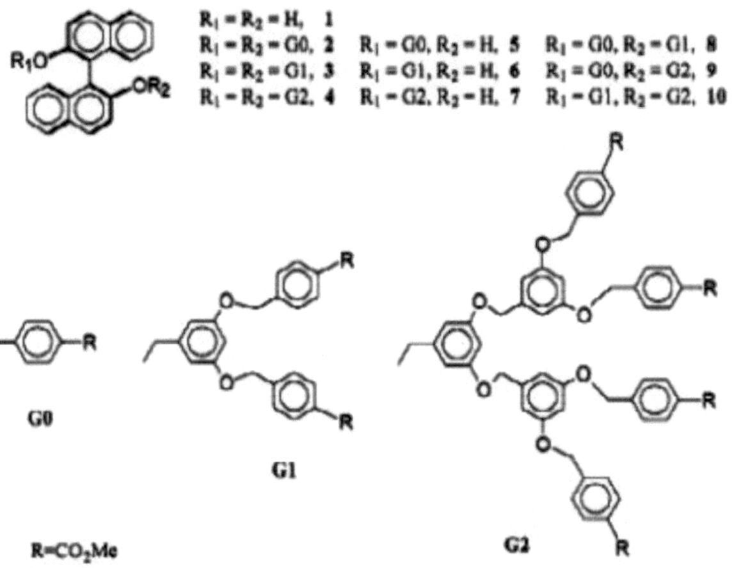

Figure 2.38. The chemical structures of the chiral dendrimers with axial chirality. Reprinted from ref. [Chen, Y.M. et al., 1998].

2.4 Applications of chiral separation systems in bioanalysis

The following examples illustrate successful EKC enantioseparations of drugs in biological samples utilizing some of the progressive chiral principles mentioned in section 2.2. and/or new chiral selectors mentioned in section 2.3. CEC and MCE applications in this field are also included.

New chiral selectors. A sensitive MEKC-MS method using poly(sodium *N*-undecenoxy carbonyl-L-leucine) sulfate was developed for enantioselective analysis of pseudoephedrine in human urine [Rizvi et al., 2007]. The permanent charge of this micelle chiral selector allows for setting separation conditions (electrolyte pH) suitable for obtaining the highest detection sensitivity maintaining sufficient enantioresolution. Other new chiral selectors and new chiral stationary phases can be also found in some applications given for the advanced electromigration modes and mechanisms below.

Countercurrent migration. Rudaz et al. [Rudaz et al., 2005] used the countercurrent migration of the negatively charged highly sulfated-γ-CD to achieve a highly effective enantioseparation of amphetamine derivatives in plasma. This strategy allowed using a low concentration (0.15%) of the chiral selector for the complete enantioseparation of seven amphetamine derivatives in analysis times of less than 6 min.

Anionic CD, the heptakis(2,6-diacethyl-6-sulfato)-β-CD, migrating in the opposite direction to the analytes, was highly effective in low concentrations (0.85 mM) for the simultaneous chiral CD-EKC-MS separation of methamphetamine, 3,4-methylenedioxyamphetamine and amphetamine in clinical human urine samples [Iio et al., 2005].

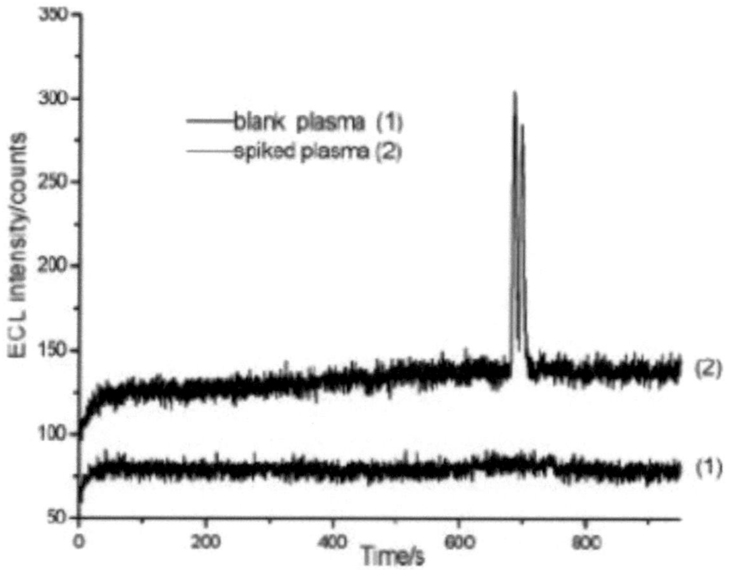

Figure 2.39. Electropherograms of extracts of blank plasma and plasma of spiked concentration of 4 μM racemic drug. Conditions: detection buffer, 5 mM $Ru(bpy)_3{}^{2+}$ in 100 mM (pH 6.5) phosphate buffer; separation buffer, 3 mg/mL of S-β-CD in 40 mM (pH 4.5) acetate buffer; applied voltage, 22 kV; injection time, 5 s. Reprinted from ref. [Fang, L. et al., 2006].

The CD-EKC method based on a combination of discontinuous buffer (separation buffer differed from detection solution, essential for chemiluminiscence detection) with low concentration (3 mg/mL) of anionic highly sulfated-β-CD was used for the baseline enantioseparation of an oppositely charged racemic antiarrhythmic drug, disopyramide, in spiked plasma samples, see Figure 2.39 [Fang, L. et al., 2006].

Naphthalene-2,3-dicarboxaldehyde (NDA) derivatized baclofen was separated in human plasma using the CD-EKC-LIF method based on a highly sulfated-β-CD [Kavran-Belin et al., 2005]. The anionic CD migrated in the opposite direction toward negatively charged baclofen (pH 9.5) transported by EOF toward the cathode.

The NACE-MS with countercurrent migration of heptakis(2,3-di-*O*-acetyl-6-*O*-sulfo)-β-CD present in acidified methanol medium was used for the separation and determination of low levels of the enantiomers of a basic chiral drug (salbutamol) in biological samples (human urine) [Servais et al., 2006].

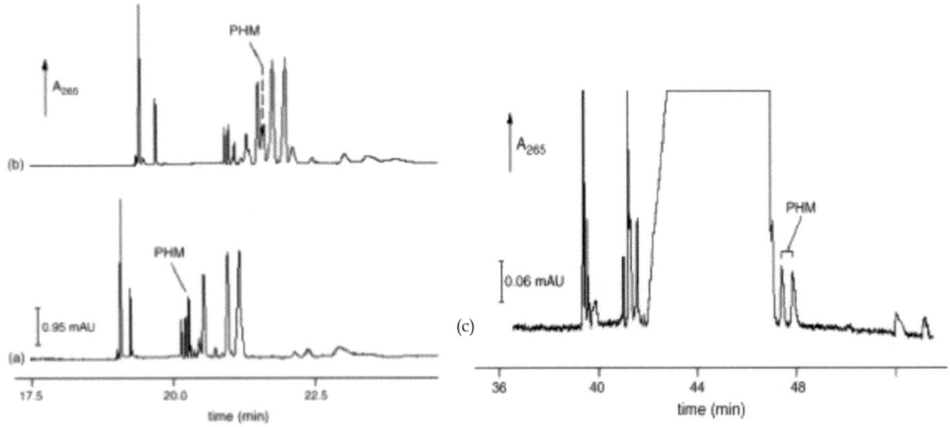

Figure 2.40. Electropherograms showing the effect of the charge of ionizable chiral selector, CE-β-CD, on the EKC separation of PHM enantiomers in a partially pretreated urine matrix. The separations were carried out with the uncharged CE-β-CD (a, b) and with the negatively charged CE-β-CD (c). Separating conditions: (a, b) EKC electrolyte system consisting of a 25mM glycine-acetic acid buffer, pH 3.2, 0.2 methylhydroxyethylcellulose as an EOF suppressor, with a 0 (a) and 15 (b) mg/mL concentration of CE-β-CD, (c) EKC electrolyte system consisting of a 25mM ε–aminocaproic acid-acetic acid buffer, pH 4.5, 0.2 methylhydroxyethylcellulose as an EOF suppressor, with a 2.5 mg/mL concentration of CE-β-CD. Sample and analyte: (a, b) PHM was present in the sample (20-times diluted urine) at a 150 ng/mL concentration. (c) PHM was present in the sample (4-times diluted urine) at a 30 ng/mL concentration. Reprinted from ref. [Mikuš et al., 2006a].

Negatively charged carboxyethyl-β-CD considerably improved enantioresolution of several oppositely charged H_1-antihistamines (pheniramine and its metabolite, dimethindene, dioxopromethazine) in comparison with native CDs [Mikuš et al., 2006a]. Countercurrent migration and enhanced complexation were responsible not only for improved chiral separation of the drugs and the metabolite, but also achiral separation allowing resolution of the drug enantiomers from their metabolic products, as well as from the sample matrix constituents when metabolic study of pheniramine in urine samples was carried out [Marák et al., 2007]. A high effectivity of the separation was demonstrated by a low concentration of the chiral selector enabling optimum separating conditions for the trace chiral analytes in concentrated biological matrices [Mikuš et al., 2006a], see Figure 2.40.

Charged chiral pseudophases/carrier systems. The enantioseparations of cyanobenz[*f*]isoindole serine (CBI) derivatives of glutamate and aspartate in squirrel brain samples were accomplished with a highly sulfated-β-CD as chiral selector at low pH and reverse polarity [Kirschner et al., 2007].

Mixed selector systems. Aspartate enantiomers (NDA derivatives) were separated in the samples prepared from tissue of the central nervous system of *A. californica* using mixed micelles composed from β-CD and SDS [Miao et al., 2005].

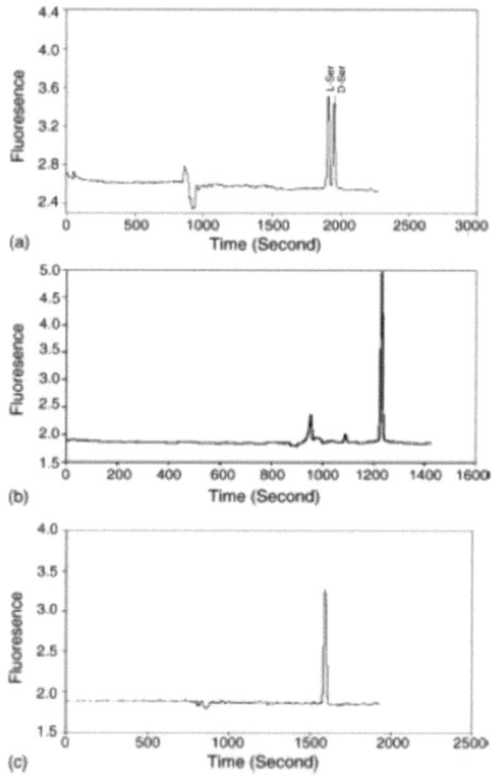

Figure 2.41. Separation of CBI-Ser enantiomers using different running buffers: (a) 100mM borate (pH 9.5), 30mM β–CD and 60mM SDC; (b) 100mM borate (pH 9.5) and 30mM β-CD; (c) 100mM borate (pH 10.0), 60mM SDC. Capillary was 50 μm i.d.×50 cm effective length. Voltage applied was 15 kV. Ser enantiomer concentration was 2.0 μM. Reprinted from ref. [Zhao, S.L. et al., 2005b].

The CD-MEKC separation of CBI-D/L-serine enantiomers was achieved by using a dual chiral selector system consisting of β-CD and chiral micelles formed by deoxycholic acid (SCD) [Zhao, S.L. et al., 2005b]. The essential role of the mixed chiral selector system for the enantioresolution in comparison with the capability of individual chiral selectors is demonstrated in Figure 2.41, compare electropherograms (a-c). In addition, an effectivity of the mixed chiral selector system in the enantioseparation of CBI-D/L-serine enantiomers in real biological matrices was demonstrated in this work. In this way, for the first time, peaks corresponding to L-serine and D-serine were completely separated in *Aplysia* ganglian (a sea mollusc widely used as a neuronal model) homogenates.

The evaluation of the enantioselectivity of glycogen-based dual chiral selector systems towards basic drugs in capillary electrophoresis is presented by Chen et al. [Chen J. et al., 2010].

Flow counterbalanced systems. Several FCCE modes have been developed and applied for enantioseparations so far, like microfluidic temperature gradient focusing [Balss et al., 2004], electric field gradient focusing [Koegler & Ivory, 1996a, 1996b, Ivory, 2000, Huang, Z. & Ivory, 1999]. Notice that these techniques have a great potential not only in enantioseparations, but also in a sample pretreatment (focusing, see chapter 3).

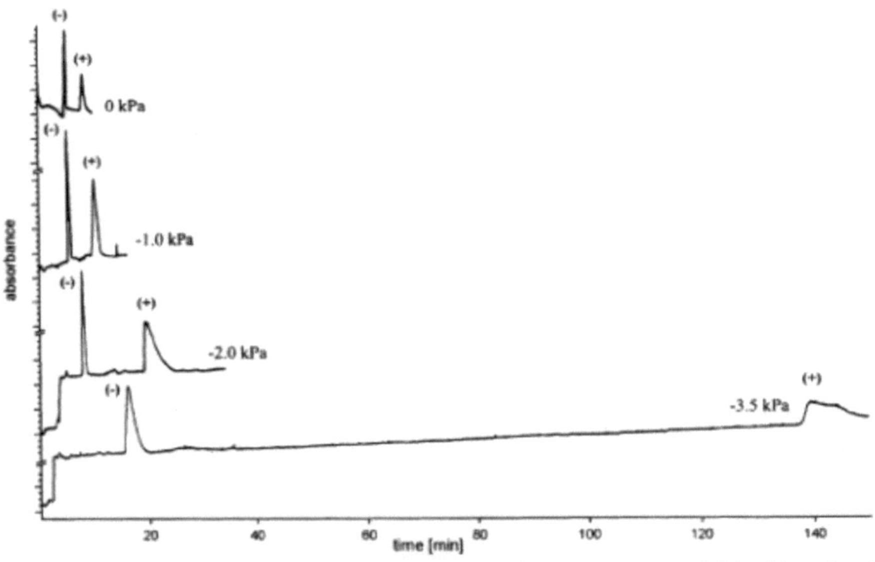

Figure 2.42. Effect of increasing counterpressure on the separation of (±)-chlorpheniramine in the presence of 2 mg/mL CM-β–CD). Reproduced from ref. [Chankvetadze et al., 1999].

The effect of increasing counterpressure on the separation of (±)-chlorpheniramine in the presence of 2 mg/mL CM-β-CD) was studied by Chankvetadze et al. [Chankvetadze et al., 1999] and remarkable results are illustrated in Figure 2.42. Applications of counterpressure techniques for the enantioseparations in complex ionic matrices, however, have not been demonstrated.

Synchronous cyclic capillary electrophoresis (SCCE) was proposed by Jorgenson's group [Zhao J. et al., 1999] as a technique which allows overcoming the dispersion problems in FCCE caused by the parabolic counterflow profile. This technique was applied for isotopic and chiral separations. In the third cycle, the chiral compound (α-hydroxybenzyl) methyltrimethylammonium with a selectivity of 1.0078 was almost baseline separated in 3.5 h [Zhao J. & Jorgenson, 1999].

CEC. CEC separations are carried out mainly in packed capillary columns. Immobilization provides an effective solution especially for the chiral selectors with problematic detection properties, such as proteins, macrocyclic antibiotics, etc., that was demonstrated on many model examples, such as vancomycin CSP vs. warfarin and various β-blockers (atenolol, metoprolol, pindolol, oxprenolol, alprenolol, propranolol, carteolol, talinolol) vs. MS detection [Zheng J. & Shamsi, 2006; Zheng J. et al., 2006].

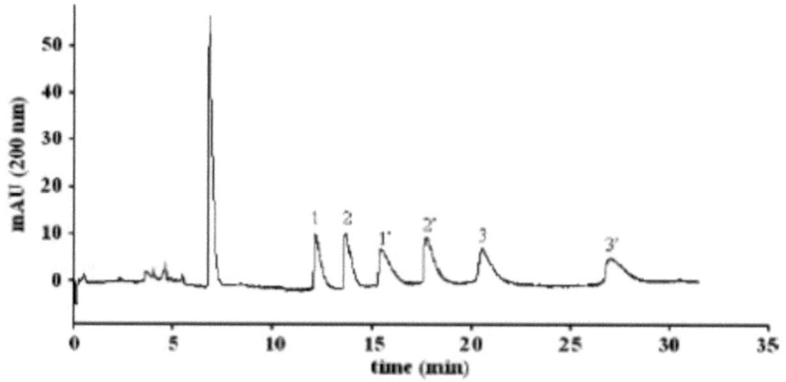

Figure 2.43. Electrochromatogram of blank urine sample spiked with 10 μg/mL of racemic MRT and 8-OH-M and 20 μg/mL of racemic DMR. Both samples were subjected to the SPE procedure. Electrochromatographic conditions: stationary phase composition, vancomycin-CSP, mobile phase, 100 mM ammonium acetate buffer (pH 6)/H_2O/MeOH/ACN (5:15:30:50, by vol.). Other CEC conditions: capillary column, 75 μm i.d., 33 cm total length, 23 cm packed length, 24.5 cm effective length; applied voltage, 25 kV; capillary temperature, 20°C; pressurized column at both ends with 10 bar; injection by pressure at 10 bar, 0.5 min, followed by a plug of mobile phase at 10 bar, 0.2 min. (1) MRT, (2) 8-OH-M and (3) DMR. Reprinted from ref. [Aturki et al., 2007].

Various new CSPs are also employed in model analyses. A new chiral capillary electrophoresis column coated by carbosilane dendrimers with peripheral Si-Cl groups and beta-cyclodextrin was prepared by Shou et al. [Shou et al., 2008]. The separation characteristics of stability and longevity of coated capillaries modified by carbosilane dendrimers were excellent. The varying of separation efficiency was less than 5%, after running for one month. The optimum conditions contained the running voltage of 12 kV, the UV detector wavelength of 214 nm, the sample injected time of 7 s and the phosphate buffer solution concentration of 40 mM. Chlortrimeton, hydrochloric promethazine and benzedrine were selected as the separation model targets. Especially, G2P columns could be used as separate chlortrimeton enantiomers effectively. Under these conditions, the column efficiency was 2.5 x 105 plates/m with a resolution of 1.43 and baseline separation.

Other examples of the CEC application are illustrated on biological samples. For example, CEC based on vancomycin CSP offered an effective solution not only for the enantioseparation of mirtazapine (MRT) and its metabolites {8-hydroxymirtazapine (8-OH-M) and *N*-desmethylmirtazapine (DMR)} in urine samples (pretreated by off-line solid-phase extraction), but also for their reliable UV absorbance detection [Aturki et al., 2007], see Figure 2.43.

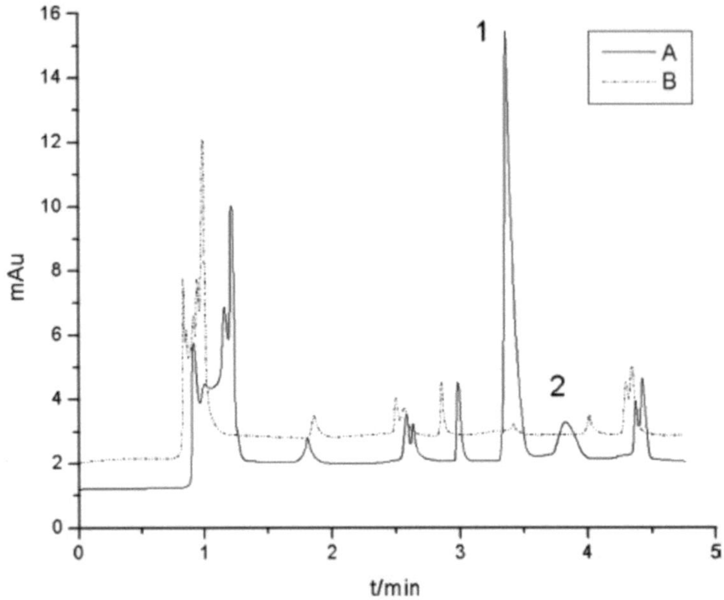

Figure 2.44. Separation of mexiletine hydrochloride in human plasma sample by Asp-β–CD fabricated monolithic column. (A) Plasma sample; (B) free plasma. 1 and 2, the enantiomers' peaks of mexiletine hydrochloride. Mobile phase: phosphate/trolamine buffer, 5mM, pH= 4.5; temperature: 20°C; voltage: −10 kV; injection: −2 kV, 2 s. Reprinted from ref. [Li Y. et al., 2010].

Very attractive applications due to rapid separations and good enantioresolutions are represented by the chiral monolithic based CEC. A monolithic column fabricated with Asp-β–CD was applied to the separation of mexiletine hydrochloride enantiomers in a human plasma sample. Because of complex matrices, as little as possible trolamine was added to the phosphate buffer to decrease absorption between the sample and the solid-phase. Figure 2.44 shows the electropherogram of mexiletine hydrochloride extracted from the plasma sample. From Figure 2.44, two enantiomers were separated by baseline, the migration times were 3.46 and 3.84 min, respectively. Some components in plasma were also determined, but they did not interfere with the determination of the enantiomers. Thus, the method was applied to the complex matrix sample, and the column had good selectivity.

MCE. MCE with (+)-18-crown-6-tetracarboxylic acid as a chiral selector was applied for the countercurrent chiral separation of gemifloxacin in urine samples after an appropriate sample pretreatment (see in 3.2.2) [Cho et al., 2004]. A successful chiral separation was achieved in ca. 3 min, with an extremely small amount of the chiral selector (50 μM), and minute amounts of both sample as well as BGE. This demonstrated significant potentialities of electromigration methods in highly effective ultraspeed microscale chiral analyses of drugs in complex matrices.

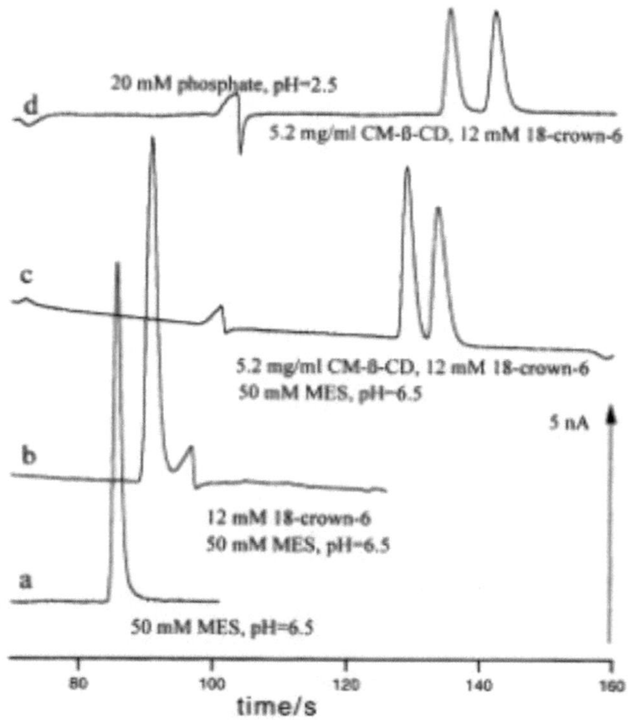

Figure 2.45. Enantiomeric separation of noradrenaline with CM-β-CD by formation of sandwich complexes with 18-crown-6 at pH 6.5 and 2.5. Separation voltage, 3 kV; detection potential, 1500 mV; injection, 1 kV (3 s); concentration of standard, 10^{-4} *M*. Reprinted from ref. [Schwarz & Hauser, 2001].

A combination of an advanced enantioseparation mechanism (dual chiral selector system) with advanced CE format (MCE) was demonstrated by Schwarz and Hauser [Schwarz & Hauser, 2001]. The separation of the enantiomers of noradrenaline in the presence of 18-crown-6 is illustrated in Figure 2.45. The crown ether on its own has a small effect on the migration, but cannot lead to a chiral separation (Figure 2.45b). In combination with the carboxymethylated β-cyclodextrin (Figure 2.45c), a chiral separation which is better than the one achieved by only carboxymethylated β-cyclodextrin is obtained. The resolution factors (*R*) were determined as 1.30 and 1.35 (5.2 mg/mL CM-β-CD, pH=6.7) with and without the addition of 12 m*M* 18-crown-6, respectively. Moreover, such an advanced system is capable of also separating multicomponent mixtures of enantiomers, as presented in Figure 2.46.

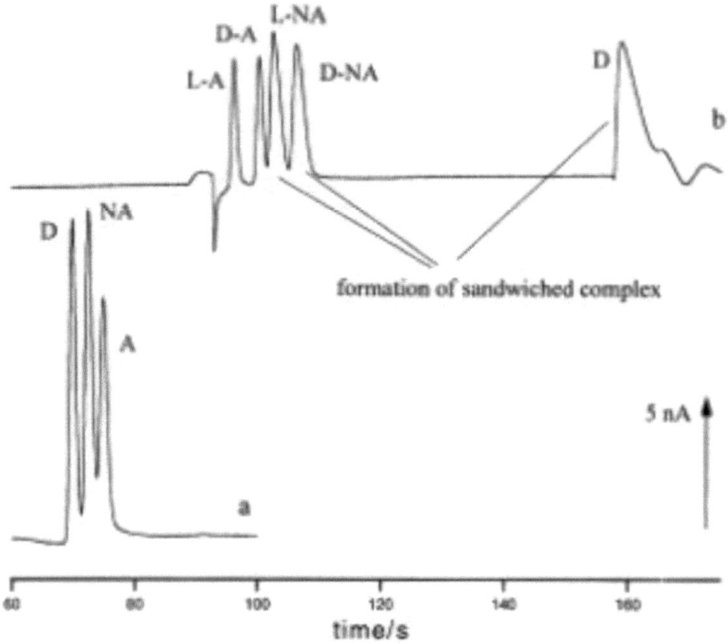

Figure 2.46. Rapid enantiomer MCE separation and amperometric detection of a mixture of adrenaline, noradrenaline and dopamine employing sandwich complexes. Buffer: (a) 50 mM MES, pH=6.7; (b) 20 mM phosphate, pH=3.0, 5.2 mg/mL CM-β-CD, 12 mM 18-crown-6. Separation voltage, 3 kV; detection potential, (a) 1300 mV, (b) 1500 mV; injection, 1 kV (3 s); concentration of standards, 10^{-4} M. Peak marks: dopamine hydrochloride, D, adrenaline, A, noradrenaline, NA. Reprinted from ref. [Schwarz & Hauser, 2001].

3

Advanced Sample Preparation

3.1 On-line sample preparation techniques in capillary electrophoresis - introduction

The importance of sample preparation is related to high demands on (i) the sensitivity of quantitative determination of trace analytes, (ii) the selectivity of monitoring of analytes in multicomponent sample matrix and (iii) the automatization and miniaturization of analysis [Mikuš & Maráková, 2010].

Sensitivity. One of the most pronounced limitations of capillary electromigration methods when compared to more traditional liquid-phase separation techniques, such as HPLC, is a poor concentration sensitivity of photometric detectors, which are the most popular among on-capillary CE detectors. The reached LODs are by two orders inferior in comparison to the HPLC technique because of a short optical pathlength and small sample injection volume. Two basic approaches can be distinguished among many efforts that have been made to improve the sensitivity of detection in CE. Either more sensitive detection schemes can displace the UV detection mode [Hernández et al., 2008, 2010; Hempel, 2000] or an increased analyte mass can be cumulated in its zone prior to detection utilizing a proper sample preparation, as it is reviewed in this section.

Selectivity. To achieve adequate separation selectivity, the analysis of real/complex samples in CE usually requires efficient sample treatment to remove interfering solutes, inorganic and organic salts, and particulate matter (as it is reviewed in this section). At the same time, the creation of a chiral environment is necessary for the separation of enantiomeric species by the electrokinetic chromatography (EKC) principle accomplished in zone electrophoretic mode simply by the addition of chiral selector molecules. In the same way, chiral selectivity can be implemented in isotachophoretic mode. Chiral separation principles in CE have been described in many review papers [Chankvetadze, 1997; Chankvetadze & Blaschke, 2001; Gübitz & Schmid, 2007, 2008; Preinerstorfer et al., 2009; Fanali, 2002; Fanali et al., 1998b; Ossicini & Fanali, 1997]. In addition to those, capillary electrochromatography (CEC) separation principles cannot be omitted for review, e.g., those by Schurig [Wistuba & Schurig, 2000a, 2000b]. On-line sample preparation and enantioseparation mechanisms should create a harmonized system, especially in chiral EKC and ITP where the chiral selector is not immobilized as it is in CEC, and all possible mutual negative interferences have to be carefully eliminated.

Automatization and miniaturization. As one moves toward small sample volumes, sample handling and preparation steps become more difficult and the concentration step is therefore preferably done on-line instead of off-line. The microfluidic devices, such as microchips, can provide several additional advantages over electromigration techniques performed in capillary format. The heat dissipation is much better in chip format compared to that in a capillary and therefore higher electric fields can be applied across channels of the microchip. This fact enables, along with a considerably reduced length of channels, significant shortening of separation time. The sample and reagent consumption is markedly reduced in microchannels. Hence, the chiral MCE can provide a unique possibility of ultraspeed enantiomeric separations of microscale sample amounts. On the other hand, the efficiency is often weak due to the shape of the chips and the quality of the injection [Guihen et al., 2009]. Until now, electrophoresis, rather than chromatography, has been the primary principle applied in microchip separations for several reasons as follows: (i) the materials typically used for microchips can barely withstand the high pressures applied for chromatographic separations; (ii) the packing of the chromatographic particles into the channels without voids can be difficult, (iii) the performance of chromatography decreases with decreased column length [Preinerstorfer et al., 2009]. Nevertheless, both electrophoretic [Gong & Hauser, 2006; Piehl et al., 2004; Belder et al., 2006], as well as electrochromatographic, modes [Weng, et al. 2006] are applicable in microchip format. Nowadays, the on-line coupling of sample treatment systems to CE or MCE are of great interest because it allows the automatization of the analytical process (from sample preparation to data treatment), which is a current trend in analytical chemistry.

Thus, the importance of on-line sample preparation is pronounced when ultratrace analytes (ng/mL and less) are determined in minute amounts (μl, μg and less) of samples with complex matrices (variable in qualitative and quantitative composition). This is a common situation in the analyses of drugs, their metabolites and biomarkers in biological samples where preconcentration of analytes, elimination of matrix interferents, and minimized sample handling is necessary to obtain relevant analytical results. Mikuš and Maráková [Mikuš & Maráková, 2010] recently provided a review on the chiral capillary electrophoresis with on-line sample preparation. The latest panorama of sample preparation methods for animal/human and plant samples given by Chen et al. [Chen Y., 2008] has been composed from almost 500 references, highlighting some promising methods which have fast developed over recent years and giving a somewhat brief introduction on most of the well-developed methods, including on-line stacking methods in CE. Wu [Wu X.Z., 2003] illustrated new approaches to sample preparation for CE and Kataoka [Kataoka, 2003] highlighted their utilization in clinical and pharmaceutical analysis. In addition to these rather general reviews, specialized reviews are included at the beginning of each following subsection. These highlight the role of electromigration effects and interactions in on-line sample preparation, and summarize basic electrophoretic (stacking) and non electrophoretic (mostly chromatographic and extraction) on-line sample preparation techniques aimed at preconcentration and purification of complex samples in chiral pharmaceutical and biomedical research. Application examples are listed in Table 3.1 showing the chiral pharmaceutical and biomedical analyses supported by on-line sample preparation procedures described in this chapter. On the other hand, conventional off-line sample preparation techniques, such as solid-phase extraction, liquid-phase extraction, solid-liquid extraction and dialysis (included in the above mentioned reviews), are not discussed here.

3.2 On-line sample preparation techniques based on electrophoretic principles

Several reviews have been published recently, focusing on the on-line sample preconcentration CE techniques based on electrophoretic principles leading to the compression of a long sample plug into a narrow band with a high concentration of analytes, so called stacking techniques [Lin C.H. & Kaneta, 2004; Gebauer et al., 2009, 2011; Silva, 2009; Ryan et al., 2009; Malá et al., 2007, 2011; Urbánek et al., 2003]. Among the latest detailed review papers are those by Lin and Kaneta [Lin C.H. & Kaneta, 2004], Simpson et al. [Simpson et al., 2008], Breadmore [Breadmore, 2007], Breadmore et al. [Breadmore et al., 2009] and Malá et al. [Malá et al., 2011], including research articles gathered in the period 2000-2011. The papers provide fundamentals and applications of basic types of on-line sample preconcentration techniques. McKibbin and Terabe [Britz-McKibbin & Terabe, 2003] emphasized on-line preconcentration strategies for trace analysis of metabolites by CE. Ruiz and Marina [Ruiz & Marina, 2006] reviewed sensitive chiral analysis by CE.

The stacking procedures, described in section 3.2.1, are modifications of the basic zone electrophoretic and/or isotachophoretic and/or isoelectric focusing separation modes (Figure 2.2). The stacking procedures are based on increasing analyte mass in its zone during the electromigration process via electromigration effects, enhancing sensitivity in this way. In all the cases, the key requirements are that there is an electrophoretic component in the preconcentration mechanism and that the analytes concentrate on a boundary through a change in velocity. Then we can recognize (i) field-strength-induced changes in velocity (field-enhanced sample stacking [Kim J.B. & Terabe, 2003; Quirino & Terabe, 2000; Chien & Burgi, 1992; Weiss et al., 2001], isotachophoresis and transient isotachophoresis [Beckers & Boček, 2000; Schwer et al., 1993; Shihabi, 2002]), and (ii) chemically induced changes in velocity (dynamic pH junction [Britz-McKibbin & Chen, 2000; Aebersold & Morrison, 1990; Kim J.B. et al., 2003], sweeping [Kitagawa et al., 2006; Palmer et al., 2001; Quirino & Terabe, 1998; Quirino & Terabe, 1999; Quirino et al., 2000]), see Table 3.2. In addition to these techniques, the counter-flow gradient focusing [Shackman & Ross, 2007], electrocapture [Horáková et al., 2007] and many others can be considered as the techniques based on a combination of field-strength and chemically induced changes in velocity offering new and interesting possibilities in on-line sample preparation (mainly preconcentration).

Some of the stacking techniques (and their combinations) can provide, besides (i) the preconcentration, other benefits, such as (ii) an effective sample purification isolating solute (group of solutes) from undesired matrix constituents [Simpson et al., 2008] or they can be combined with (iii) the chemical reaction of the analyte(s) [Ptolemy et al., 2005, 2006], in this way simplifying the overall analytical procedure. On the other hand, great attention must be paid to the selection of the type of chiral selector as its charge can interfere with a sample preparation technique that employs electrophoretic principles.

Analyte	Sample	Chiral selector[a]	Sample preparation: type and main purpose[b]	Detection and LOD	Application	Ref.
Fenoprofen and amino acid derivates	River water	vancomycin	LVSEP-ASEI/on preconcentration (~10^3)	UV, 0.38-2.10 ng/mL	Spiked real samples	Wang Z.Y. et al., 2011
Cimaterol, clenbuterol, terbutaline	Human urine	β-CD	t-ITP and FESI/on preconcentration (250x)	1 ng/mL		Huang L. et al., 2011
Amlodipine	Plasma and urine	HP–α–CD	EME/ preconcentration (124x)	3 ng/mL		Nojavan & Fakhari, 2010
Primary amine drugs (amphetamine)	Human urine	(+)-(18-crown-6)-tetracarboxylic acid	SDME/in preconcentration (~10^3) + clean-up	UV, 0.5 ng/mL	Spiked real samples	Choi et al., 2009
Trihexyphenidyl	Serum	CM–β–CD	LLE/off clean-up, FESS/on preconcentration (490x)	DAD, 0.92 ng/mL	Spiked real samples	Li H. et al., 2008
Pheniramine and its metabolites, dimethindene, dioxopromethazine	Human urine	CE-β-CD	ITP-EKC; ITP/on preconcentration (~10^2) + clean-up	UV, 1.1-4.8 ng/mL	Spiked real samples and metabolic study	Mikuš et al., 2006a
Pheniramine and its metabolites	Human urine	CE-β-CD	ITP-EKC; ITP/on preconcentration (~10^2) + clean-up	DAD, 5.2-6.8 ng/mL	Metabolic study	Marák et al., 2007
Amlodipine	Human urine	HP-β-CD	ITP-EKC; ITP/on preconcentration (~10^2) + clean-up	DAD, 9.3-10.4 ng/mL	Pharmacokinetic study	Mikuš et al., 2008a
Metoxamine, carvedilol, terbutaline, metaproterenol	Serum	β-CD	PP/off clean-up, LVSS/on preconcentration (100-1000x)	DAD, <300 ng/mL	Spiked real samples	Denola et al., 2007
Gemifloxacin	Urine, saliva	CWE	EK clean-up, MCE with coupled channels/on clean-up	UV, LIF, 3-4x10^{-6} M	Spiked real samples	Cho et al., 2004

New adrenoreceptors antagonists	Plasma	HP-β-CD	SPE/off clean-up, FESI/on preconcentration (180x)	UV, MS, 3 ng/mL	Spiked real samples	Grard et al., 2002
Lorazepam and its metabolites	Urine	HP-β-CD, SDS micelles	EH/off, SPE/off clean-up, SWP/on preconcentration	UV, ESI-MS	Metabolic study	Baldacci & Thormann, 2006
S-timolol, 1R,2S-ephedrine	Infusion solution	Ketopinic acid and diisoproylidenek etogulonic acid (NACE)	EK + tITP/on preconcentration	DAD, 0.2 % S-timolol, 0.033% 1R,2S-ephedrine	Enantiomeric purity testing of pharmaceuticals	Hedeland et al., 2007
CBI-amino acids	Squirrel brain samples	S-β-CD	HD + LVSS-SWP/on preconcentration	LIF, 10^{-10} M	Biomedical study	Kirschner et al., 2007
Muramic acid and diaminopimelic acid	Bacterial cultures	OPA/NAC	HD + SPCD/on derivatization + preconcentration, DPJ/on preconcentration (100x)	UV, 2 and 0.2×10^{-6} M	Biomedical study	Ptolemy et al., 2005
Amino acids	Bacterial cultures	OPA/NAC, β-CD	EH, SPCD/on derivatization + preconcentration	UV, 0.4-0.6×10^{-6} M	Biomedical study	Ptolemy et al., 2006a
DL-Glutamic acid, baclofen	urine	γ-CD	CFGF/on preconcentration (1200x)	DAD (glutamic acid), LIF (baclofen)	Spiked samples	Balss et al., 2004
Dexbrompheniramine	Pharmaceutical preparations	CE-β-CD	ITP-EKC; ITP/on preconcentration (~10^2) + clean-up	DAD, 2.5 ng/mL	Enantiomeric purity testing of pharmaceuticals	Marák et al., 2008
Terbutaline	Plasma, water matrices	DM-β-CD	EK + SPE/on preconcentration (7000x)	UV, 0.6×10^{-9} M	Spiked real and model samples	Petersson et al., 1999
Ephedrine derivatives	Urine	β-CD	SPME/on clean-up, FESI/on preconcentration	DAD, 3-5 ng/mL	Spiked real samples	Fang, H.F. et al., 2006b

(1*R*, 2*R*)-pseudoephedrine, (1*R*, 2*S*)-ephedrine, (1*S*, 2*S*)-pseudoephedrine, (*S*)-(+)-methamphetamine	Urine, serum	β-CD	LLE/on clean-up, FESI/on preconcentration (3800x)	DAD, 0.15 to 0.25 ng/mL	Spiked real samples	Fang, H.F. et al., 2006a
Aspartate	Tissue samples from rats	β–CD	Microdialysis/on clean-up, Derivatization/on	LIF, 9x10^{-7} M (D-aspartate)	Biomedical study	Thompson et al., 1999
D-serin + other neurotransmitters	Tissue homogenates	β–CD, HP–β-CD, HP-γ-CD	Microdialysis/on clean-up, Derivatization/on	LIF, 270x10^{-9} M; LIF (sheath flow detection cell), 21x10^{-9} M	Biomedical study	O'Brien et al., 2003
Isoproterenol	Intravenous dialysed samples	M-β-CD	Microdialysis/on clean-up, pH-mediated sample stacking/on preconcentration	Amperometric detection, 0.6 ng/mL	Pharmacokinetic study	Hadwiger et al., 1996
Bambuterol	Plasma		SLM/on + MLC/on clean-up, double stacking/on preconcentration (40 000x)	UV, 2.5x10^{-10} M		Pálmarsdóttir et al., 1996
Terbutaline, but also brompheniramine, propranolol, ephedrine	Plasma, synthetic samples	Alkyl- or hydroxyalkyl-β-CDs	SLM/on + MLC/on clean-up, double stacking/on preconcentration (400x)	UV, 5x10^{-9} M	Spiked real and model samples	Pálmarsdóttir et al., 1995

FMOC-carnitine	Synthetic samples	HDM-β–CD	FI/on derivatization	DAD, $5x10^{-6}$ M	Enantiomeric purity testing in model samples	Mardones et al., 1999
Fenoxy acid herbicides	Water matrices	Octyl-β-D-maltopyranoside	FESS/on preconcentration, derivatization/off	LIF, $0.5x10^{-9}$ M	Spiked model samples	Mechref & El Rassi, 1997
Ephedrine, amphetamine and related compounds	Hair	β–CD	LLE/off clean-up, FESS/on preconcentration	DAD, 25-75 ng/mL	Forensic analysis	Tagliaro et al., 1998
β–blockers	Serum	CM–β–CD	PP/off clean-up, FESI/on preconcentration (5-25x)	UV, 10-50 ng/mL	Spiked real samples	Huang L. et al., 2008
3-carboxyadipic acid	Minerals	Vancomycin	FESS/on preconcentration (1000x)	DAD, 10^{-7} M	Environmental analysis	Castro-Puyana et al., 2008
Sulindac and its metabolites	Plasma	DM-β-CD	LLE/off clean-up, FESI/on preconcentration (500x)	UV, $1\text{-}3x10^{-7}$ M	Pharmakokinetic study	Chen, Y.L. et al., 2006
Glufosinate	River water sample	γ-CD	SPE/off clean-up, LVSS/on preconcentration	LIF, $2x10^{-9}$ M	Environmental analysis	Asami & Imura, 2006
Flavins	Bacterial cell extracts, plasma and urine	β-CD, SDS	PP/off clean-up, DPJ-SWP/on preconcentration (60x)	LIF, $4x10^{-9}$ M	Spiked real samples, biomedical study	Britz-McKibbin et al., 2003b
Propiconazol	Grape	HP-γ-CD, SDS micelles	SPE/off clean-up, SWP/on preconcentration (100x)	DAD, 90-100 ng/mL	Spiked real samples	Ibrahim et al., 2007
Triadimenol	Methanol matrices	HS-β-CD, HP-γ-CD	SRMP/on preconcentration (10x)	DAD, 0.8-3.8 ng/mL	Spiked model samples	Otsuka et al., 2003

Tryptophan	Urine	α–CD	ITP-EKC; ITP/on preconcentration + clean-up (~99%)	UV, 1.5 ng/mL	Spiked real samples	Danková et al., 1999
Isoxyzolylpenicilines	Milk	HP–β–CD	LLE/off clean-up, LVSS/on preconcentration	DAD, 2 ng/mL	Food analysis	Zhu et al., 2003
Clenbuterol	Acetic acid matrices	DM–β–CD	tITP/on preconcentration	UV, 10^{-6} M	Spiked model samples	Toussaint et al., 2000

Table 3.1. Chiral CE determinations of biologically active compounds in various biological matrices employing advanced (on-line) sample preparation.

[a] Or derivatization agent creating diastereomeric products.

[b] An on- or off-line mode is given behind slash, preconcentration factor or amount of removed interfering compounds are given in brackets

ITP = isotachophoresis, tITP = transient isotachophoresis, EKC = electrokinetic chromatography, CFGF = counter-flow gradient focusing, CWE = crown ether, NACE = non-aqueous capillary electrophoresis, MCE = electrophoresis on microchip, SPCD = in-capillary sample preconcentration with chemical derivatization, OPA/NAC= *ortho*-phthalaldehyde/*N*-acetyl l-cysteine, S-β–CD = sulphated-β-CD, HS-γ-CD = highly sulphated-γ-CD, M-β-CD = methyl-β-CD, DM-β-CD = dimethyl-β-CD, CM-β-CD = carboxymethyl-β-CD, CE-β-CD = carboxyethyl-β-CD, HP-β-CD = hydroxypropyl-β-CD, HP-γ-CD = hydroxypropyl-γ-CD, HDM-β-CD = heptakisdimethyl-β-CD, EH = enzymatic hydrolysis, HD = hydrodynamic injection, EK = electrokinetic injection, FI= flow injection, DPJ= dynamic pH junction, SRMP=stacking with reverse migrating phase, FESS = field-enhanced sample stacking, LVSS = large volume sample stacking, FESI= field-enhanced sample injection, SPE = solid-phase extraction, LLE = liquid-liquid extraction, LPME = liquid-phase microextraction, LVSEP-ASEI=large volume sample stacking with EOF as a pump plus anion-selective exhaustive injection, PP = protein precipitation, CME = centrifuge microextraction, SDME = single drop microextraction, SLM = supported liquid membrane technique, DAD = diode array detection, UV-ultraviolet (absorbance detection), LIF = laser induced fluorescent detection, MS = mass spectrometry, LOD = limit of detection, SDS = sodium dodecylsulphate, FMOC = 9-fluorenylmethyl chloroformate, EME=electro membrane extraction.

Technique	Principle	Characteristic features
Electrophoretic (stacking)		
FESS: NSM, LVSS, FESI	Analyte from a low-conductivity sample solution zone is concentrated at the boundary of a high-conductivity separation solution zone. Concentration effect is related to conductivity ratio of these two zones ($c_{stacked} \sim G_{separation\ solution} / G_{sample\ solution}$). Water plug is injected prior to the injection of the analyte in FESI.	Advantages. Easy to perform by simply optimizing concentrations or electrical conductivities of the sample and separation solutions. Possibility to inject a selectively large amount of charged analyte from the sample with electrokinetical injection (FESI) with simultaneous preconcentration and purification aspect. Preconcentrations: NSM ~10-fold; LVSS ~100-fold; FESI >1000-fold Limitations. Limited applications {charged analytes, separations only cations or anions in one run, samples with a low-conductivity matrix (can be overcome by pH mediation)}. Requirements {removing of sample matrix (LVSS), EOF suppression}. Reproducibility with FESI (injecting amount is biased by electrophoretic mobility, time depletion of the analyte in the sample solution).
tITP	Temporary ITP action being replaced later by zone electrophoretic regime. Analyte migrates between the highest (leading ion) and lowest (terminating ion) electrophoretic mobility zones of electrolyte solution. The concentration of each separated zone is adjusted to that determined by the concentration of the ion in the foregoing neighbour zone ($c_{analyte\ ion} \sim c_{leading\ ion}$) resulting in the preconcentration of diluted sample zones.	Advantages. Flexible. Directly applicable to samples with a significant matrix ion (acting as a leader). Applicable for low-conductivity (diluted) samples with the aid of added leading ion (inserted in capillary or in sample). Direct analysis of water soluble supernatants of precipitated proteinic samples. Precipitation agent (e.g., acetonitrile) serves simultaneously as terminating ion (transient pseudoisotachophoresis). Sample purification aspect (neutral and oppositely charged compounds do not interfere). Preconcentration: more than three orders. Limitations. Preconcentration only cations or anions in one run. Analysis of neutral compounds is not possible.

DPJ	Based on significant changes in electrophoretic velocities of the analytes between different pH values (BGE solution vs. sample solution with a suppressor of analyte ionization). Long plug of sample zone is gradually titrated by the ion from the BGE solution and the analyte will be ionized in the neutralized zone. The analyte is focused at the neutralization boundary during the neutralization of the sample zone.	Advantages. Selective concentration of the analytes having a narrow range of p*K*a. Useful for the concentration of weakly acidic or basic analytes. Limitations. Electrokinetic dispersion plays an important role in this technique. Only for ionizable analytes (weak acids/bases). Analysis of neutral compounds is not possible.
SWP	Analytes are picked up and accumulated by the appropriate pseudostationary phase (e.g., micelles) that penetrates the micelle free sample zone. The length of the analyte zone after sweep is inversely proportional to the retention factor of the analyte (the ratio of the analyte amounts present in micelle and in solution), $L_{sweep} \sim 1 / k$.	Advantages. Electrokinetic dispersion is minimized by homogeneous electric field strength throughout the whole capillary. High concentration efficiency, possibly up to 5000-fold (according to the affinity analyte vs. pseudophase), or even up to several million-fold (when the length to the detection point is very short and very narrow detection window is employed, e.g., in MCE), or even more (with electrokinetic injection). Suitable for charged as well as neutral analytes. Sample purification aspect (migrate only analytes interacting with sweeping pseudophase), useful for complex matrices. Combinable with nearly every other stacking mechanism. Limitations. The narrow analyte zone created by sweeping tends to broaden quickly according to the diffusion along the capillary (separation efficiency significantly decreases with the length of capillary). Application is limited by availability of appropriate pseudophase.
CFGF	Counter-flow gradient focusing (CFGF) methods can focus the analyte into a concentrated plug via simultaneous acting an electrophoretic velocity and the opposite bulk solution flow so that the total velocity (the sum of both velocities) is equal to zero at a unique point (characteristic for the analyte).	Advantages. CFGF approaches are a potentially simple and versatile way in which to simultaneously concentrate and separate charged and neutral analytes. See also Pressure flow section in this table. Limitations. Specific electrolytes must be used in some of these techniques. See also Pressure flow section in this table.

EOF	Electroosmotic flow (EOF) is the motion of liquid induced by an applied potential across a porous material, capillary tube, membrane, microchannel, or any other fluid conduit. Electroosmotic velocity is dependent of the charge in the electrical double layer, solid surface vs. liquid.	Advantages. EOF enables movement of compounds regardless on their charge. Therefore analysis of neutral compounds is possible, and separation of neutral, positively and negatively charged compounds in one run is possible too. EOF enables an implementation of the countercurrent migration effects (EOF vs. analytes vs. selector) for an enhancement of the separability. A flat EOF profile is favourable for a high separation efficiency. Limitations. An EOF velocity depends of a solid surface area and charge, therefore a precise control of the EOF velocity can be difficult. Hence, the reproducibility of the EOF based systems is lower than the systems with suppressed EOF. It is very pronounced in e.g., CEC systems. EOF cannot be applied in the hydrodynamically closed electrophoretic systems.
Nonelectrophoretic		
Chromatography	The separation is based on a distribution of the analytes between the stationary and mobile phase according to the different interactions of these analytes with the stationary phase. This mechanism differentiates migration velocities of the analytes. Separations are based on chemical principles.	Advantages. An alternative separation mechanism to the electrophoretic one that enables to increase selectivity of the system. The stationary phase serves as an immobilized selector that eliminates any interferences of the selector with the detection. CEC represents a single column chromatographic implementation with EOF as a driving force. Limitations. The chromatographic systems do not provide a concentration of the analytes. Therefore, a chomatographically pretreated sample must be further treated before the electrophoretic separation. A coupling of the pressure driven chromatographic techniques with electrophoresis is difficult in terms of the instrumentation as well as the compactibility of the electrophoretic and chromatographic systems (mobile phase vs. electrolyte).

Extraction	The analytes are trapped on/in a suitable solid/liquid-phase according to the affinities. The distribution constant of the analytes in the sample vs. extraction phase system determines the extraction recovery. Separations are based on chemical principles. The concentration factor depends on the ratio of sample volume : extractor volume.	Advantages. An important sample purification (clean-up) and preconcentration method. The extraction selectivity can be easily modified by the type of extractor and a specific or more universal extraction can then be reached. Limitations. The whole analytical procedure is complex (extraction requires conditioning, loading/sorption, washing, labelling, if necessary, elution/desorption). In the single capillary systems, the entire sample must pass through the capillary, which can lead to fouling or clogging of the separation capillary and significant decreasing of reproducibility of the analyses when particularly problematic samples (like biological ones) are used. A hyphenation of the extraction techniques with electrophoresis is difficult in terms of the instrumentation, however, SPE can be implemented to the electrophoresis easier than LLE.
Membrane techniques	Separations are based on physical principles, i.e., size exclusion. In the microdialysis or filtration, small molecules are able to diffuse across the membrane while large molecules, such as proteins and cell fragments, are excluded. This is the principle of the sample cleanup. Moreover, large molecules are preconcentrated on the membrane in this way.	Advantages. Microdialysis is a widely accepted sampling and infusion technique frequently used to sample small molecules from complex, often biological, matrices. Filtration can be applied directly in electrophoresis avoiding a sample collection. Both techniques can concentrate large molecules, and purify large as well as small molecules. Limitations. Do not concentrate small molecules. In the microdialysis, the minimum volume required for analysis often determines the rate at which the dialysate can be sampled. The whole analytical procedure is complex (dialysis requires preconcentration of the analyte from dialysate). Single column filtration systems are relatively simple but less flexible and versatile. On the other hand, a hyphenation of the membrane techniques with electrophoresis is more difficult in terms of the instrumentation.

Pressure flow	Driving pressure or counter-pressure based flows are provided simply by the pumps and they are controlled electronically. This is important tool also in CFGF.	Advantages. One of the basic tools in the advanced systems enabling a controlled transfer of solutes in various segments of the hyphenated systems (e.g., electrophoretic and non electrophoretic). A counter-flow enables to increase virtually the effective length of the capillary or channel and, by that, increase the separability. Limitations. Fluctuations of these non selective flows decrease the reproducibility of the analysis. An additional instrumentation (pumps and auxiliaries) must be implemented into the analytical system. Dead volumes (tubing and connections) decrease the separation efficiency.

Table 3.2. The most important electrophoretic and nonelectrophoretic techniques and tools applicable in electrophoresis.
FESS = field-enhanced sample stacking; NSM = normal stacking mode; LVSS = large volume sample stacking; FESI = field-enhanced sample injection; tITP = transient isotachophoresis; DPJ = dynamic pH junction; SWP = sweeping; EOF = electroosmotic flow; CEC = capillary; SPE = solid-phase extraction; LLE = liquid-liquid extraction

3.2.1 Single column (in-capillary) electrophoretic techniques

3.2.1.1 Field-enhanced sample stacking

The field-enhanced sample stacking (FESS) is easy to perform in a zone electrophoretic mode (Figure 2.2a) by simply optimizing the sample solution and the separation solution, mainly in their concentrations or electrical conductivities, to constitute different electrical field strengths between the two solutions. To perform preconcentration, the discontinuous zones having different electrical conductivities (G) must be constructed along the capillary axis. The analyte from a low-conductivity sample solution zone is concentrated at the boundary of a high-conductivity separation solution zone. The concentration effect is related to the conductivity ratio of these two zones according to Equation 3.1 [Simpson et al., 2008]:

$$c_{stacked} = c_{injected} \cdot \gamma \qquad 3.1$$

where $c_{stacked}$ is the concentration of the analyte concentrated by FESS, $c_{injected}$ is the concentration of the analyte in the sample solution injected, γ is the ratio of the electrophoretic velocities of the ions between the two discontinuous zones (sample zone and BGS, *1* and 2) having different conductivities (the ratios can be written for velocities, v_1/v_2, intensities of electric field, E_1/E_2, as well as resistivities, ρ_1/ρ_2). From this it is obvious that the sample solution should be prepared in a low-conductivity matrix (as in other stacking modes) that is limiting in terms of application, see Figure 3.1. This technique requires suppressing EOF as EOF velocity is also proportional to the field strength and mixing of the two solutions can occur at the boundary, causing broadening of the focused zone. In practice, we often stack in the presence of EOF, albeit at lesser enrichment. In fact, at high pH, stacking occurs for anions at the rear zone boundary as opposed to the front boundary for cations at low pH. The suppression (reduction) of EOF is more important when electrokinetic injection is employed. The FESS approach is useful for charged analytes, while neutral analytes cannot be directly concentrated (with the exception of their charged complexes) [Kim J.B. & Terabe, 2003]. The FESS can be carried out in the CZE or MEKC mode where the stacking action (see below) is the same while the final separation is based on the CZE or MEKC principles [Lin C.H., 2004; Kim J.B. & Terabe, 2003]. In fact, when a chiral separation is required, the final step following stacking procedure must be principally based on the EKC (chiral MEKC, CDEKC, etc.) mechanism, see chapter 2.

Several techniques have been developed by utilizing the FESS for sample preconcentration [Lin C.H. & Kaneta, 2004; Quirino & Terabe, 2000; Chien R.L. & Burgi, 1992].

(i) Normal stacking mode is the simplest mode, it requires a rather low amount of the injected sample, the EOF must be suppressed and ca. 10-fold concentration can be easily achieved. For schematic diagrams of the normal FESS model carried out in CZE or MEKC modes see Figure 3.2 and Figure 3.3a, respectively. The schemes of FESS with CZE or MEKC separation in Figure 3.2 and Figure 3.3 can be easily modified to the chiral EKC regime implementing chiral selector into the system. Then, the final step after stacking is a chiral EKC separation (i.e., FESS-EKC). For example, the scheme of FESS with MEKC separation in Figure 3.3 can be changed from the achiral (with achiral micelles) to the chiral one (with chiral micelles). Such chiral modification can also be done for other stacking techniques with the zone electrophoresis separation step (see the techniques described below). Depending on the charge of chiral selector and polarity of electric field the normal or reversed stacking EKC models can be created that offer different separation selectivities. For example, depending on the charge of micelles and the polarity of the electric field, the normal (Figure 3.3a) or reversed stacking MEKC models (Figure 3.3b) can be created.

(ii) Large volume sample stacking (LVSS) requires removing the sample matrix. This can be done with polarity switching where the analysed anion has higher velocity in the opposite direction than the velocity of EOF, or without polarity switching where EOF has to be suppressed as the cations migrate oppositely to EOF. It is possible to separate only cations or anions in one run and more than 100-fold concentration can be achieved. For schematic diagrams of the LVSS model see Figure 3.4.

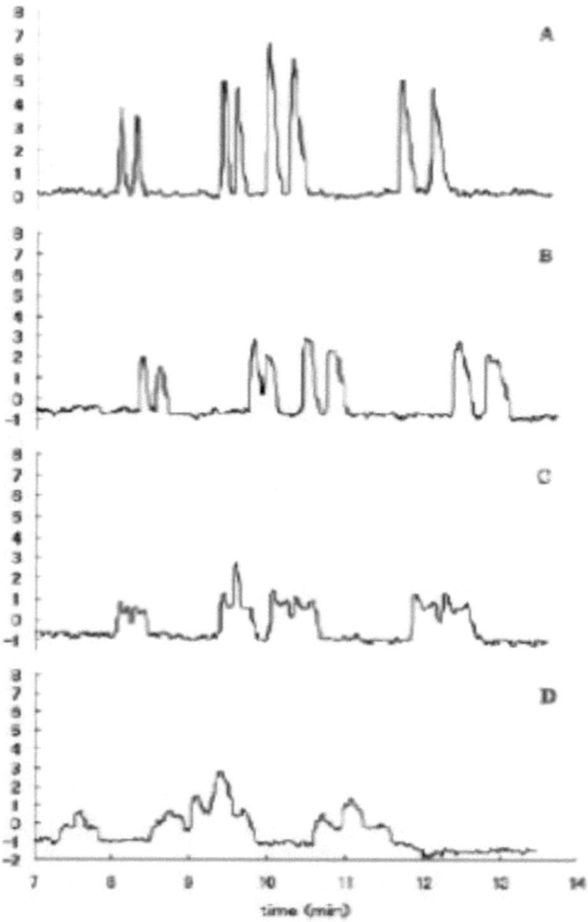

Figure 3.1. Effect of sample matrix on LVSS. Effect of NaCl on the stacking and enantioseparation of the analytes studied. Analytes 0.01 mg/mL in 20% ACN with [NaCl] in A = 0%, B = 0.1%, C = 0.2% and D = 0.4% w/v. Injection length: 20% capillary volume. Reprinted from ref. [Denola et al., 2007].

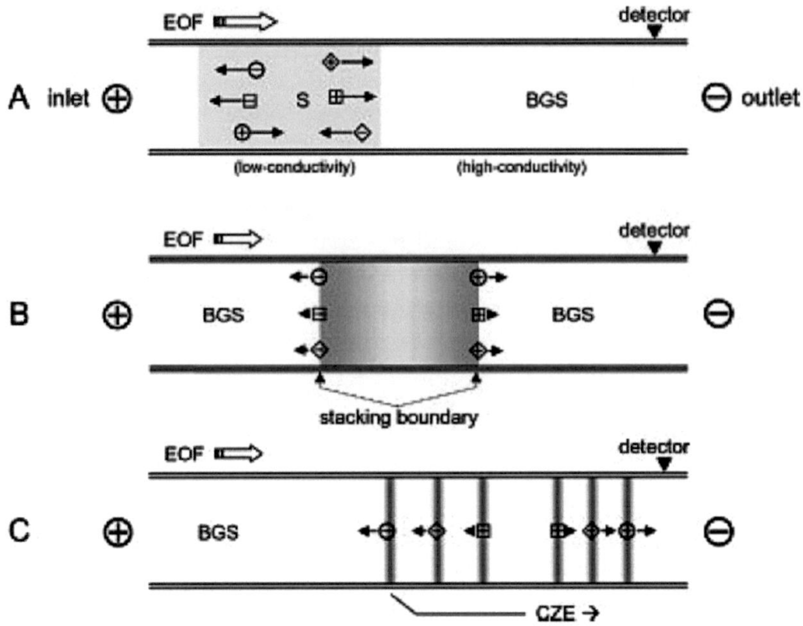

Figure 3.2. Schematic diagrams of the normal FESS model. (A) The capillary is conditioned with a BGS (a high-conductivity buffer), the sample, prepared in a low-conductivity matrix, is then injected to a certain length, and a high positive voltage is applied; (B) focusing of the analytes occurs near the boundaries between the sample zone and the BGS because of its mobility changes; (C) stacked analytes migrate and are separated by the CZE mode. Reprinted from ref. [Lin C.H. & Kaneta, 2004].

(iii) Field-enhanced sample injection (FESI) is based on the injection of a short (usually 2-3 mm, i.e., ca. 0.5% of the effective capillary length) water plug prior to the electrokinetical injection of the analyte. The EOF has to be reduced. Injection of a larger amount of the sample than in (ii) is possible. The injected amount is biased by the electrophoretic mobility. More than 1000-fold concentration is possible, however, injection reproducibility is influenced by depletion of the analyte in the sample solution. Selective injection is given by the charge of the sample constituents.

It should be highlighted that some of the above mentioned electrophoretic on-line preconcentration approaches can be utilized simultaneously also for on-line sample purification. For example, the use of the FESI technique can eliminate potential interfering compounds from the matrix via electrokinetic injection being selective to the sample constituents according to their charge. The selectivity of the electrokinetic injection can be easily influenced by the pH of the sample solution (adjusted by an appropriate buffer if necessary) where the solute of interest has unconditionally to be ionized while the ionization of potential interfering compounds should be suppressed. The FESI can be used for the exhaustive sample injection, e.g., almost all of the ions in a sample can be injected when the volume is small. This is a real advantage to the off-line solvent extraction, evaporation to dryness and redissolving of the analyte in a small amount of dilute buffer.

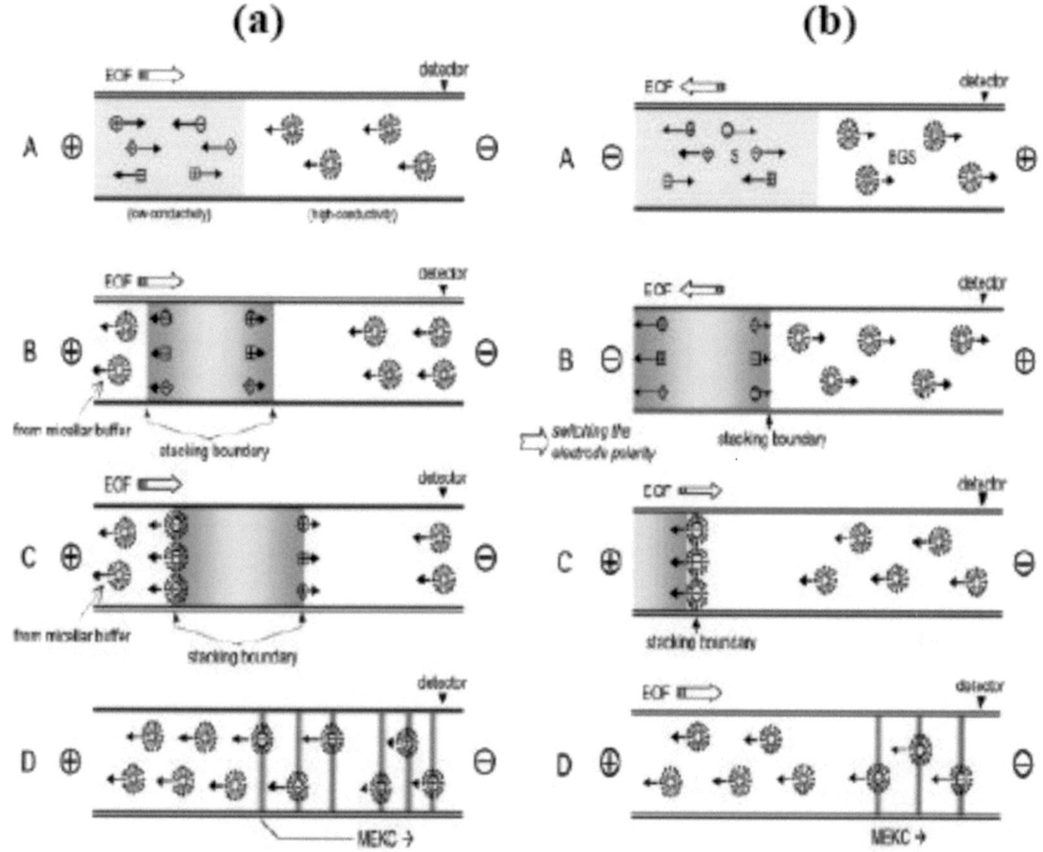

Figure 3.3. Schematic diagrams of stacking MEKC models. (a) A normal stacking MEKC model. (A) The sample is dissolved in a low-conductivity buffer, BGS, consisting of SDS to form the micelles; after the background and sample solution are injected, respectively, a positive voltage is applied; (B) the SDS micelles from the inlet enter the sample zone and then permit the analytes to migrate and become stacked; (C) then the SDS-analytes are separated by the MEKC mode. (b) A reversed stacking MEKC model. (A) The sample and BGS are prepared as described in Figure 3.3aA but a negative polarity is applied; (B) the EOF moves toward the inlet, the anionic analytes move toward the outlet and stack at one side of the boundary; (C) the electrophoretic current reaches approximately 95–99% of its original value, the polarity is quickly returned to positive, reversing the EOF; (D) then the SDS-analytes are separated by the MEKC mode. Reprinted from ref. [Lin C.H. & Kaneta, 2004].

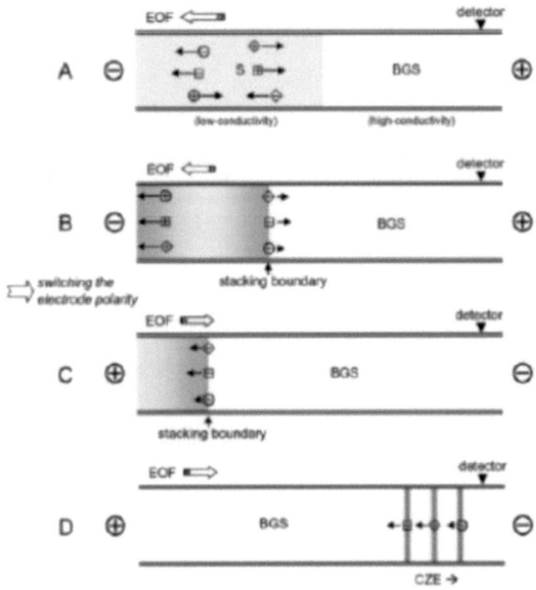

Figure 3.4. Schematic diagrams of the LVSS model. (A) The capillary is conditioned with a BGS (a high-conductivity buffer), the sample, prepared in a low-conductivity matrix, is then injected to a certain length, and then a high negative voltage is applied (EOF is toward the inlet); (B) the anionic analytes move toward the detection end (outlet) and stack at one side of the boundary, whereas the cations and neutral species move and exit the capillary at the injection end (inlet); (C) the electrophoretic current is carefully monitored until it reaches approximately 95–99% of its original value, and the polarity is then quickly returned to positive (EOF is reversed); (D) the following separation occurs by CZE mode. Reprinted from ref. [Lin C.H. & Kaneta, 2004].

However, the FESS methods suffer generally from poor applicability to real samples. (i) For optimal precision, hydrodynamic injection is preferred since we start with the correct number of ions in the capillary. On the other hand, sample depletion and injection reproducibility could be a problem when making more than one electrokinetic injection from a vial. In a practical sense, there is a balance between the degree of enrichment and the stability of the system. This is a significant problem when performing extreme enrichment from real samples. (ii) Poor applicability to real samples is primarily because the complicated (high-conductivity) matrices increase the conductivity of the sample and reduce the efficiency of stacking. This is typical for urine or blood samples which contain salts as matrix macroconstituents. Therefore, they are usually applied in conjunction with off-line sample pretreatment. A pH-mediated FESS method was introduced by the group of Lunte and is an indirect way of changing a high-conductivity sample into a low-conductivity sample to allow field-enhanced sample stacking [Weiss et al., 2001]. Schematic diagrams are shown in Figure 3.5. In the initial step, the sample is prepared in a high-ionic strength medium and is electrokinetically injected into the capillary. Then, a plug of strong acid is electrophoretically injected and a positive separation voltage is applied. The strong acid titrates the sample solution to create a neutral zone (a high-resistance zone). Thus, a proportionally greater field will develop across the neutral zone, causing the ions to migrate faster. As a result, the analytes are stacked at the boundary between the low-conductivity zone (prepared by on-line titration of the sample solution zone, e.g., by a strong acid plug) and the high-conductivity BGS. A (chiral) separation by the zone electrophoresis mode then occurs. This is a simple and attractive approach for high-conductivity samples, which is growing in popularity. Another strategy introducing a sample with a higher ionic strength than the running buffer has been proposed by Landers et al. [Palmer et al., 1999]. For example, using sodium cholate as the pseudostationary phase and simply adding sodium chloride (or other ions) to the sample matrix, a reasonable enhancement in sensitivity has been achieved for a series of corticosteroids. In the first step the micelles, and not the analytes, are stacked at the boundary between the sample and buffer zone. Subsequently, the analytes migrating with the EOF are enriched in the zone with the high micelle concentration as the micelles are negatively charged and migrate in the opposite direction (Figure 3.6). Summarizing, the stacking effect is dependent on the affinity of the analytes to the micelles that were stacked before, at the boundary between the sample (with increased conductivity, e.g., by adding salt) and the buffer zone. This approach is attractive due to its robustness towards other sample constituents. Although these last two procedures have not been used for chiral analysis so far, their potential in this field is apparent. Other strategies for samples with high ionic strengths, also used in the chiral field, are based on appropriate combinations of different stacking techniques as briefly discussed, inter alia, in section 3.2.1.5.

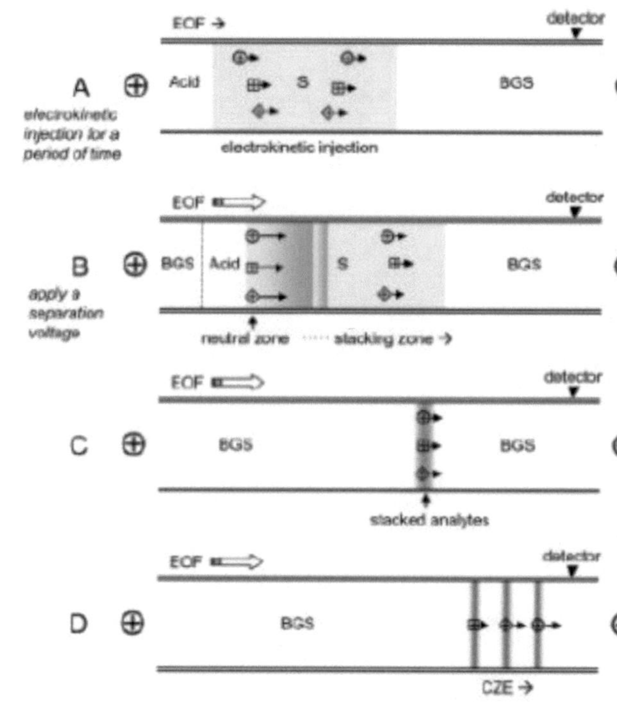

Figure 3.5. Schematic diagrams of a pH-mediated stacking model. (A) The capillary is conditioned with a high-conductivity BGS, the cationic analytes dissolved in a low-conductivity buffer are electrokinetic injected into the capillary, and then a plug of strong acid is also electrokinetically injected; (B) a positive separation voltage is applied; (C) the strong acid titrates the sample solution to create a neutral zone causing the ions to migrate faster and become stacked; (D) the subsequent separation occurs by the CZE mode. Reprinted from ref. [Lin C.H. & Kaneta, 2004].

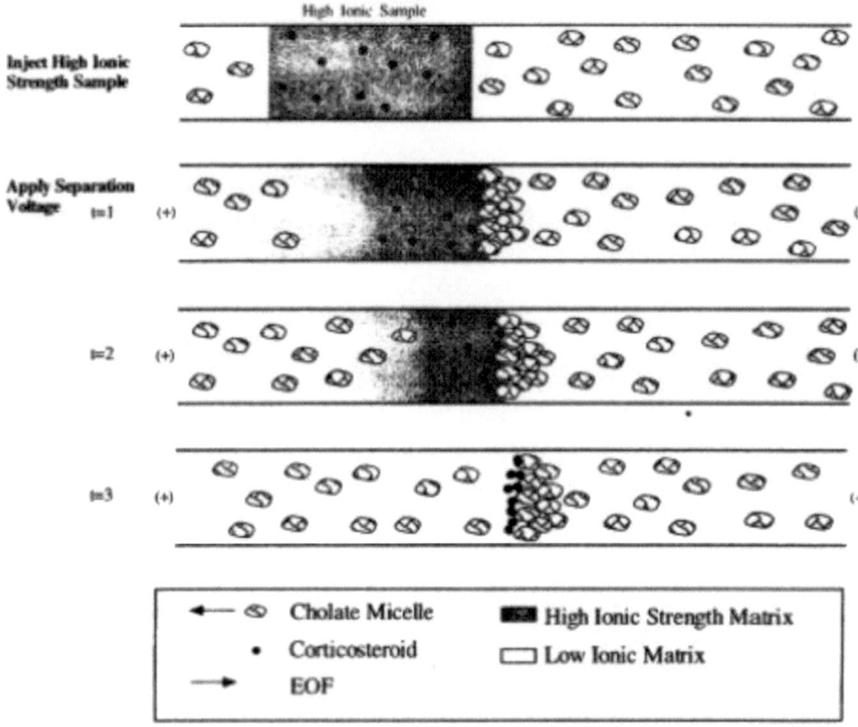

Figure 3.6. Mechanism for stacking in MEKC with a high ionic strength matrix. Reprinted from ref. [Palmer et al., 1999].

3.2.1.2 Isotachophoresis and transient isotachophoresis

Analytes are separated in isotachophoresis (ITP) as adjoining successive zones in the order of decreasing electrophoretic mobilities, migrating between the leading (the highest electrophoretic mobility) and terminating (the lowest electrophoretic mobility) electrolyte solution zones (Figure 2.2b). In the presence of voltage applied, the concentration of each separated zone is automatically adjusted to that determined by the concentration of the ion in the foregoing neighbour zone according to Equation 3.2 [Simpson et al., 2008]:

$$c_A = \frac{c_L \mu_A (\mu_L + \mu_Q)}{\mu_L (\mu_A + \mu_Q)} \tag{3.2}$$

resulting in the preconcentration of diluted sample zones. In this equation, $\mu_L > \mu_A$ and c_A, c_L are concentrations of analyte ion, A, in the adjoining zone to the leading ion, L, zone and μ_A, μ_L, μ_Q electrophoretic mobility of A, that of L, and that of the counter ion Q (assumed the same ion for A and L), respectively. ITP is a flexible and powerful method for on-line concentration. It is directly applicable to samples with a significant matrix ion and can also provide very high enrichment factors for low-conductivity samples.

The principle of ITP can be applied to preconcentration in zone electrophoresis techniques (CZE, EKC), which is termed as transient ITP (tITP) [Beckers & Boček, 2000; Schwer et al., 1993]. Schematic diagrams of tITP are shown in Figure 3.7. There are several modifications in tITP to perform sample preconcentration, such as the following configurations (i) a low electrophoretic mobility background solution (e.g., borate) is inside the capillary, a leading electrolyte (e.g., chloride ion) solution is injected as the first plug, the sample solution is injected as the second plug, sample solution zones are preconcentrated by the tITP mechanism and further migrate as zones in zone electrophoresis, (ii) as in (i) but the sample and leading solutions are mixed and then injected as one plug. It is particularly suited to the analysis of trace components in samples with a significant matrix ion in which that matrix ion functions as a leader. This is called 'sample self-stacking' in the literature. (iii) Transient pseudoisotachophoresis is a modification of previous tITP modes, based on the addition of a water miscible organic solvent (e.g., acetonitrile, acetone, methanol, 2-propanol) serving as a pseudoterminating ion [Shihabi, 2002]. Of course, it cannot be a terminating ion in the true sense. The organic solvent serves as a zero mobility low-conductivity zone. This approach is attractive for the analysis of biological fluids because acetonitrile added 2:1 to the sample (making 66% acetonitrile) is used for protein precipitation and it is therefore possible to directly inject the supernatant and achieve a 20-30 fold improvement in sensitivity.

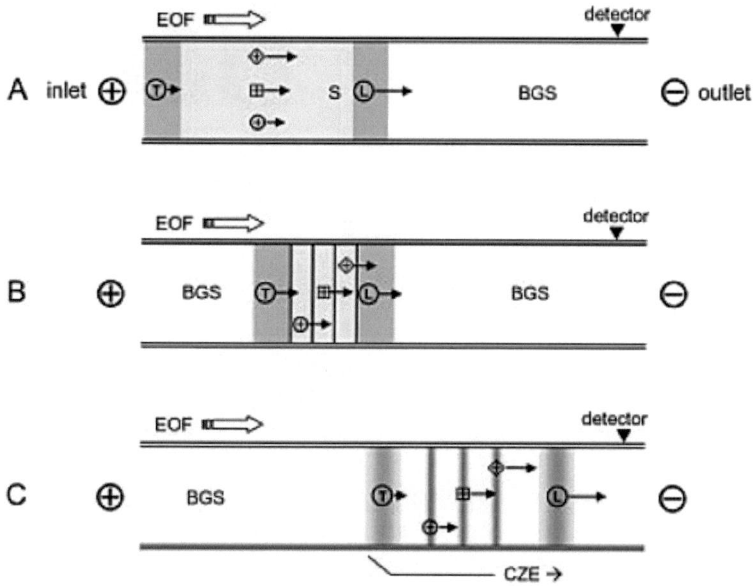

Figure 3.7. Schematic diagrams of a tITP model for cations. (A) The capillary is conditioned with a BGS, the leading electrolyte and sample solution, and terminating electrolyte are then injected in turn - a high positive voltage is also applied; (B) concentration of the analytes occurs between the leading and the terminating ions during tITP migration; (C) the concentrated analyte zones are separated by the CZE mode. Reprinted from ref. [Lin C.H. & Kaneta, 2004].

Like FESI, tITP and ITP is adversely affected by changes in sample conductivity. The ITP and tITP techniques are applicable to charged analytes only and simultaneous analysis of oppositely charged analytes is not possible. On the other hand, this limitation can be understood as an advantage in terms of selective removal of neutral or oppositely charged sample matrix constituents.

3.2.1.3 Dynamic pH junction

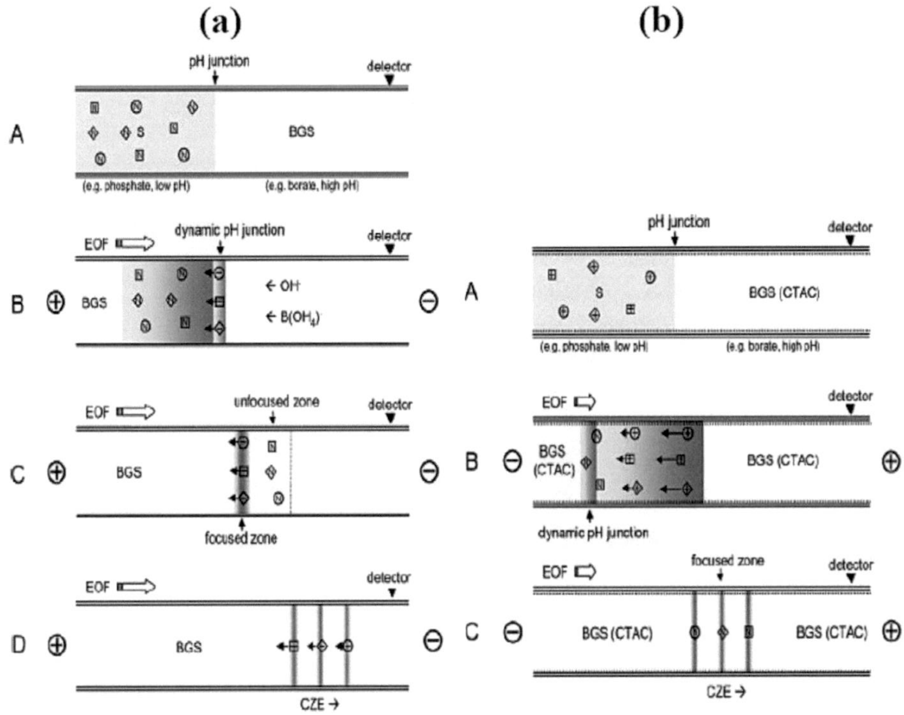

Figure 3.8. Schematic diagrams of dynamic pH junction models. (a) The normal and (b) reversed dynamic pH junction models. (a) (A) The capillary is filled with a high pH-BGS and a section of sample solution (prepared in a lower-pH buffer); (B) a high positive voltage is applied, resulting in a discontinuous electrolyte zone; (C) the anionic analytes are focused on the boundary of the pH junction; (D) separation of the analytes occurs by the CZE mode. (b) (A) The capillary is filled with BGS (prepared in a higher-pH buffer containing CTAC) and sample solution (prepared in a lower-pH matrix); (B) a negative voltage is applied because of the addition of CTAC the EOF moves toward the outlet; the cationic analytes move toward the inlet and change to neutral at the rear boundary due to the change in pH; (C) separation of the analytes occurs by the CZE mode. Reprinted from ref. [Lin C.H. & Kaneta, 2004].

The dynamic pH junction (DPJ) technique utilizes significant changes in ionization states of the analytes or electrophoretic velocities between different pH values [Britz-McKibbin & Chen, 2000; Aebersold & Morrison, 1990]. Possible configuration is as follows: the capillary is filled with an alkaline background solution (high concentration, low electrophoretic mobility), a long plug of a weakly acidic analyte dissolved in an acidic matrix (high concentration, high mobility) is injected, a positive voltage is applied at the injection end, the acidic sample zone is gradually titrated by the hydroxide ion in the alkaline background solution from the cathodic side and the analyte will be ionized in the neutralized zone. The negatively ionized analyte will migrate toward the anode, but if it enters into the acidic sample zone it will be protonated again to neutral and stop the electrophoretic migration. Thus, the weakly acidic analyte can be focused at the neutralization boundary during the on-line neutralization of the sample zone. Two modes of the DPJ can be used for the analyte preconcentration, namely the normal (Figure 3.8a) and reversed (Figure 3.8b) DPJ model, providing conditions for preconcentration of anionic or cationic analytes, respectively. This focusing technique is different from sample stacking since the conductivity of the sample matrix is not of great importance; it can be less than or greater than that of the BGS. The electrokinetic dispersion plays an important role in this technique [Kim J.B. et al., 2003]. The DPJ technique can selectively concentrate analytes having a narrow range of p*Ka* and it is useful for the concentration of weakly acidic or basic analytes, as well as zwitterionic analytes. This technique has been used in the chiral field in appropriate combinations with other on-line preconcentration techniques, see section 3.2.1.5.

3.2.1.4 Sweeping

Sweeping (SWP) can be defined as a phenomenon whereby analytes are picked up and accumulated by the appropriate pseudostationary phase (micelles, microemulsions, charged cyclodextrins) that penetrates the sample zone. The homogeneous electric field strength is given by the similar conductivity of the nonmicelle sample zone (provided by the addition of salt if needed) and the running micelle solution. Homogeneous electric field strength is assumed throughout the whole capillary under SWP conditions different from field-enhanced stacking techniques. The schematic diagrams of SWP preconcentration are shown in Figure 3.9. The length of the analyte zone after sweep, L_{sweep}, is inversely proportional to the retention factor of the analyte, k (the ratio of the analyte amounts present in micelle and in solution), according to Equation 3.3. [Simpson et al., 2008]:

$$L_{sweep} = L_{inj}\left[\frac{1}{(1+k)}\right] \qquad 3.3$$

where L_{inj} is the length of the sample solution injected. It is apparent that the analyte having a higher k value is more efficiently concentrated. According to the affinity of the analyte to the pseudostationary phase the concentration efficiency can be very high, possibly up to 5000-fold. The narrow analyte zone created by SWP, however, tends to broaden quickly according to the diffusion along the capillary (CE) or channel (MCE). Therefore, when the length to the detection point is very short and a very narrow detection window is employed, very high concentration efficiency, up to several million-fold, can be observed [Kitagawa et al., 2006]. Electrokinetic injection in combination with SWP has made it possible to inject a large volume of samples, and, by that, additionally increase sensitivity [Palmer et al., 2001]. However, commonly used SWP pseudophases do not provide specific interactions with the analyte and many interfering compounds from the sample matrices with affinity to the pseudophase can be swept (enriched) together with the analyte. Therefore, a sample clean-up technique along with the SWP technique can be required to introduce into analytical protocol too, especially when analysing biological samples [Hempel, 2000; Baldacci & Thormann, 2006].

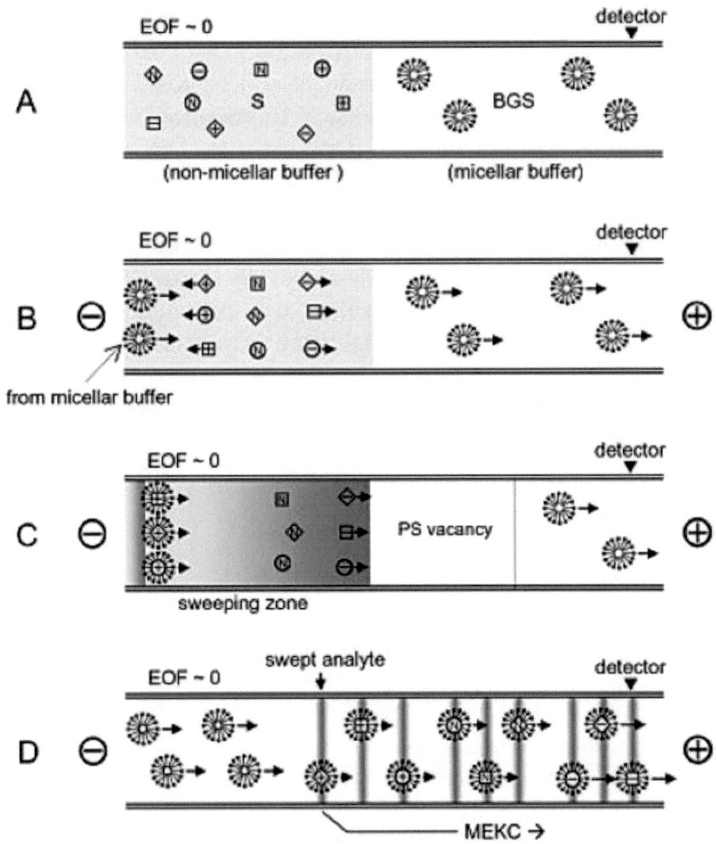

Figure 3.9. Schematic diagrams of a reversed sweeping MEKC model. (A) The BGS consists of a surfactant (for example, SDS, a negatively charged surfactant) and electrolytes to form a micelle buffer, but the samples are dissolved in a nonmicelle buffer; (B) after the injection of the BGS and the sample solution, a negative polarity is applied to power the CE separation; (C) the cations and anions move toward the inlet and outlet , respectively, and anionic SDS micelles enter the capillary sweeping the analytes; (D) the analytes are completely swept by SDS, the subsequent separation occurs by the MEKC mode. Reprinted from ref. [Lin C.H. & Kaneta, 2004].

SWP was originally developed for the on-line concentration of neutral analytes for MEKC separation [Quirino & Terabe, 1998]. The SWP approach is suitable also for charged analytes, regardless of the charge of the analyte and the direction of EOF. Strong Coulomb interactions between oppositely charged analytes and the pseudophase can be reflected in a higher k value and, subsequently, more efficient preconcentration [Quirino & Terabe, 1999; Quirino et al., 2000]. SWP is a perfect combination for nearly every other stacking mechanism. Its complementarity so far has really only been used for sensitivity enhancement, but it could also be used to selectively enrich specific analytes. This will become increasingly important as more integrated methods are developed for the analysis of more complex samples with less off-line sample pretreatment (clean-up).

3.2.1.5 Single column combinations of sample preparation techniques based on electrophoretic principles

A combination of two of the electrophoretic on-line sample preconcentration techniques described in sections 3.2.1.1-3.2.1.4 can be more efficient in increasing detection sensitivity, preconcentration selectivity and spreading application capabilities (i.e., analysis of a wider range of analytes, differing by their charge, polarity, etc., in one experiment), according to particular demands. It can also overcome some limitations of these methods when used separately.

Most of these combinations have been used only in achiral analyses so far, however, their potential in the chiral field is apparent. As it is believed that they will appear in the chiral field in the near future, it is useful to list them (corresponding schemes of these techniques can be found in the cited references or in ref. [Lin, C.H. & Kaneta, 2004]):

(i) FESI + tITP (i.e., electrokinetic supercharging, EKS): 3000-fold concentration, analysis of ionic analytes in diluted samples [Fang L. et al., 2006]. Compared with conventional electrokinetic injection, the enhancement factors can be greatly improved, e.g., to be 250-fold [Huang, L. et al., 2011].

(ii) pH-mediated FESS + DPJ: only for ionisable analytes [Chou Y.W. et al., 2008]. This technique has been developed to enhance analyte focusing for CE for the analysis of physiological samples. The process results in ultra-narrow peak widths and no dilution of the sample to lower ionic strength is necessary. In comparison with normal base stacking and electrokinetic injection, mass loading capacity can be increased with this technique without degradation in peak shape and resolution is dramatically improved.

(iii) tITP + DPJ: 50-fold increase in sensitivity, nM LODs of cationic metabolites [Hou J. et al., 2007]. The authors depict three major transitions experimentally observed in the process: (a) initial tryptophan (Trp) focusing at the back end of the sample-BGE boundary, (b) partial focusing of Trp with residual peak fronting and (c) complete focusing of Trp within the original sample plug. The authors demonstrated that CE could serve as an effective preconcentrator, desalter and separator prior to ESI-MS, while providing additional qualitative information for unambiguous identification among isobaric and isomeric metabolites. The proposed strategy is particularly relevant for characterizing yet unknown biologically relevant metabolites that are not readily synthesized or commercially available.

(iv) FESI + SWP: up to million-fold increase in sensitivity [Rudaz et al., 2005; Servais et al., 2006]. This technique has two modes. (a) The cation selective exhaustive injection (CSEI) + SWP. The CSEI-SWP-MEKC method provides for a more sensitive detection than sweeping and is sufficiently flexible to offer the potential for achieving an increase in the detection limit of more than 100 000-fold, for positively chargeable analytes [Rudaz et al., 2005]. (b) Alternatively, anion selective exhaustive injection (ASEI)-SWP-MEKC, using a cationic surfactant, offers under optimized conditions an approximately 1000 to 6000-fold improvement in LODs of negatively chargeable analytes [Servais et al., 2006]. Applications of the CSEI-SWP-MEKC method: (methamphetamine, ketamine, morphine and codeine in hair, LODs of 50–200 pg/mg hair) [Huang Y.S. et al., 2003], (amphetamine, methamphetamine and hydroxymethamphetamine in urine, LODs of 15–20 ppm) [Theurillat & Thormann, 2008], (amphetamine, methamphetamine and methylenedioxymethamphetamine, 6–8 ppt LODs, several 1000-fold improvement in detection sensitivity compared with typical injection) [Tsimachidis et al., 2008; Theurillat et al., 2007].

(v) Electrocapture. Horáková et al. [Horáková et al., 2007] presented a novel approach which they called 'electrocapture'. This technique makes possible the determination of nanomolar concentrations of weak acidic analytes in CE. The method consists of long-running electrokinetic sample injection and stacking (electrokinetic immobilization) of the analytes at a boundary of two electrolytes with different pH values (pH 9.5 and 2.5), and consequent mobilization of the stacked uncharged analytes in a micelle system (containing SDS micelles). The micelle system can provide for further concentrating the analytes by sweeping. An approximate 4600-fold increase of the sample concentration (in comparison with the standard CZE) can be achieved during the preconcentration step.

Some of the techniques based on combined electrophoretic principles in a single column arrangement have also been used for chiral analyses, or, at least, a chiral separation environment has been utilized in these techniques. These are the following methods:

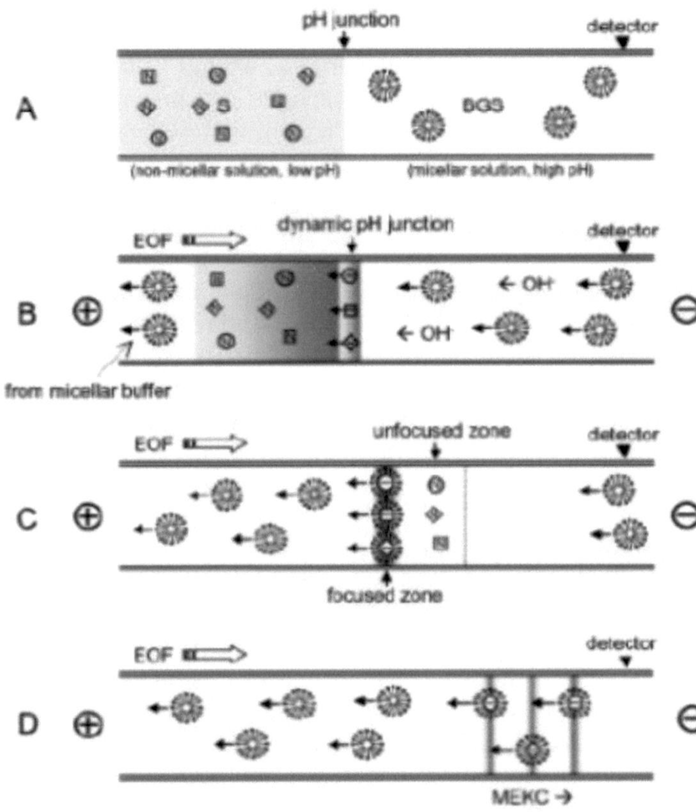

Figure 3.10. Schematic diagrams of the DPJ-SWP model. (A) The micelle (such as SDS) BGS and the sample solution (a nonmicelle buffer) are injected into the capillary, respectively; (B) when the injection is complete, a positive polarity is applied (if a negatively charged SDS surfactant is used) to power the CE separation; (C) the neutral analytes are converted to anions and are swept by the SDS micelles; (D) separation occurs by the MEKC mode. Reprinted from ref. [Lin C.H. & Kaneta, 2004].

(i) SWP + DPJ: suitable for a mixture of neutral and weakly acidic/basic analytes [Britz-McKibbin et al., 2002], for illustrative scheme see Figure 3.10. This method is very effective for overcoming the often poor band-narrowing efficiency of conventional SWP (using anionic micelles) and the DPJ for hydrophilic and neutral analytes, respectively, even if the migration time needed for separation is much longer than that of a conventional DPJ or SWP. This method was applied for plasma and urine samples. A picomolar detectability can be achieved by CE-LIF detection without the need for laborious off-line preconcentration and clean-up [Britz-McKibbin et al., 2003].
(ii) LVSS (a combination of field-enhanced stacking and pH-mediated stacking) + SWP: LODs up to 10^{-10} M with LIF detection, applied for animal tissues [Kirschner et al., 2007], for illustrative scheme see Figure 3.11.
(iii) FESI + tITP: applied for the simultaneous on-line preconcentration and enantioseparation of drugs in urine samples. The detection limits in ng/mL levels can be easily obtained [Huang, L. et al., 2011].

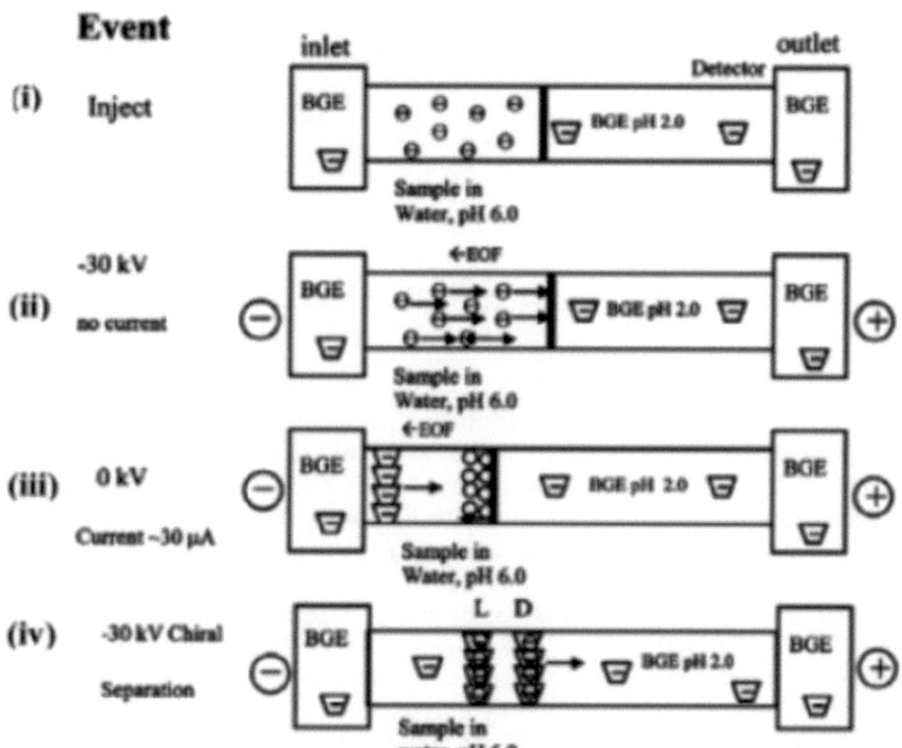

Figure 3.11. Schematic diagram of the stacking/sweeping: (i) hydrodynamic injection of large volume (1/3 of the capillary) of the CBI–amino acids in water at pH 6.0; (ii) migration toward the pH junction at the outlet side of the injection plug of the anionic CBI–amino acids; (iii) pumping water out of the capillary and movement of the stacked analyte band toward the inlet by the EOF; (iv) sweeping of the HS-β-CD through the stacked band of analyte. Adapted from ref. [Kirschner et al., 2007].

3.2.1.6 Single column combination of sample preparation techniques based on electrophoretic principles with chemical reaction

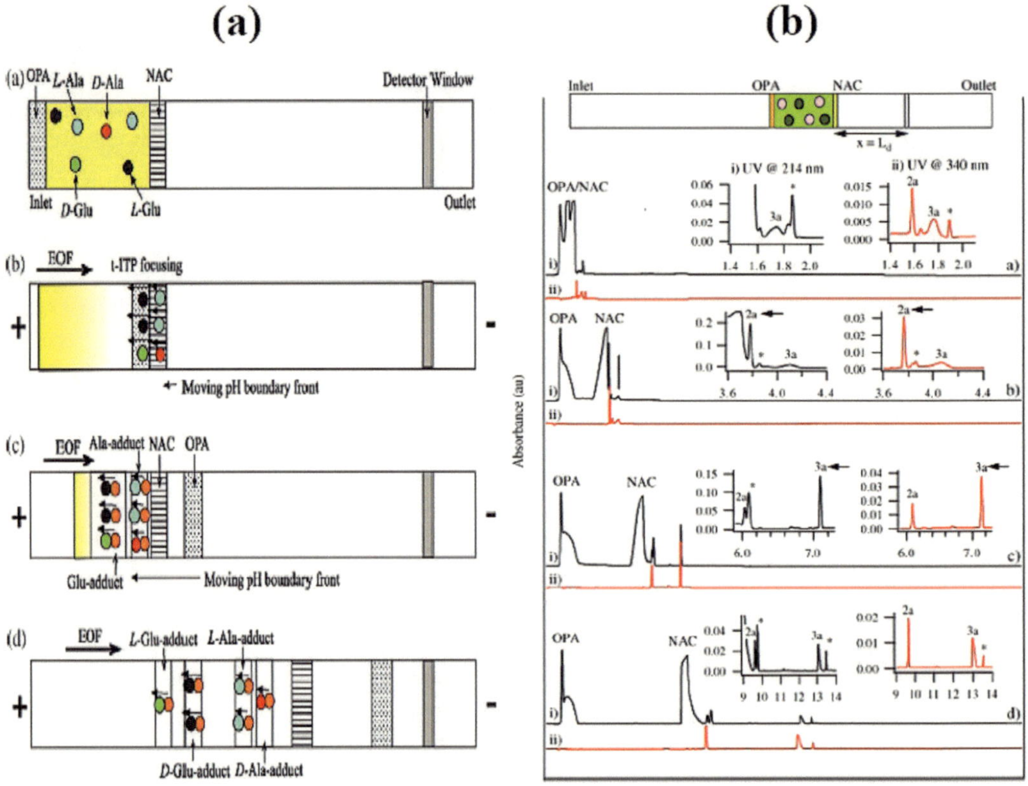

Figure 3.12. SPCD-CE method. (a) Proposed mechanism and kinetics of analyte electrokinetic focusing with in-capillary derivatization of amino acid enantiomers by SPCD-CE using OPA/NAC based on time-resolved electrophoretic experiments depicted in Figure 3.12b. Note the rapid analyte focusing with labelling of the long sample plug via tITP with subsequent zone passing of reagents, as well as the distinct time-dependent electrokinetic focusing of labelled amino acid-adducts at later stages by the moving pH boundary. (b) Series of electropherograms showing the distinct time-dependent processes of electrokinetic focusing and in-capillary OPA/NAC derivatization by SPCD-CE. Electropherograms were monitored with UV absorbance: (i) 214 nm and (ii) 340 nm. Arrows note time-delayed analyte electrokinetic focusing mediated by a dynamic pH junction. All samples contained 20 µM D-Ala and D-Glu in 40mM phosphate, pH 6.0. A long sample plug (6.1 cm, using a sample injection of 100 s) was placed at different positions from the capillary window using a low pressure rinse (0.5 psi or 3.5 kPa) in order to change the effective capillary length (Ld) from (a) 0 cm, (b) 11.4 cm, (c) 22.8 cm and (d) 30.5 cm. Other conditions: 140mM borate buffer, pH 9.5; voltage 25 kV; capillary length 67 cm; internal diameter; 50µm; UV 340 nm. Analyte peak number corresponds amino acid-isoindole adducts, where 2a: D-Ala, 3a: D-Glu. Reprinted from ref. [Ptolemy & Britz-McKibbin, 2006].

In-capillary sample preconcentration with chemical derivatization (SPCD) is included as an innovative strategy [Ptolemy et al., 2005, 2006; Ptolemy & Britz-McKibbin, 2006]. The general principles of SPCD–CE for single-step enantioselective analysis of submicromolar levels of analytes are: (i) multiple hydrodynamic injection sequence (appropriate arrangement of sample and derivatization reagent(s) zones); (ii) on-line sample preconcentration (electrokinetic focusing); (iii) in-capillary chemical labelling by zone passing of derivatization reagent(s); (iv) chiral separation of diastereomeric analyte adducts formed, see illustrative schemes in Figure 3.12a and corresponding electropherograms in Figure 3.12b.

3.2.1.7 Single column combination of electrophoretic migration with counter-flow

Counter-flow gradient focusing (CFGF) approaches [Shackman & Ross, 2007] are a potentially simple and versatile way in which to simultaneously concentrate and separate charged and neutral analytes. These types of techniques have the potential to concentrate each sample component in a uniquely different place in the separation space (similarly to the IEF where each component is concentrated at its pI region, see Figure 2.2c). Over the last decade a number of new approaches that can focus analytes at positions according to their electrophoretic mobility (electric field gradient focusing, temperature gradient focusing) and interaction with a pseudophase (micellar affinity gradient focusing) have been developed. It is worthwhile noting that counter-flow gradient focusing methods are exceptionally flexible: they can be used as an analytical method in itself or as an electrophoretic equivalent to solid-phase extraction (SPE), whereby analytes can be selectively captured and/or released in a well-defined and controlled manner.

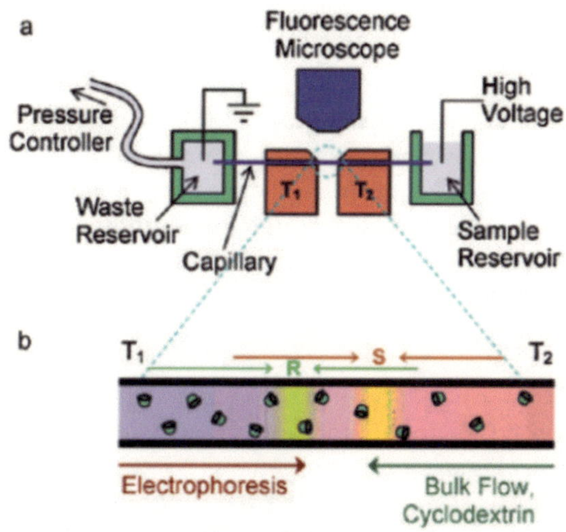

Figure 3.13. TGF method. (a) Schematic illustration of the TGF apparatus. A linear temperature gradient is formed along the capillary in the 2-mm space between the copper blocks regulated at temperatures T1 and T2. (b) Schematic of chiral TGF separations. T1, 13°C (left side in image); T2, 40°C; +1000 V/cm; BGS,10 mM γ-CD in 1 M Tris–borate (pH 8.3). The D-enantiomer peak is to the left in the figure; the L-enantiomer is to the right. Reprinted from ref. [Balss et al., 2004].

The method termed temperature gradient focusing (TGF) [Ross & Locascio, 2002; Balss, 2004; Danger & Ross, 2008; Kitagawa & Otsuka, 2011], applied also in the chiral field, relied upon the use of a buffer with a temperature-dependent ionic strength (such as tris-borate) so that application of a temperature gradient would result in an electrophoretic velocity gradient. For the scheme of the TGF apparatus and separation mechanism see Figure 3.13. For real-time chiral TGF separation see an application example in section 3.5. The advantages of the TGF method included easier implementation than electric-field gradient focusing (EFGF), as well as the ability to focus wider classes of analytes, see review [Shackman & Ross, 2007]. The maximum reported concentration enhancement was 10 000-fold in 100 min. A disadvantage of TGF can be the limited variety of buffers having the necessary temperature-dependent ionic strength.

3.2.2 Column-coupled (hyphenated) electrophoretic techniques

The theory and analytical potentialities of the column coupled electrophoretic techniques carried out in the capillary, as well as channel (microchip), formats and applied in the field of advanced pharmaceutical and biomedical analysis are comprehensively presented in the latest monograph chapter of the authors [Mikuš & Maráková, 2011]. On the other hand, in the present book/section the theory and potentialities of the column-coupled electrophoresis with chiral aspect are given.

The CE performed in a hydrodynamically closed separation system (hydrodynamic flow is eliminated by semipermeable membranes at the ends of the separation compartment) can be easily implemented into advanced CE systems, e.g., into those operating with coupled columns [Kaniansky & Marák, 1990; Kaniansky et al., 1993, 1994a, 1994b]. In addition to the single column (in-capillary) sample preconcentration and purification approaches (section 3.2.1), an on-line column combination of two CE methods can effectively solve problems of sample preparation and final analysis in one run in a well-defined way, i.e., producing high reproducibility of analyses. The Kaniansky group has been carrying out detailed research on the basic aspects, instrumentation and utilization of on-line coupled CE techniques for many years with interesting results. The proposed and commercially available CE-CE systems have a modular composition that provides a high flexibility in arranging particular modules in the separation unit, creating desirable CE-CE combinations (e.g., ITP-ITP, ITP-EKC, EKC-EKC, small or large volume injection) capable of solving a wide range of advanced analytical problems.

One pioneering work [Kaniansky & Marák, 1990] demonstrates the analytical potential of on-line coupling of ITP with CZE in the trace analysis of multicomponent ionic mixtures, see the instrumental scheme in Figure 3.14 for a general point of view. The ITP stage serves for the sample preparation and CZE stage for the final separation and detection of the analyte, and the following benefits can be recognized: (i) the ITP technique is useful for the separation of only cations or only anions in one run and this can be considered as an in-column ITP sample clean-up. (ii) ITP provides preconcentration of the sample constituents along with the analyte (see 3.2.1.2). (iii) In the column coupling separation system the post-column ITP sample clean-up (removing of undesired zones migrating in ITP) is performed via a proper switching of the direction of the driving current to the counter-electrodes. This enables transfer of an ITP zone of the concentrated analyte with only minimum interfering compounds (up to 99% or even more interfering compounds can be isolated [Danková et al., 1999]) into the second CE stage for the final separation and detection. It should also be mentioned that the use of tubes with larger internal diameter in CE analysis (300-800μm, typical in hydrodynamically closed separation systems) is favourable for their enhanced sample load capacities (30μl sample injection volumes are then common) linked with lower LODs [Kaniansky et al., 1997]. Using an ITP-CZE method, it is possible to analyse directly ultratrace charged analytes (lower ng/mL regions even with conventional detectors, e.g., UV absorbance detector) in complex ionic matrices (e.g., biological fluids) with minimum sample handling (e.g., only dilution) and to improve the LOD commonly more than 100-fold (depending on ionic matrix composition/concentration) in comparison with single column CE.

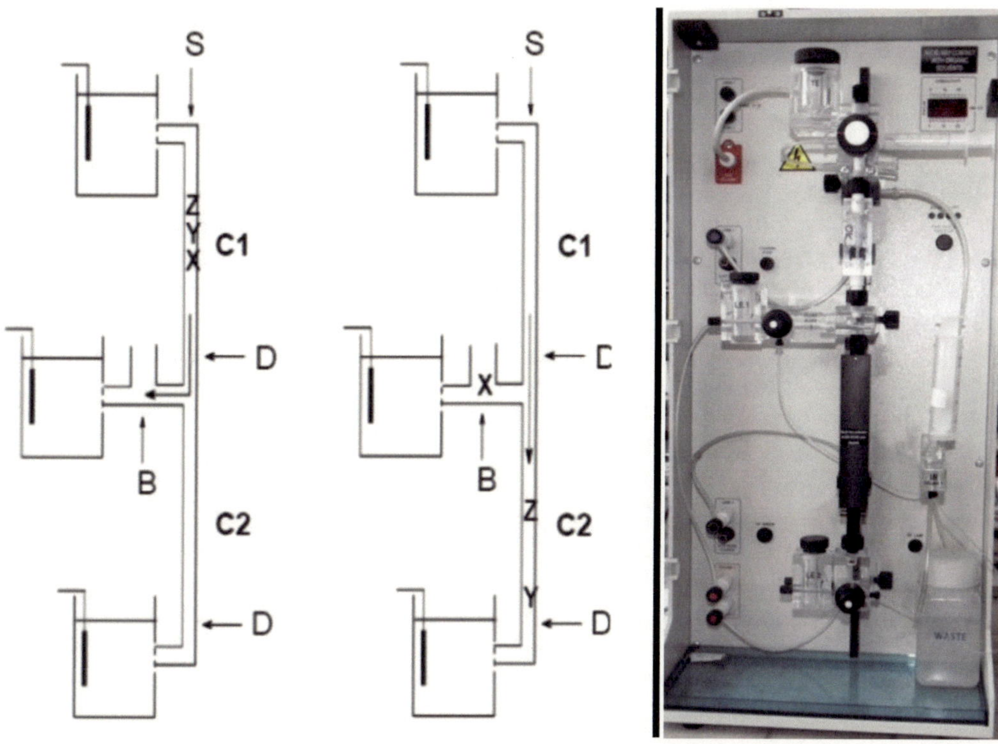

Figure 3.14. ITP-EKC technique in the capillary format and column coupling configuration of the separation units for the direct analysis of samples with the unpretreated complex matrices. The instrumental schemes (left and middle) and the photo of the corresponding commercial equipment, capillary electrophoresis analyser EA-102 (Villa-Labeco, Spišská Nová Ves, Slovakia), (right). On-line sample preparation: removing matrices X, preconcentration of enantiomers Y, Z in the first ITP stage (column C1). Final separation: enantioseparation of Y and Z in the second EKC stage (column C2). C1 - ITP column, C2 - EKC column, B - bifurcation block for coupling C1 and C2, D - positions of detectors. The instrumental schemes are adapted from ref. [Tekel' & Mikuš, 2005].

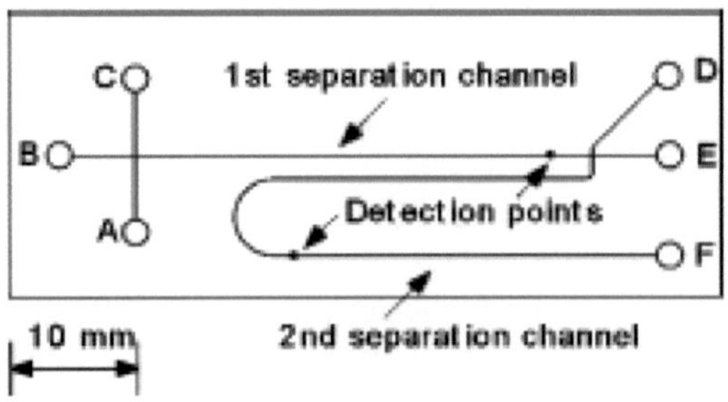

Figure 3.15. Schematic layout and dimensions of the microchip with on-line coupled separation channels. Reservoirs are labelled as: (A) run buffer; (B) sample; (C) sample waste; (D) buffer waste; (E) run buffer containing a chiral selector; and (F) buffer waste containing the chiral selector. The channel depth was 35 μm and width at a half-depth was 60 μm. The dots represent the detection points, which are located at 32 and 38 mm from the first and second injection crosses, respectively. Reprinted from ref. [Cho et al., 2004].

The CE-CE methodology is easily adaptable to chiral analysis. ITP-EKC is the most popular combination for the ultrasensitive determinations of chiral analytes present in complex matrices, see the schematic separation of electrophoretic zones in Figure 3.14 and several application examples in section 3.5. Neutral, as well as charged, chiral selectors are usually implemented in the EKC stage of the ITP-EKC combination [Danková et al., 1999; Fanali et al., 2000; Mikuš et al., 2006a, 2008a, 2008b; Marák et al., 2007]. Nevertheless, an ITP-ITP combination is also applicable for chiral analyses as the implementation of both neutral and charged chiral selectors in the ITP is possible [Ölvecká et al., 2001, Mikuš et al., 2006b; Kubačák et al., 2006a, 2006b, 2007].

On-line combinations of the electrophoretic techniques performed on chip (coupled channels), see Figure 3.15, offer additional advantages of microscale analysis as they are described in the introduction part of chapter 3 and section 2.2.3 (and references given therein) and also provide good possibilities for speed chiral analyses of drugs in minute amounts of sample with the model [Ölvecká et al., 2001], as well as complex matrices [Cho et al., 2004], as illustrated by an application example in section 3.5.

3.3 On-line sample preparation techniques based on nonelectrophoretic principles

The on-line sample preparation can be carried out advantageously also combining CE with other than electrophoretic techniques. Most of these approaches are based on extraction or chromatographic principles, but also other techniques, such as membrane filtration or microdialysis (separations based on physical principles), can be used. Electrophoresis and nonelectrophoretic on-line sample preparation techniques can be properly combined to achieve a desired effect. Lately several such approaches have been introduced, as illustrated by application examples in section 3.5.

On the other hand, attention must be paid when on-line sample preparation based on sorption-desorption or distribution mechanism is combined with a chiral system, as chiral molecules can influence these mechanisms through competitive complexing equilibria. For example, a partial filling of the separation capillary with chiral electrolyte can be employed to avoid the elution of the enriched solutes during flushing of the sorbent with chiral electrolyte [Petersson et al., 1999].

3.3.1 Chromatographic techniques

A microcolumn liquid chromatography (MLC) can be used in an on-line arrangement with the CE for sample purification and concentration allowing the injection of microlitre volumes into the electrophoresis capillary [Bushey & Jorgenson, 1990; Pálmarsdóttir et al., 1995]. For the instrumental scheme of the MLC-CE see Figure 3.16. The combined system has a much greater resolving power and peak capacity than either of the two systems used independently of each other. The selectivity and sensitivity gain of combining MLC with CE for determination of low concentrations of chiral drugs in biosamples is exemplified in section 3.5. However, the MLC-CE coupling is technically much more difficult than the CE-CE because it has to be accompanied by collection, evaporation and reconstitution of fraction isolated by MLC.

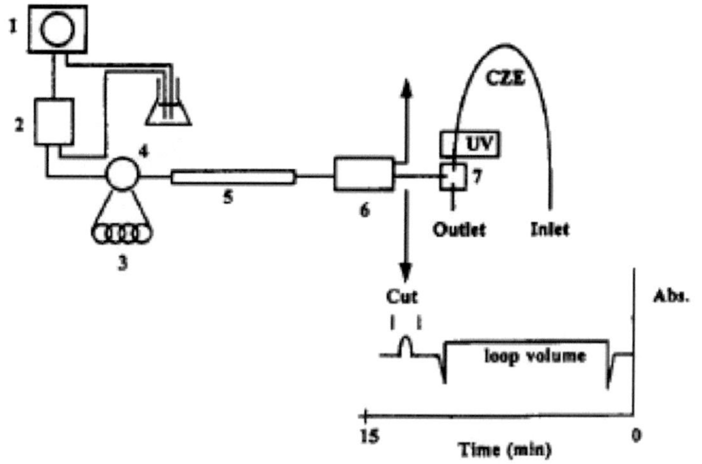

Figure 3.16. Experimental set-up of MLC coupled on line with CE. (1) Pump; (2) flow processor; (3) loop; (4) valve; (5) analytical column; (6) p.-dumper interface; (7) Tee adapter. Reprinted from ref. [Pálmarsdóttir et al., 1995].

3.3.2 Extraction techniques

Extraction techniques now play a major role in sample preparation in CE. These techniques can be used not only for reconstitution of the sample from small volumes, but also for sample clean-up in complex matrices and desalting for very saline samples that would interfere with the electrophoretic process. Considerable progress has been made towards the coupling of solid-phase extraction (SPE) with subsequent electrophoresis, while coupling of liquid-phase extraction (LLE) with electrophoresis is less used. The review by Breadmore et al. [Breadmore et al., 2009] gives attention to on-line or in-line extraction methods that have been used for electrophoresis.

3.3.2.1 Solid-phase extraction / microextraction

Solid-phase extraction (SPE) is the most attractive way of coupling extraction with CE and, especially, MCE. This is in particular because it can provide significant improvements in sensitivity without the use of electrokinetic injection [Puig et al., 2007a, 2008; Bertoncini & Hennion, 2004]. Depending on the nature of the adsorbent chemistry, this can be specific for certain analytes, such as through the use of a biopolymeric phase (see a generalized mechanism in Figure 3.17), or more generic for the extraction of a range or classes of compounds, such as a C18 reverse phase material, ion-exchanger resins, etc. These solid phases can be present in various formats, such as particles, parallel open channels and monoliths.

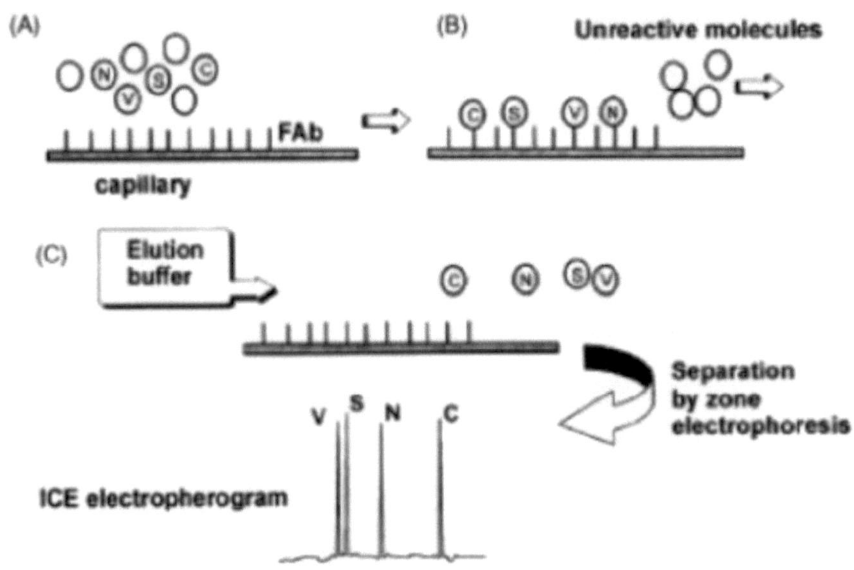

Figure 3.17. Diagrammatic representation of the 3-D biospecific extraction employing biopolymer coupled to CE technique. (A) Analyte percolation and capture phase. (B) Washing of non-retained compounds. (C) Acid elution of the analytes and separation by CE. V, S, N, C = chiral analytes. Adapted from ref. [Phillips, 1998].

In-line systems are created inserting solid-phase column into capillary (see Figure 3.18a, b) and they are attractive thanks to their low cost and easy construction. The whole analytical procedure includes conditioning, loading/sorption, washing, (labelling, if necessary), filling (by electrolyte), elution/desorption, separation and detection, see an example in Figure 3.18c. One of the main limitations of performing in-line SPE is that the entire sample, washing and elution solvents must pass through the capillary, which can lead to fouling of the separation capillary, particularly when problematic samples are used.

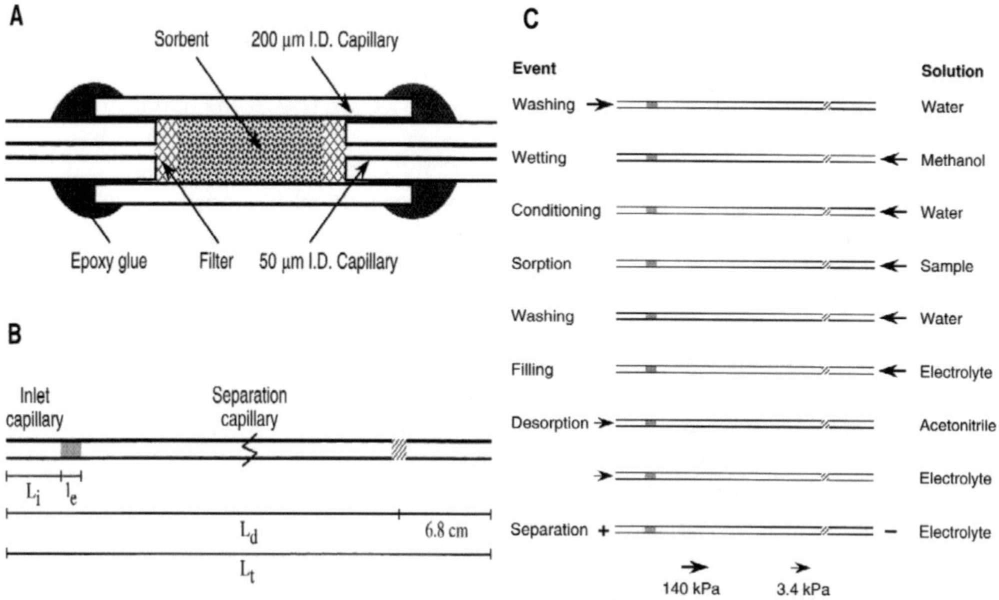

Figure 3.18. Miniaturised on-line SPE for enhancement of concentration sensitivity in CE. Cross-section of (A) the extractor and (B) the enrichment capillary where L_t (28–58 cm) is the enrichment capillary total length, L_d (21.2–51.2 cm) is the length to the detector, L_i (5.4 cm) is the length of the inlet capillary and l_e (1-3 mm) is the extractor length. (C) Sample enrichment procedure for terbutaline dissolved in water. Arrows indicate flow directions. The post-sorption washing with water is optional, as the electrolyte filling, in which non-retained solutes are flushed out of the capillary, usually is enough for rather clean samples. Reprinted from ref. [Petersson et al., 1999].

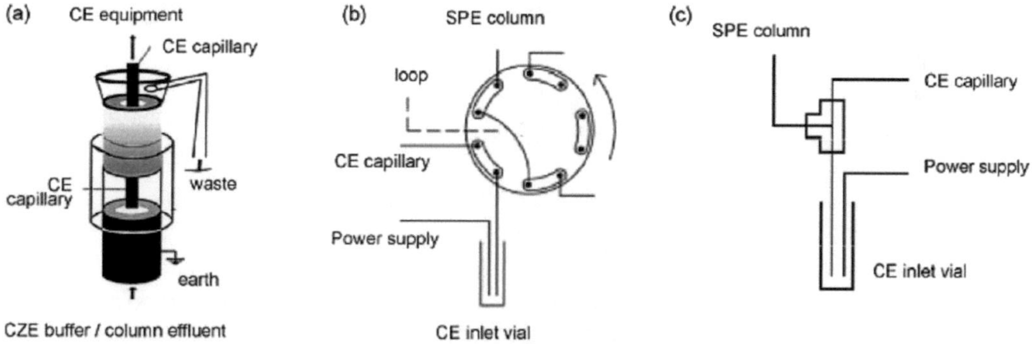

Figure 3.19. Schematic diagram of the three types of interfaces for on-line SPE–CE coupling: (a) vial interface; (b) valve interface; (c) T-split interface. Reproduced from refs. (a) [Stroink et al., 2003], (b) [Tempels et al., 2007] and (c) [Puig et al., 2007b].

In order to overcome this issue, on-line methods may be used, although care must be taken to ensure that no efficiency is lost in the transferral (e.g., dead volume must be minimized). Nowadays, the most used on-line SPE interfaces are the vial-type, the valve-type and the T-split-type [Bonneil & Waldron, 2000; Tempels et al., 2006; Puig et al., 2007b; Jiménez & de Castro, 2008]. Figure 3.19 shows a schematic representation of these interfaces. On-line SPE interface ensures that during the extraction waste solvents from the wash step are redirected, providing a cleaner extract for analysis. However, one of the major limitations of this approach is that because of the dead volume of the system, the entire eluate is not injected for separation, hence, some of the sensitivity gain is lost. Zhang and Wu [Zhang L.H. & Wu X. Z., 2007] presented a novel and conceptually simple approach to overcome this by creating a small hole in the capillary just after the SPE phase. The hole in the capillary allowed sample and wash solutions to be redirected to waste away from the separation capillary, while ensuring that the entire volume of solution used to elute the analytes was used for electrophoretic separation. While the integration level is impressive and the improvement in the LOD is sufficient (more than 10 000-fold is not unusual), practical analyses can be limited by the loading times in some cases (injection time can even be several hours). With respect to shortening analysis time, microchips offer a more attractive way of integrating SPE with electrophoresis, see examples in the review paper by Breadmore et al. [Breadmore et al., 2009]. However, unlike capillary format (SPE-CE), on-line coupled SPE-MCE has not been applied in chiral analysis so far.

Solid-phase microextraction (SPME) is an increasingly used technique because it is simple, can be used to extract analytes from very small samples and provides a rapid extraction and transfer to the analytical instrument. Moreover, it can be easily combined with other extraction and/or analytical procedures, improving to a large extent the sensitivity and selectivity of the whole method [Pawliszyn, 1997; Lord & Pawliszyn, 2000; Ouyang & Pawliszyn, 2006; Saito & Jinno, 2003]. As an example, an interface for SPME–CE–MS coupling is given in Figure 3.20. The on-line coupling of microextraction with the chiral CE has been described in the literature. For example, a direct chiral analysis of primary amine drugs in human urine by single drop microextraction in-line coupled to CE was demonstrated by Choi et al. [Choi K et al., 2009]. Examples on sensitive chiral analyses by means of microextraction-CE are stated in section 3.5. However, such coupling has not been widely used in practice because of its inherent drawbacks regarding the low injection volumes typically required in the CE (which are crucial to obtaining a good separation efficiency) and also because the different sizes of the separation capillaries usually used for CE and the SPME fibres [Liu Z. & Pawliszyn, 2006].

A general problem with the SPE/SPME-CE is the poisoning of the concentrator by matrix components and also their adsorption on the capillary wall. The use of coated capillaries, like poly(vinyl alcohol) (PVA), can decrease problems involved with protein adsorption. However, PVA capillaries are not available in the dimensions often required. Washing with sodium hydroxide is excluded due to incompatibility with the silica-based sorbent. Alternatives, then, are the use of polymer-based sorbents [Knudsen & Beattie, 1997] or a detergent such as SDS [Lloyd & Wätzig, 1995].

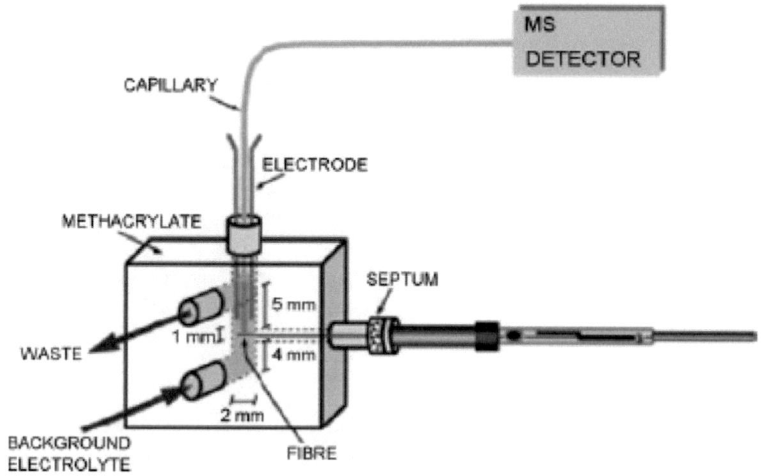

Figure 3.20. Interface for SPME–CE–MS coupling. Reproduced from Santos et al. [Santos et al., 2007].

3.3.2.2 Liquid-phase extraction

The miniaturization of liquid-phase (or liquid-liquid) extraction (LLE) has benefits in minimizing organic solvent consumption and sample amount requirements. Moreover, it simplifies and (partially) automates the extraction process. However, there are a number of technical issues that must be overcome for the development of an on-line integrated system. Recent progress covering the whole field of liquid-phase microextraction can be found in reviews on the subject by Bjergaard and Rasmussen [Bjergaard & Rasmussen, 2008], Lee et al. [Lee et al., 2008] and Xu et al. [Xu L. et al.; 2007]. The authors summarize miniaturized and highly flexible formats for LLE combinable with separation techniques, including CE, and they also gives views on environmental and bioanalytical applications of this coupled technique.

Integration of LLE with CE is based on an on-line back extraction system with FESI [Fang H.F. et al., 2006a]. In this approach the weak bases are first extracted into an organic solvent following a conventional off-line LLE protocol. The organic solvent containing the analytes is then placed in the sample vial and a small amount of water is placed on top. The analytes distribute between the organic phase (donor solution) and aqueous phase (acceptor solution), where they are partially protonated. Electrokinetic injection of the charged analytes depletes the analytes from the aqueous layer, disrupting the equilibrium, and more analytes are transferred from the organic phase into the water plug. Upon entering the capillary, analytes stack by normal FESI principles. Using this approach, a several thousand-fold increase in sensitivity can be obtained accompanied with sample purification. Other modifications of this approach are based on the use of a Teflon micromembrane [Almeda et al., 2007] or propylene hollow fibre [Nozal et al., 2007] filled with an acceptor solution and placed between the capillary and sample vial, see a scheme of LLE-CE equipment in Figure 3.21. For a detailed illustration, a schematic description of the construction of the liquid-phase microextraction unit can be seen in Figure 3.22.

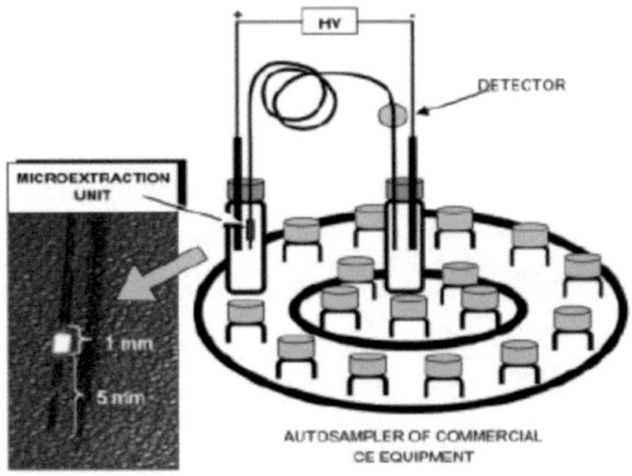

Figure 3.21. In-line liquid-phase microextraction – capillary electrophoresis (LLE-CE) arrangement for the determination of nonsteroidal antiinflammatory drugs in urine. Reprinted from ref. [Nozal et al., 2007].

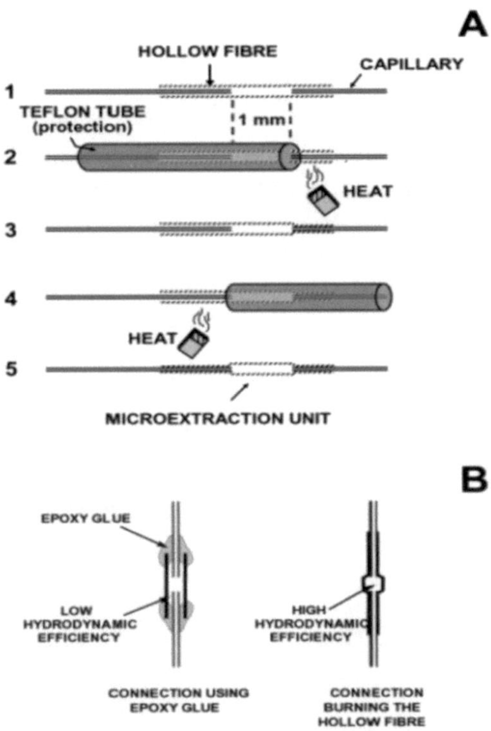

Figure 3.22. (A) Description of the construction of the liquid-phase microextraction unit. (1) Capillaries lining up and insertion in the hollow fibre; (2) protection of the hollow fibre with a Teflon tube and burning of the free part for capillary-hollow fibre connexion; (3) system with one connexion; (4) performance of the second connexion and (5) microextraction unit integrated into the capillary. (B) Comparison of connexions performed with epoxy glue and by burning the hollow fibre. Reprinted from ref. [Nozal et al., 2007].

3.3.3 Membrane filtration, microdialysis

Analytes can also be concentrated by inducing a velocity change due to their size by physically restricting their movement, so called concentration by physically induced changes in velocity. This has traditionally been most easily performed with large molecules, such as proteins and DNA [Yu C.J. et al., 2008]. Implementation of nanoporous media (nafion membrane, anionic hydrogel plug, etc.) in microchips (MCE is dominant in this field) has led to a number of interesting developments where the concentration of much smaller molecules is possible [de Jong et al., 2006; Holtzel & Tallarek, 2007; Dhopeshwarkar et al., 2008; Long et al., 2006]. Sensitivity enhancements of 4–6 orders of magnitude make this method powerful for sensitivity enhancement. A small piece of membrane (e.g., with 10 nm pores) can be integrated into a microchip also for the isolation of small molecules from crude samples. The potential of this approach was demonstrated with the analysis of biomarkers in blood without any off-line protein removal [Long et al., 2006]. A scheme of membrane - preconcentration/purification device implemented on-line into the CE is given as an example in Figure 3.23, where the detail of membrane insertion can be clearly seen.

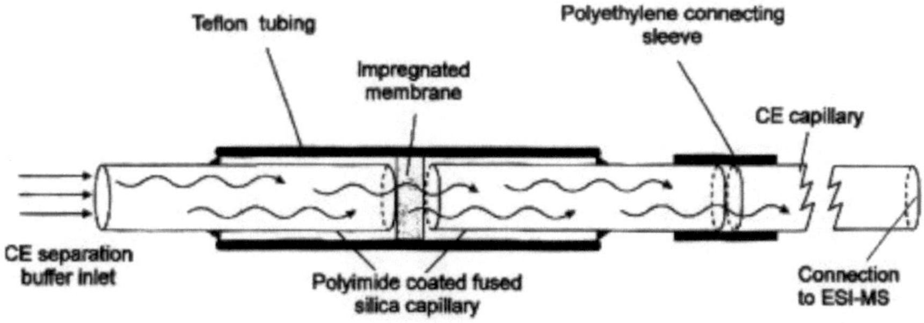

Figure 3.23. Membrane - preconcentration device with styrene-divinyl-benzene membrane to concentrate samples on-line in CE. Reprinted from ref. [Barroso & de Jong, 1998].

A microdialysis is frequently used to sample small molecules from complex, often biological, matrices [Adell & Artigas, 1998; Robinson & Justice, 1991; Chaurasia, 1999]. For example, some amino acid neurotransmitters are heterogeneously distributed in the brain and colocalized with *N*-methyl-D-aspartate (NMDA) receptors, suggesting a role in neurotransmission. In this analytical field, initial tissue assays for D-serine and D-aspartate biomarkers were based on a somewhat labour-intensive clean-up procedure followed by, e.g., a 70 min HPLC separation and LIF detection [Hashimoto et al., 1992, 1995]. On the other hand, in microdialysis, small molecules are able to diffuse across the dialysis membrane into the probe, while large molecules, such as proteins and cell fragments, are excluded. The clean-up provided by the microdialysis can allow analysing for neurotransmitters in tissue (e.g., brain) homogenates directly [Thompson, J.E. et al., 1999]. In the microdialysis, the minimum volume required for analysis often determines the rate at which the dialysate can be sampled. On-line microdialysis-CE-LIF assays (for the instrumental scheme see Figure 3.24) eliminate fraction collection. This elimination of fraction collection, combined with the high mass sensitivity of LIF or electrochemical detectors, makes sampling rates on the order of seconds possible [Thompson, J.E. et al., 1999; Hogan et al., 1994; Zhou S.Y. et al., 1995, 1999; Lada & Kennedy, 1995, 1997; Lada et al., 1998]. On-line microdialysis-CE assays for neurotransmitters to date have been most successful for easily resolved analytes such as glutamate and aspartate [Thompson, J.E. et al., 1999; Zhou S.Y. et al., 1995; Lada et al., 1997, 1998; Lada & Kennedy, 1996]. Efficiency and peak capacity of high-speed CE separations are often not high enough to resolve complex mixtures. Recently, improvements in injection technique and detection limits have improved separation efficiency, e.g., allowing singly charged amine derivatives, such as γ–amino-*n*butyric acid (GABA), to be analysed [Bowser & Kennedy, 2001]. Recently, on-line microdialysis-CE has been adapted to chiral determinations of neurotransmitters in multicomponent amino acid mixtures, as well as biological matrices [O'Brien et al., 2003], as shown in section 3.5.

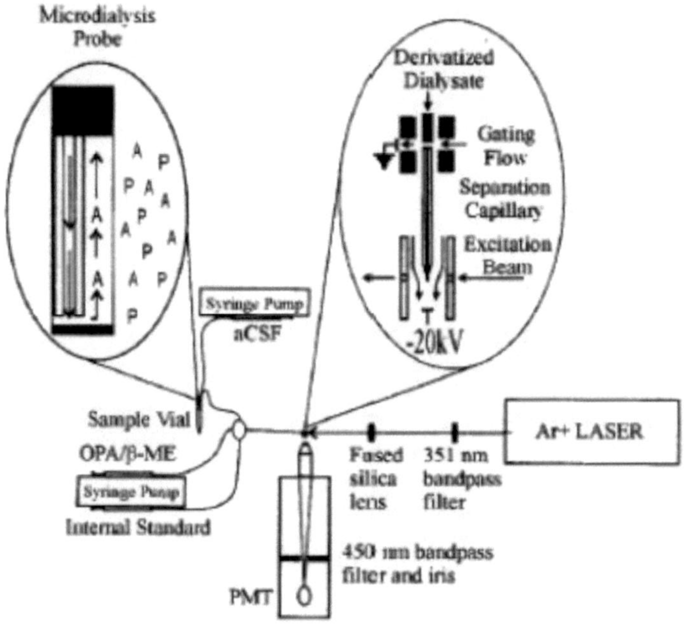

Figure 3.24. Diagram of the microdialysis-CE-LIF instrument. The whole automated procedure consists of following steps/modules performed on-line: (i) Microdialysis, (ii) derivatization, (iii) Flow-gated injection interface, (iv) High-speed CE with LIF detection. Reprinted from ref. [O'Brien et al., 2003].

3.3.4 Combination of electrophoretic stacking with nonelectrophoretic techniques

The electrophoretic stacking and nonelectrophoretic on-line sample preparation principles can be properly combined with each other to achieve the desired effect. Lately several such hybrid on-line sample preparation techniques have been introduced into the CE that offer excellent solutions, especially, for the sample clean-up (often accomplished by nonelectrophoretic principles) and analyte preconcentration (often accomplished by electrophoretic principles) in one experiment. Some of them, namely (i) extraction + stacking [Fang H.F. et al., 2006a, 2006b], (ii) dialysis + stacking [Hadwiger et al., 1996], (iii) chromatography + stacking [Pálmarsdóttir & Edholm, 1995; Pálmarsdóttir et al., 1996, 1997], were successfully applied also in chiral analyses of biologically active compounds in biological samples as presented in section 3.5.

The great potential with the hybrid on-line sample preparation techniques lies in their complementarity that enables the accumulation of positive effects and/or overcoming the weak points of the individual sample preparation techniques (discussed in sections 3.2 and 3.3). For example, the extraction used as the first step of the sample preparation can simplify the sample matrix (e.g., removing major interfering ionic constituents from the sample matrix) that is essential for some of the stacking modes (e.g., FESS requires a low-conductivity sample) used as the second step.

3.4 Flow injection

A combination of on-line sample preparation techniques based on electrophoretic and nonelectrophoretic principles can be performed in a single column or column coupling arrangement. Another interesting possibility with how to implement various sample preparation procedures on-line is a combination of the flow injection (FI) with electrophoresis. The combination of FI with electrophoresis using capillaries and chips is reviewed by Lü et al. [Lü W.J. et al., 2009]. Here, the basic principles, instrumental developments (including newly designed interfaces for FI-CE) and applications of FI-CE system from 2006 to 2008 are reviewed. The technique of combined flow injection CE (FI-CE) integrates the essential favourable merits of FI and CE. It utilizes the various excellent on-line sample pretreatments and preconcentration (such as cloud point extraction, SPE, ion-exchange, DPJ and head-column FESS technique, analyte derivatization) of FI, which has the advantages of high-speed, accuracy, precision and avoiding manual handling of sample and reagents. Therefore, the coupling of FI-CE is an attractive technique; it can significantly expand the application of CE and has achieved many publications since its first appearance. The significant potential of the FI-CE method in the automatization of sample derivatization and chiral separation was demonstrated by Mardones et al. [Mardones et al., 1999], and the proposed FI-CE scheme is shown in Figure 3.25.

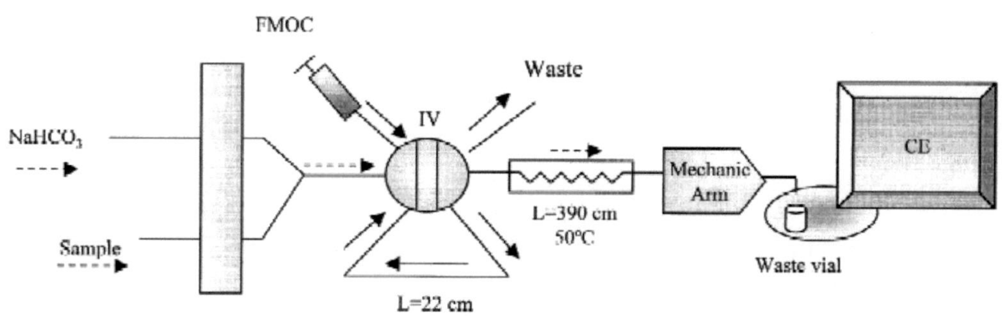

Figure 3.25. FI manifold used for the derivatization of the carnitine enantiomers and their on-line introduction into the CE system. Reprinted from ref. [Mardones et al., 1999].

3.5 Applications

The sample preparation techniques on-line combined with the CE, described in sections 3.2-3.4 (see for the theory and schemes), have been applied in many models, as well as real situations. In a lesser extent, given by (i) the higher complexity of experimental arrangement with chiral additive(s), as well as (ii) the natural proportion between currently solved chiral and achiral analytical problems, these techniques have been on-line combined with chiral CE systems.

Chiral CE determinations of biologically active compounds in various real matrices, e.g., environmental, food, beverage and mainly biological (clinical, forensic), as well as pharmaceutical samples, employing an on-line sample preparation, are listed in Table 3.1.

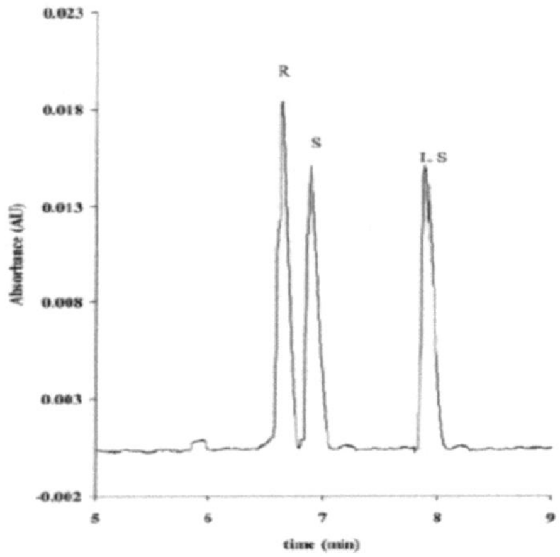

Figure 3.26. Analysis of plasma extracts containing 50 ng/mL of drug enantiomers and internal standard by CE with optimized FESI injection. Capillary column, 57 cm x 50 μm) i.d.; applied voltage, +20 kV; temperature 25°C; buffer, formic acid-ammonia (pH 4, ionic strength 50 mM) and 3.5 mM HP-β-CD. FESI, hydrodynamic injection of water plug (5 s) then electrokinetic injection (+10 kV, 20 s) of racemic drug dissolved in a water-methanol (10/90 v/v) and 80 μM H_3PO_4 mixture. SPE pretreatment of plasma sample was carried out before FESI-CE. Reprinted from ref. [Grard et al., 2002].

In this Table we tried to emphasize briefly the most important features of the methods and purpose of sample preparation, i.e., sample clean-up, analyte preconcentration, analyte derivatization. Here, the selectivity and sensitivity gain of combining on-line sample preparation procedures with chiral CE for the determination of low concentrations of drugs in complex matrices was clearly exemplified.

From among those examples, selected applications in biological and model (presented here for a given sample preparation method only in the case when no bioapplication is available) samples are described in the text of this section in detail, emphasizing the practical aspects of the proposed methods via their performance parameters (precision, recovery, etc.). In this way, the usefulness of the various techniques in routine analysis can be clearly ascertained.

Field-enhanced sample stacking. The FESI-CE-UV method has been developed for the quantification of cationic enantiomers of the new adrenoreceptor antagonists in plasma samples, for the illustrative electropherogram see Figure 3.26 [Grard et al., S., 2002]. An excellent accuracy on retention times and peak efficiencies was found with relative standard deviations (RSDs) being generally less than 1% and 2%, respectively. The FESI method also provided good reproducibility of ratio between the corrected areas of enantiomer and of the internal standard, since the RSD never exceeded 3%. These experimental results attest to the reliability of the FESI method in analysing chiral drugs by CE.

The increase of sensitivity by applying a FESS procedure was necessary for the analysis of amphetamine and its metabolic products (3,4-ethylenedioxymethamphetamine, MDMA, 3-4-methylenedioxyamphetamine, MDA, 3,4-methalenedioxyethylamphetamine, MDE) in hair samples [Tagliaro et al., 1998]. The FESS-CE-DAD method allowed the chiral determination of the metabolites at concentrations occurring in real samples from ecstasy users, with the possibility of recording UV spectra of the peaks. The analytical precision was characterized by relative standard deviation values <0.8 % (≤0.15% with internal standardization) for migration times intra-day and <2.0% (≤0.54% with internal standardization) day-to-day; linearity, in the range 0.156-40 μg/mL, and accuracy were also satisfactory. Even when evaluated at the lowest concentration of the standard curve, 0.156 pg/mL (with a signal-to-noise ratio of 5 for MDMA and 3 for amphetamine), the between-days area reproducibility was acceptable, ranging from 7.93% RSD for MDMA, to 16.07% RSD for amphetamine. The intra-day RSDs of migration times were always <0.8%, while the between-days RSDs were <2.0%; for relative migration times, RSDs were ≤0.15% and ≤0.54%, respectively. Absolute peak area reproducibility was still acceptable at 20 pg/mL (RSD was about 5% intra-day and ≤8% inter-days), but at 0.2 pg/mL the variability was relevant (RSDs between 9 and 12%). The area normalization on the basis of an IS (D-methamphetamine) was helpful, but for MDMA, MDA and MDE, RSDs remained around 10%.

FESI as an on-line sample stacking method was employed in order to increase the detection sensitivity for six β-blockers, namely (±) carteolol, (±) atenolol, (±) sotalol, (±) metoprolol, (±) esmolol and (±) propranolol, in human serum samples [Huang L. et al., 2008]. The final serum sample solution had to be diluted before injection since the ion concentration in the sample solution strongly influenced the signal enhancement. When the human serum sample was not diluted, the signal enhancement was not great because of the matrix effect. For validation of the FESI-CE-UV method, sensitivity (Table 3.1), linearity and precision were evaluated. The study showed that the repeatabilities of migration times (intra-day RSD 5.5-6.1%, inter-day RSD 4.4-5.2%) and peak heights (intra-day RSD 1.5-12.9%, inter-day RSD 3.6-5.2%) for the enantiomers of β-blockers were satisfactory. Recoveries (calculated using the 5 mg/mL racemic standard solutions) ranged from 82.1 to 98.2%.

The FESI-CE-UV method was used to determine the concentration of sulindac (SU) and its two active metabolites, sulindac sulfide (SI) and sulindac sulfone (SO), in human plasma [Chen Y.L. et al., 2006]. During method validation, calibration plots were linear ($r > 0.994$) over a range of 0.3–30.0 μM for SU and SO, and 0.5–30.0 μM for SI. During intra- and inter-day analysis, relative standard deviations (RSD) and relative errors (RE) were all less than 16%. Compared to the peak area ratio of the standard analytes, the absolute recoveries for SU, SO and SI were about 82, 81 and 60%, respectively. This method was feasible for the investigation of a pharmacokinetic profile of SU in plasma after oral administration of one SU tablet (Clinoril, 200 mg/tab) to a female volunteer.

The LVSS-CE-DAD method was applied for the sensitivity enhancement of four basic racemic drugs (methoxamine, metaproterenol, terbutaline and carvedilol) in serum samples [Denola et al., 2007]. Accuracy ranges were 96.4–103.4% for the hydrodynamic injection and 102.3–115.5% for the electrokinetic injection. Better recovery values were achieved with hydrodynamic injection wherein values ranged from 62.8–74.5% as compared to that of the electrokinetic injection in which recovery values were all lower (31.1–69.4%). The deviations in the resolution values were higher for the electrokinetic (RSD 3.6–6.0%) than for the hydrodynamic injection (RSD <1.9%). However, the repeatability of migration times was better when control samples were loaded electrokinetically (RSD 0.6–0.8%) rather than hydrodynamically (RSD 2.1–2.6%). Migration times do not vary significantly from those obtained with the control samples. Good repeatability in terms of migration times and enantioresolution was evident in the very low RSD values (migration time RSD ≤0.5; enantioresolution RSD ≤5.5) in both types of injections.

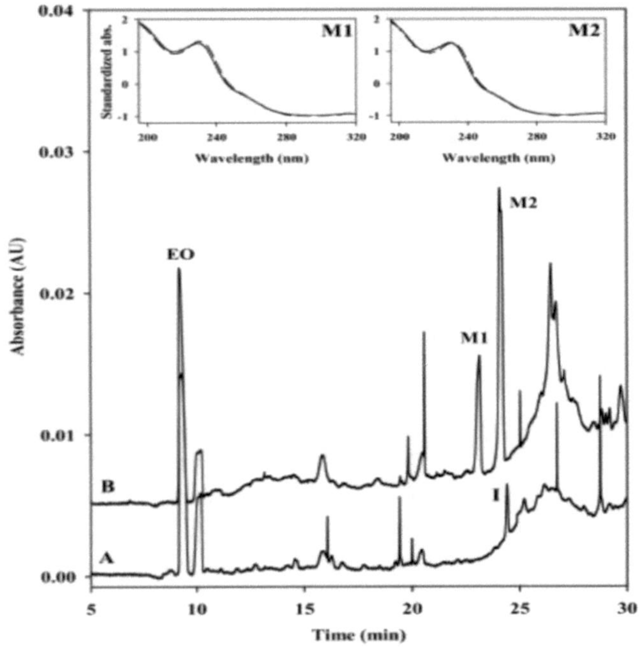

Figure 3.27. SWP-MEKC electropherograms obtained from a 30 psi x s injection of four pooled human liver microsomes incubations (A) without lorazepam (blank) and (B) with 50 μM lorazepam. Two insets show the comparison of blank subtracted, standardized spectra of lorazepam metabolites M1 and M2 (broken lines), and lorazepam (full line). Analytical conditions: detection was effected at 200 nm and, for solute identification purpose, the fast scanning mode (range: 195-320 nm, scanning interval: 5 nm) was employed, temperature 25°C, applied voltage 20kV (current about 28 μA). Separation electrolyte: 6 mM $Na_2B_4O_7$, 10 mM Na_2HPO_4, and 75 mM SDS, pH 9.1 (before addition of SDS). Reprinted from ref. [Baldacci & Thormann, 2006].

Transient isotachophoresis. tITP was used for the preconcentration of timolol and ephedrine in standard solutions and dosage forms [Hedeland et al., 2007]. tITP served for peak sharpening of S-timolol and therefore, the tITP-CE-DAD determination of the enantiomeric impurity (R-timolol) was possible with sufficient enantioresolution, as illustrated in Figure 3.28. For ephedrine, the tITP-CE-DAD method was validated. The intermediate precision for the quality control (QC) samples was in the interval 4.2–5.6% and the precision for each set of samples was equal or less than 5.6% (for seven out of nine values), which is considered as acceptable for the application. The accuracy at 1.9% of the enantiomeric impurity for three different BGEs where the composition was varied (±1%) was in the range 91.3–99.7% and the precision was 1.7–8.7% (n = 2). Thus, the method is robust and small differences in the BGE composition should not have any major influence in the determination of the 1R,2S-ephedrine impurity.

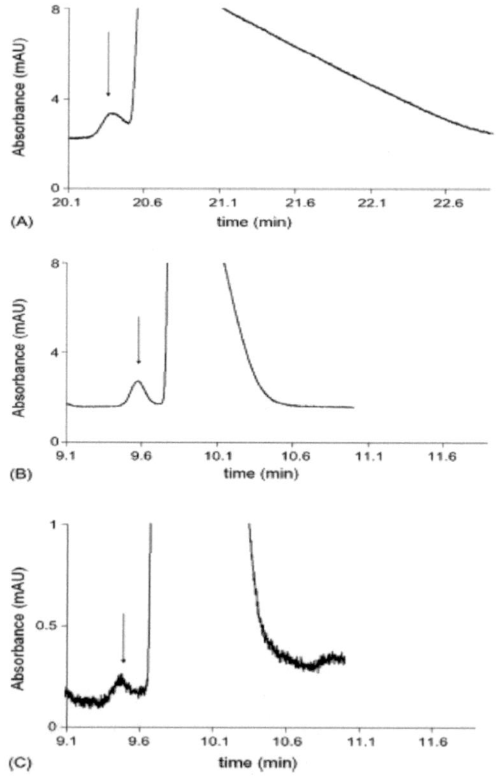

Figure 3.28. Peak sharpening of S-timolol by tITP. BGE: 100mM (+)-ketopinic acid and 40mM KOH in methanol:ethanol (3:2, v/v). 30 kV, L_{det} 23 cm. Sample: 2mM *S*-timolol and 0.05mM *R*-timolol (2.4%) dissolved in methanol. (A) Normal injection pressure injection at 35 mbar over 5 s, (B) tITP, leading electrolyte: 100mM sodium acetate in methanol (25 mbar over 1 s). Terminating electrolyte: 200mM triethanolamine in methanol (anodic vial). (C) tITP at LOD (0.2% *R*-timolol). Conditions as in (B). The arrow in the electropherograms (A–C) points out the position of the *R*-timolol peak. Reprinted from ref. [Hedeland et al., 2007].

Combined stacking techniques. A combination of LVSS and SWP, where LVSS involves a subcombination of field-amplified stacking and pH-mediated stacking, provided a very high sensitivity for the anionic cyanobenz[*f*]isoindole (CBI)-amino acids [Kirschner et al., 2007]. Average and standard deviation in peak area ratios (CBI-amino acid/ internal standard) for nine injections of 2.4 μM CBI-amino acid were as follows: CBI-L-Glu 0.461±0.070, CBI-D-Ser 0.400±0.085, CBI-L-Asp 0.358±0.036. A procedure for the LVSS-SWP-CE-LIF determination of CBI-D-Ser was applied for squirrel brain samples. This preconcentration technique was also applied to multicomponent mixtures of CBI amino acid derivatives without loss of resolution, see electropherogram in Figure 3.29.

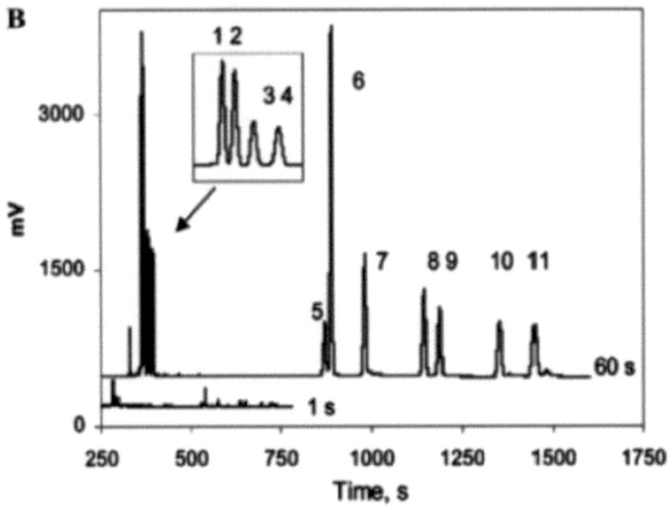

Figure 3.29. Electropherogram showing the potential of stacking/sweeping-EKC combination to the enantioseparation of a complex sample of CBI–amino acids (0.5 μM each). Electrophoretic conditions: fused-silica capillary, 70 cm total length (45 cm detector length) and 25 μm i.d.; separation buffer, 25 mM phosphate buffer (pH 2.0) containing 2% HS-β-CD; applied voltage, 230 kV; hydrodynamic injection, 380 mbar for 180 s. LIF detection with l_{exc} at 420 nm. Peak identification: 1, CBI-D-Arg; 2, CBI-L-Arg; 3, CBI-D-His; 4, CBI-L-His; 5, CBI-Gly; 6, CBI-L-Tyr; 7, CBI-L-Glu; 8, CBI-D-Ser; 9, CBI-L-Ser; 10, CBI-L-Glu; 11, CBI-D-Glu. Adapted from ref. [Kirschner et al., 2007].

Sensitive CE methods are required for emerging areas of biochemical research such as the metabolome. In ref. [Britz-McKibbin et al., 2003], DPJ-SWP-CE-LIF was applied as a robust single method to analyse trace amounts of three flavin derivatives, riboflavin, flavin mononucleotide (FMN) and flavin adenine dinucleotide (FAD), from several types of samples including bacterial cell extracts, recombinant protein and biological fluids. For the separation of flavins a chiral selector mediated CE separation system was needed. Submicromolar amounts of flavin coenzymes were measured directly from formic acid cell extracts of *Bacillus subtilis*. This method was also applied to the analysis of free flavins in pooled human plasma and urine without the need for laborious off-line sample preconcentration (e.g., SPE). The method was validated in terms of reproducibility, sensitivity (Table 3.1), linearity and specificity. The linearity of the method within a 100-fold concentration range was excellent as reflected by the correlation coefficient (R^2) of 0.999 for all three flavin calibration curves. However, significant nonlinearity was observed to occur at concentrations above 0.1 μM. Because of the lack of native fluorescent species in most biological matrices, the method is considered to be extremely specific with few chemical interferences. Reproducibility of the CE method was assessed by analysis of five replicate injections of formic acid cell extract (malate) sample performed on two consecutive days. Inter-day coefficients of variance (CV, n=10) for migration time and peak area of flavin coenzymes were determined to be 0.68 and 3.8%, respectively. The low reproducibility of this technique may be attributed in part to the long injection time (60 s) used for analysis, whereas precision in CE is often limited by short hydrodynamic injections. Anyway, flavin analysis by DPJ-SWP-CE-LIF offers a simple, yet sensitive way to analyse trace levels of flavin metabolites from complex biological samples.

Transient isotachophoresis with field-enhanced sample injection, using β-CD as the chiral selector and tetrabutylammonium hydroxide (TBAOH) as the additive, was applied for on-line preconcentration and enantioseparation of three beta-agonists, namely, cimaterol, clenbuterol and terbutaline. Under the optimum conditions, the detection limits (defined as S/N = 3) of this method were found to be 1 ng/mL for all three pairs of beta-agonists enantiomers. Compared with conventional electrokinetic injection, the enhancement factors were greatly improved to be 250-fold. The proposed method has been applied for the analysis of human urine samples [Huang, L. et al., 2011].

Stacking techniques with derivatization. An on-line sample preconcentration approach coupled with in-capillary derivatization (SPCD-CE) has recently been applied, among others, to the (indirect) chiral separation of amino acids, whereby a special application represents the detection of D-amino acids as biomarkers in connection with bacterial growth, see Figure 3.30 [Ptolemy et al., 2006; Ptolemy & Britz-McKibbin, 2006]. In comparison with conventional CE, SPCD-CE provided a 100-fold improvement in concentration sensitivity, reduced sample handling and shorter analysis time. The reproducibility (n = 5) of the integrated SPCD-CE-UV technique was acceptable with average coefficients of variation of approximately 7.4 and 1.2% for quantitation (peak height) and apparent migration time, respectively [Ptolemy et al., 2006].

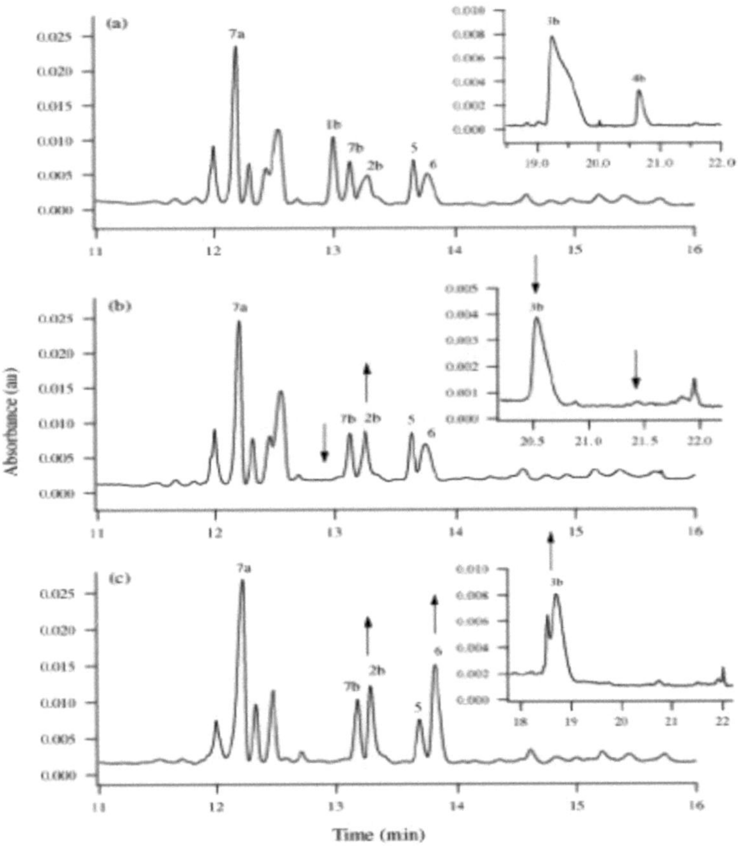

Figure 3.30. Direct enantioselective amino acid flux analyses in the extra-cellular medium of *E. coli* by SPCD-CE. Electropherograms represent the extra-cellular media with 5% seeding volume incubated for (a) 0 h (control), (b) 3 h and (c) 5 h. Other conditions: sample solutions contained 25 and 50μM of the D and L-amino acids, respectively, prepared in 40mM phosphate, pH 6.0 using a sample injection of 100 s. Conditions: 140mM borate buffer, pH 9.5; voltage 25 kV; capillary length 67 cm; internal diameter; 50μm; UV 340 nm. Analyte peak number corresponds amino acid-isoindole adducts, where 1a: D-Ser, 1b: L-Ser, 2a: D-Ala, 2b: L-Ala, 3a: D-Glu, 3b: L-Glu, 4a: D-Asp, 4b: L-Asp, 5: taurine (6 μM, internal standard), 6: Gly and 7a,b: L-Lys side-product. The direction of arrow indicates a net release (↑) or uptake (↓) of amino acid has been observed in the extra-cellular medium during bacterial growth. Note the rapid uptake of L-Ser and L-Asp and the steady-state enantioselective release of L-Ala. There was no detection of net efflux of D-Ala and D-Glu from *E. coli* into extra-cellular matrix during bacterial growth. Reprinted from ref. [Ptolemy & Britz-McKibbin, 2006].

Counter-flow gradient focusing. TGF has been shown to be effective for a 1200-fold concentration enrichment in 30 min for the baseline-separated enantiomers of glutamic acid, as illustrated in Figure 3.31 [Balss et al., 2004]. No validation data are available for this method.

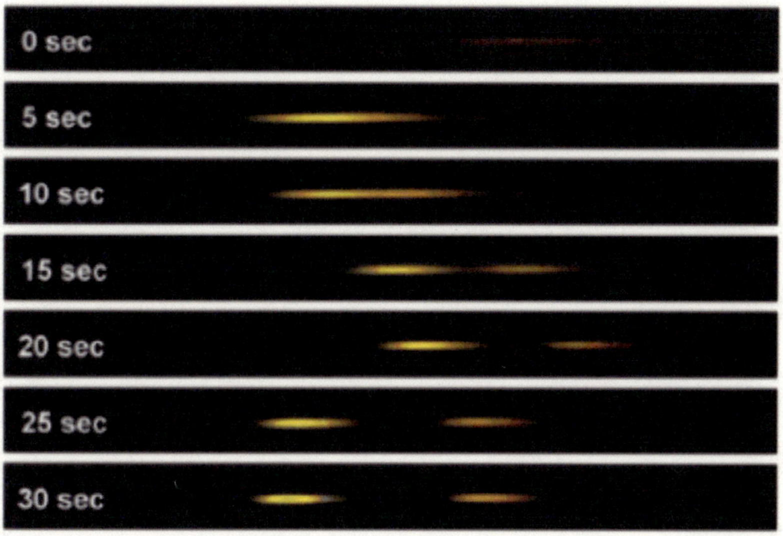

Figure 3.31. Example of TGF focusing and separation. Total image length is 1.9 mm. Real-time chiral TGF of DNS-D,L-Glutamic acid. Working conditions as in Figure 3.13. The D-enantiomer peak is to the left in the figure; the L-enantiomer is to the right. Reprinted from ref. [Balss et al., 2004].

Column-coupled electrophoretic techniques. An ITP-EKC-UV method was successfully applied for the determination of trace enantiomers of various drugs and their biodegradation products (pheniramine and its metabolites, dioxopromethazine, dimethindene, amlodipine) in model complex ionic matrices and clinical samples [Mikuš et al., 2006, 2008a, 2008b; Marák et al., 2007], see an example in Figure 3.32. RSD values of migration times were lower than 2.0%. The concentrations of the analytes in tested samples, corresponding to the quantitation limits, were determined with acceptable precisions (RSD values ranged in interval 3.95–4.54%, n = 5) and accuracies (relative errors ranged in interval 5.84–6.22%, n = 5) under the stated conditions. The mean relative errors (REs) indicated by the recovery tests, characterizing accuracy of the chiral method for pheniramine, dimethindene and dioxopromethazine, were 4.5, 4.8 and 3.6%, respectively [Mikuš et al., 2006a].

The ITP-EKC-DAD method was shown to be a powerful tool in enantioselective pharmacokinetic studies of the β-blocker drug, amlodipine, in clinical urine samples [Mikuš et al., 2008a] and the enantioselective metabolic study of cationic H_1-antihistamine, pheniramine, present in clinical urine samples [Marák et al., 2007]. Performance parameters of the ITP-EKC-UV/DAD methods were sufficient for the routine enantioselective biomedical analyses of unpretreated biological samples. Besides all the benefits of the ITP-EKC combination, as mentioned above, speed spectral evaluation of separated zones enabled preliminary characterization of their homogeneity (presence of mixed zones) and preliminary indication of structurally (spectrally) similar compounds (potential metabolites of the drugs) in unknown electrophoretic peaks. To complete the evaluation of the performance parameters, the selectivity of the ITP-EKC separation method can be examined by the spectral evaluation of purity of analyte zones.

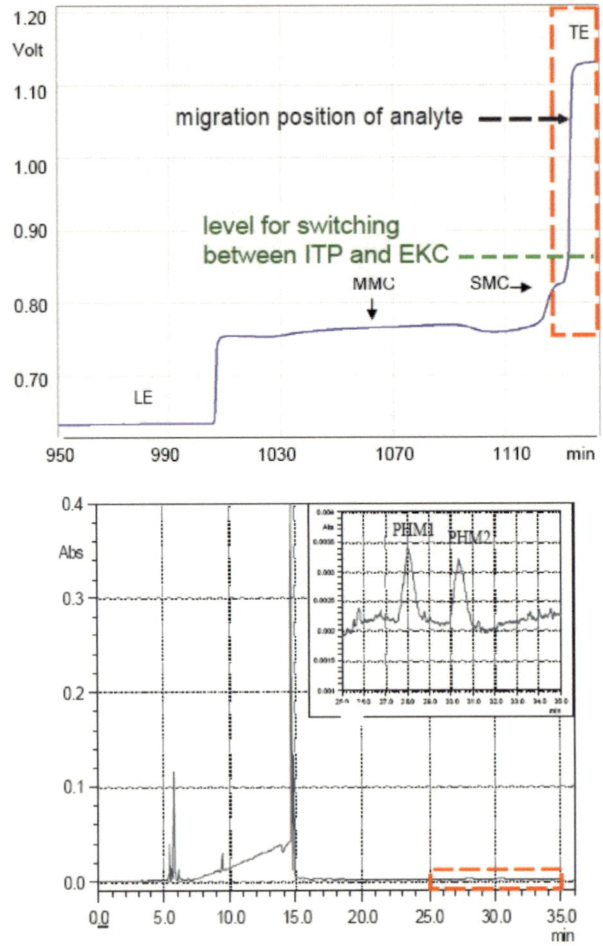

Figure 3.32. ITP-EKC method in column coupling configuration of the separation units for the direct analysis of unpretreated complex matrices sample; electrophoretic traces. Determination of pheniramine enantiomers in model urine sample demonstrates the effectivity of on-line sample preparation (removing matrices, preconcentration of enantiomers) in the first ITP stage (upper trace) and countercurrent separation mechanism (enantioseparation) in the second EKC stage (lower trace) of the ITP-EKC method. The separations were carried out using 10 mM sodium acetate - acetic acid, pH 4.75 as a leading electrolyte (ITP), 5 mM ε-aminocaproic acid - acetic acid, pH 4.5 as a terminating electrolyte (ITP), and 25 mM ε-aminocaproic acid - acetic acid, pH 4.5 as a carrier electrolyte (EKC). 0.1% (w/v) methyl-hydroxyethylcellulose served as an EOF suppressor in leading and carrier electrolytes. Carboxyethyl-β-CD (5 mg/mL) was used as a chiral selector in carrier electrolyte. Concentration of pheniramine was 7.10^{-8} M in the injected sample (a 10 times diluted spiked urine). The detection wavelength in EKC stage was 261 nm. The driving currents in the ITP and EKC stages were 200 μA and 80 μA, respectively. LE – leading cation; TE – terminating cation; PHM1, PHM2– migration positions of the first and second pheniramine enantiomer, respectively, MMC – major matrix constituents, SMC – semiminor matrix constituents. Reprinted from ref. [Mikuš et al., 2008b].

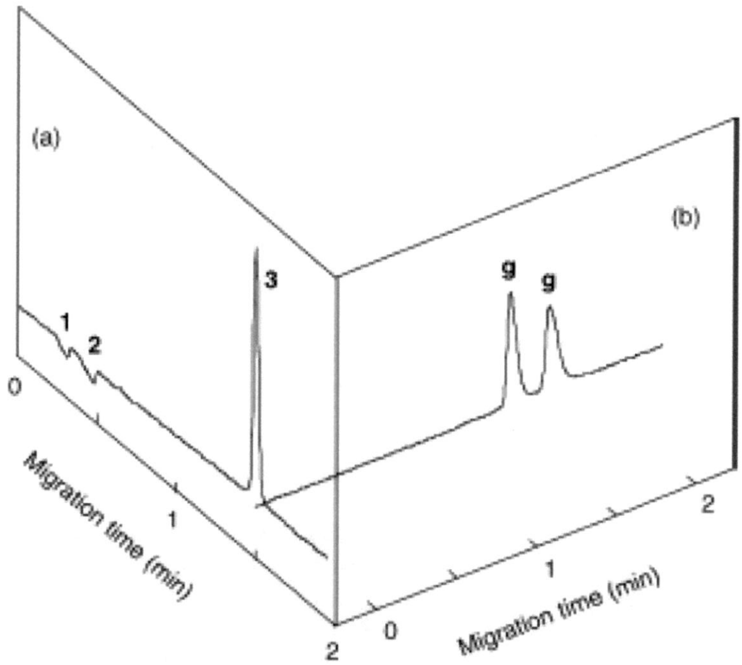

Figure 3.33. Chiral separation of gemifloxacin dissolved in a urinary solution with microchip electrophoresis. Peaks: (1) K^+; (2) Na^+; and (3) gemifloxacin racemate. Peaks for gemifloxacin enantiomers are denoted by 'g'. (a) The removal of metal ions was performed in the first separation channel. Run buffer: (50mM Bis–Tris + 10 μM quinine)/Citric acid of pH 4.0. (b) The chiral separation was performed in the second separation channel using a run buffer of 50mM Bis–Tris/Citric acid containing 50 μM 18C6H4 (pH 4.0). A urinary solution was five-fold diluted using 50mM Bis–Tris/Citric acid (pH 4.0). Gemifloxacin was 100 μM in five-fold diluted urinary solution. Gemifloxacin was injected into the second separation channel by floating reservoir D, with reservoir F grounded, for 15 s right after the analyte passed the first detection point to ensure that all gemifloxacin was introduced into the second channel. For the analysis in the second channel, the applied voltage was 3.0 kV at reservoir E with reservoir F grounded and all other reservoirs floating. For the instrumental scheme, see Figure 3.15. Light source: He–Cd laser (325 nm); indirect laser-induced fluorescence detection at 405 nm using a photomultiplier tube. Analytes were detected at 32 and 38mm from the first and second injection crosses, respectively. Reprinted from ref. [Cho S.I. et al., 2004].

A channel-coupled microchip electrophoresis device was designed to clean-up alkaline metal ions (interfering with chiral selector) from a sample matrix for the chiral analysis of gemifloxacin in urine, see Figure 3.33 [Cho S.I. et al., 2004]. The total analysis time of directly injected urine samples was less than 4 min with micromolar amounts of chiral selector (50 μM CWE). No validation data are available for this method.

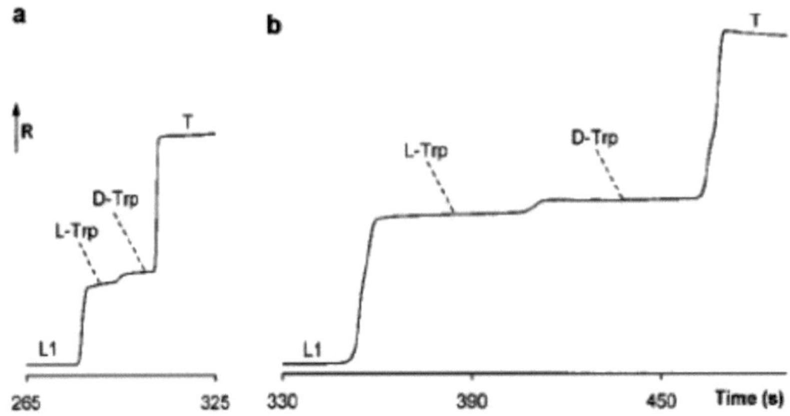

Figure 3.34. Isotachopherogram from the separations of racemic mixture of tryptophan enantiomers on the CC chip. (a) Single-column separation in the first channel using C1 to monitor the situation. The separation was carried out in the electrolyte system L1 with 8.5 A driving current. The injected sample contained the racemate at a $6x10^{-4}$ M concentration. (b) Separation in the tandem-coupled separation channels using C2 to monitor the separation. The separation was carried out in the electrolyte system L1 placed in both separation channels. The driving current was 8.5 A during the run in the first channel and it was reduced to 5 μA during the separation in the second channel. The injected sample contained the racemate at a $1.5x10^{-3}$ M concentration. R, increasing resistance; L1 leading anion (propionate), T, termination anion (ε-aminocaproate). Reprinted from ref. [Ölvecká et al., 2001].

The use of a poly(methylmethacrylate) chip, provided with a pair of on-line hyphenated separation channels and on-column conductivity detectors, to isotachophoresis (ITP) separations of optical isomers was investigated by Ölvecká et al. [Ölvecká et al., 2001]. Single-column ITP, ITP in the tandem-coupled columns, and concentration-cascade ITP in the tandem-coupled columns were employed in this investigation using tryptophan enantiomers as model analytes, see Figure 3.34. Although providing a high production rate (about 2 pmol of a pure tryptophan enantiomer separated per second), single-column ITP was found suitable only to the analysis of samples containing the enantiomers at close concentrations. The best results in the respect of the resolution were achieved by using a concentration-cascade of the leading anions in the tandem-coupled separation channels.

Extraction. A miniaturized SPE (1-3 mm capillary of 200 μm internal diameter packed with C18 alkyl-diol silica and capped by glass-fibre filters for the sorbent retaining) coupled on-line with CE significantly enhanced the concentration sensitivity for terbutaline [Petersson et al., 1999]. Experimental arrangement of the extractor and speed (10 min) sample enrichment procedure for the terbutaline enantioselective analysis are illustrated in Figure 3.18. The chiral application of the SPE-CE-UV method for model sample, as well as achiral application of the same method for plasma sample, is shown in Figure 3.35 [Petersson et al., 1999].

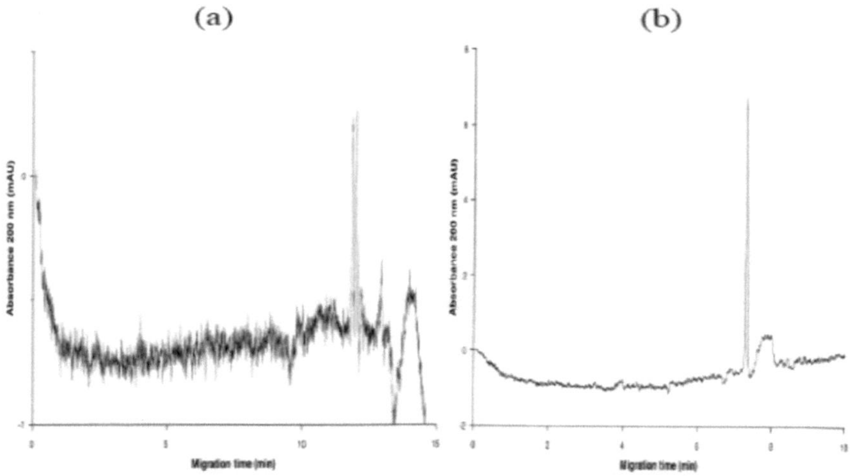

Figure 3.35. Miniaturized on-line SPE for enhancement of concentration sensitivity in CE. (a) Terbutaline enantiomer separation with on-line enrichment. A resolution of 1.6 and a separation efficiency of 300 000 plates were obtained. Enrichment capillary: L_t 58.0 cm, L_d 51.2 cm, L_i 5.5 cm, l_e 2.5 mm, wash: water x 1.6 min x 140 kPa, wetting: methanol x 2.4 min x 140 kPa, conditioning: water x 2.4 min x 140 kPa, injection: 100 nM *rac*-terbutaline in water x 1.0 min x 140 kPa, wash/ filling: 40 mM potassium phosphate (pH 6.4) x 0.1 min x 140 kPa, 15 mM dimethyl-β-CD in 40 mM potassium phosphate (pH 6.4) x 0.7 min x 140 kPa, desorption: acetonitrile x 40 s x 3.4 kPa followed by 15 mM dimethyl-β-CD in 40 mM potassium phosphate (pH 6.4) x 4.0 min x 3.4 kPa, voltage: 14 kV, detection wavelength: 200 nm, temperature: 25°C. (b) Direct injection of terbutaline in plasma with on-line enrichment. The enrichment capillary had not been subjected to plasma samples before this run. Enrichment capillary: L_t 58.0 cm, L_d 51.2 cm, L_i 5.4 cm, l_e 1.25 mm, wash: water x 1.4 min x 140 kPa, 200 mM SDS in 100 mM sodium borate (pH 9.0) x 3.5 min x 140 kPa, wetting: methanol x 7.0 min x 140 kPa, conditioning: water x 2.1 min x 140 kPa, injection: 2 mM terbutaline in water–bovine plasma (3:1) x 0.1 min x 140 kPa, wash: water x 1.4 min x 140 kPa, filling: 40 mM potassium phosphate (pH 6.4) x 0.8 min x 140 kPa, desorption: acetonitrile x 30 s x 3.4 kPa followed by 40 mM potassium phosphate (pH 6.4) x 3.0 min x 3.4 kPa, voltage: 20 kV, detection wavelength: 200 nm, temperature: 25°C. Adapted from ref. [Petersson et al., 1999].

The separation efficiency was 300 000 plates. The relative average deviation from the mean was 17% for the enrichment capillaries. Within each enrichment capillary the relative average deviation from the mean was below 2% (n=6). Fouling of the capillary wall with plasma protein during the analysis was prevented by an SDS washing step. However, partial clogging of the enrichment capillary was observed after repeated plasma injections.

Electro membrane extraction as a new microextraction method was applied for the extraction of amlodipine (AML) enantiomers from biological samples [Nojavan & Fakhari, 2010]. During the extraction time of 15 min AML enantiomers migrated from a 3 mL sample solution through a supported liquid membrane into a 20 μl acceptor solution presented inside the lumen of the hollow fibre. The driving force of the extraction was 200 V potential with the negative electrode in the acceptor solution and the positive electrode in the sample solution. 2-Nitro-phenyl octylether was used as the supported liquid membrane. Using 10 mM HCl as background electrolyte in the sample and acceptor solution, enrichment up to 124 times was achieved. Then the extract was analysed using the CD modified CE method for separation of AML enantiomers. The best results were achieved using a phosphate running buffer (100 mM, pH 2.0) containing 5 mM hydroxypropyl alpha CD. The range of quantitation for both enantiomers was 10-500 ng/mL. Intra- and inter-day RSDs (n = 6) were less than 14%. The limits of quantitation and detection for both enantiomers were 10 and 3 ng/mL respectively. Finally this procedure was applied to determine the concentration of AML enantiomers in plasma and urine samples.

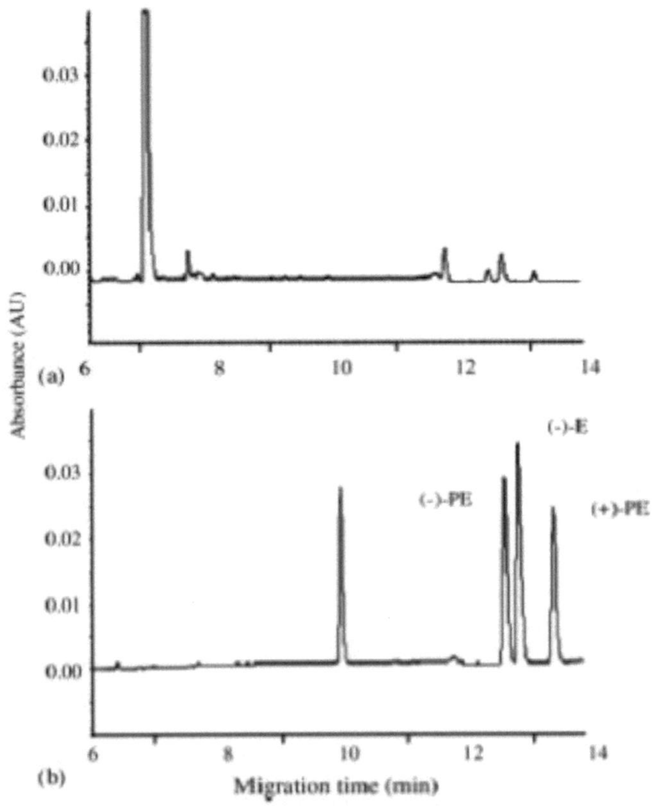

Figure 3.36. Separation of spiked urine sample (a) with directly injected (concentration of each analyte: 5.00 μg/mL); (b) after SPME-FESI (concentration of each analyte: 0.25μg/mL) followed by CE separation. The optimized SPME conditions: temperature of 90°C, time of 30 min, 2.00 g sodium hydroxide and 0.50 g sodium chloride for headspace extraction; 20% acetonitrile aqueous phase solvent with desorption time of 20 min for desorption. CE conditions: the run buffer contained 17.5mM β-CD and 150mM phosphate (pH 2.5) in the running voltage 25 kV at 20°C. Sample injection: 7 kV×10 s. (1R,2S)-ephedrine ((−)-E), (1R,2R)-pseudoephedrine ((−)-PE) and (1S,2S)-pseudodephedrine ((+)-PE). Reprinted from ref. [Fang H.F. et al., 2006b].

Extraction + stacking. A sufficient selectivity and sensitivity enhancement of two orders of magnitude was achieved for ephedrine derivatives {(1R,2S)-ephedrine, (1R,2R)-pseudoephedrine, (1S,2S)-pseudoephedrine} in human urine samples using an on-line combination of headspace SPME with FESI, see ref. [Fang H.F. et al., 2006b]. Electropherogram from the SPME-FESI-EKC method applied on spiked urine samples is shown in Figure 3.36. The intra-assay relative standard deviations were between 4.38 and 7.76% (concentration of analytes: 0.3 µg/mL; n = 5). Recovery was in range 88.7-97.5%. The performance parameters indicate a good potential of the SPME-FESI-CE-DAD method for its routine use.

The back LLE integrated with FESI and supported by centrifuge microextraction (CME) was applied for a significant increase in sensitivity for (1*R*, 2*R*)-pseudoephedrine, (1*R*, 2*S*)-ephedrine, (1*S*, 2*S*)-pseudoephedrine and (*S*)-(+)-methamphetamine in spiked serum [Fang H.F. et al., 2006a]. In this method, the CME effectively combined removal of macromolecular contaminants and other interfering components, desalting and preconcentration into one single step. Performance parameters of the CME-LLE-FESI-CE-DAD method indicate good potential of the proposed method for its routine use. The relative standard deviations (RSD, n=6) of all of the analytes were between 8.7-17.7% on the basis of peak areas. Utilizing (-)-pseudoephedrine as an internal standard, RSD results showed significant improvement (5.3-8.9%). For a 0.1 µg/mL concentration of the ephedrine derivates, recoveries were in the range of 97-114%. Relative recoveries, defined as a ratio of CE peak areas of two different sets of spiked urine extracts, were calculated to evaluate the effect of the matrix. The relative recoveries for all target drugs were from 90-112%. This means that the matrix had little effect on the method, particularly on the CME step.

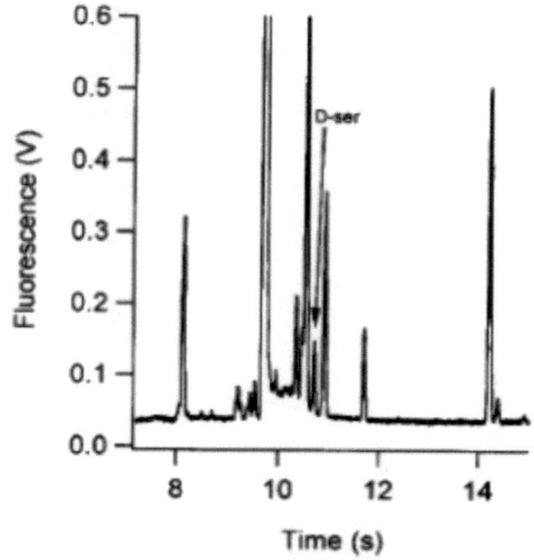

Figure 3.37. On-line microdialysis-CE-LIF analysis of the supernatant over an intact larval tiger salamander retina. A single salamander retina was incubated for 3 h in 50 µL Amphibian Ringers solution. D-Serine (5.2±2.1 µM, standard error, *n* = 4) was detected in the supernatant. Separation buffer, 50 mM borate, 20 mM HP-β-CD, pH 10.5. Separation distance, 8 cm. Reprinted from ref. [O'Brien et al., 2003].

Dialysis. A microdialysis coupled on-line with CE has been used for the rapid determination of Asp enantiomers in tissue samples from rats [Thompson, J.E. et al., 1999]. Filtration and deproteination was carried out inserting a microdialysis probe into a homogenized tissue sample. The variability that was observed by the microdialysis-CE method was due to variations in the sample as the same sample analysed repeatedly gave a RSD of 2.6%. A similar set-up for the on-line microdialysis-CE was used for the enantioselective analysis of Ser (separated from other primary amines commonly found in biological samples) in tissue homogenates [O'Brien et al., 2003], see electropherogram in Figure 3.37. Recovery was in the range of 71.5-86.8%.

Dialysis + stacking. An EKC analysis method designed for use with microdialysis sampling and electrophoretic sample stacking has been developed for the determination of isoproterenol enantiomers [Hadwiger et al., 1996]. The half-life of isoproterenol is less than 10 min, therefore, a 1 min sampling frequency, with a dialysis perfusion flow-rate of 500 nL/min, was needed to sufficiently define the pharmacokinetic curve. The optimized chiral CE method was applied to the analysis of intravenous microdialysis samples collected following administration of racemic isoproterenol. A typical electropherogram of a microdialysis sample collected over the first 5 min after dosing is shown in Figure 3.38. The enantiomers of isoproterenol are resolved from each other and from all endogenous compounds. Unfortunately, the detection limits were not sufficient to follow the concentration of isoproterenol for long enough to establish pharmacokinetic parameters. However, no off-line sample preconcentration was possible because of very low sample volumes for the analysis. Using an on-column concentration technique (*pH-mediated peak stacking,* i.e., injecting a plug of acidic solution directly after the sample) essential for analysing highly ionic sample, i.e., the microdialysis perfusate of plasma, the pharmacokinetic data/curve for the enantioselective elimination of isoproterenol could be obtained. A five-fold increase in sensitivity was achieved inserting an in-capillary stacking preconcentration of microdialyzed plasma samples, as shown in Figure 3.39. Using a catecholamine-based internal standard with similar electrochemistry (important for the electrochemical detection, EC) to isoproterenol, the precision of analysis increased from 3.2% RSD to 1.4%. This example illustrated a practical situation where the on-line sample preparation essentially replaced an off-line procedure.

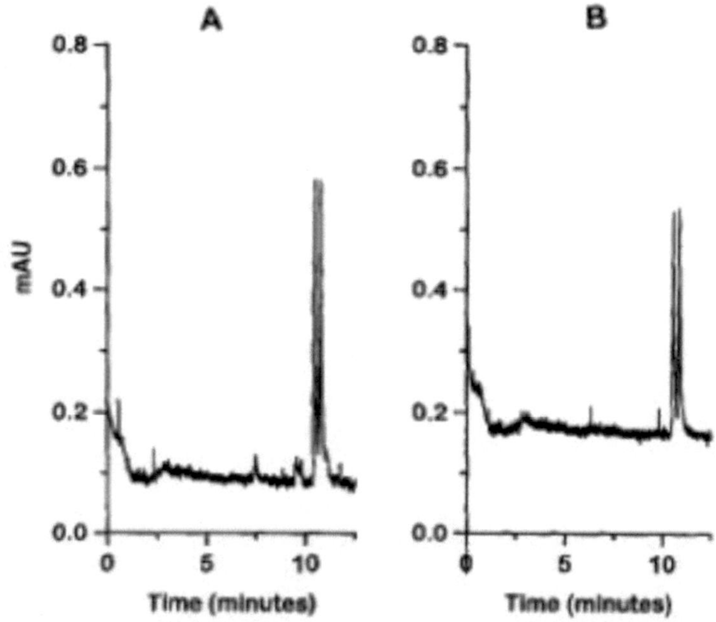

Figure 3.38. CE-UV electropherograms of isoproterenol obtained with CE and CE-microdialysis method. (A) Standard containing 100μM of (-)- and (+)-isoproterenol (ISP) bitartrate dissolved in Ringers-8.0 mM Na_2EDTA-97 μM $NaHSO_3$; (B) Microdialysate acquired from a rat 5 min after dosing. Reprinted from ref. [Hadwiger et al., 1996]

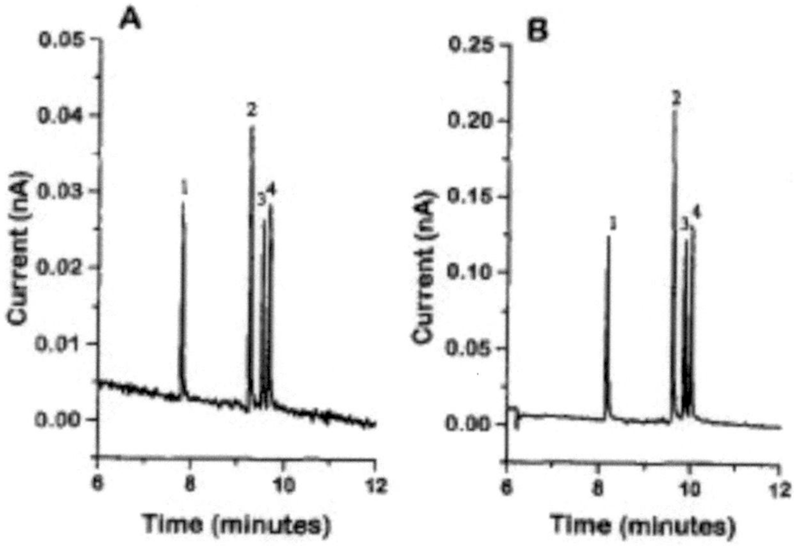

Figure 3.39. CE-EC electropherograms of standard solutions using normal electrokinetic injection (A) and acid stacked electrokinetic injection (B). Peaks: I=DHBA; 2=5NMHT; 3=(-)-iso -proterenol (ISP); 4=(+)-ISP. Reprinted from ref. [Hadwiger et al., 1996].

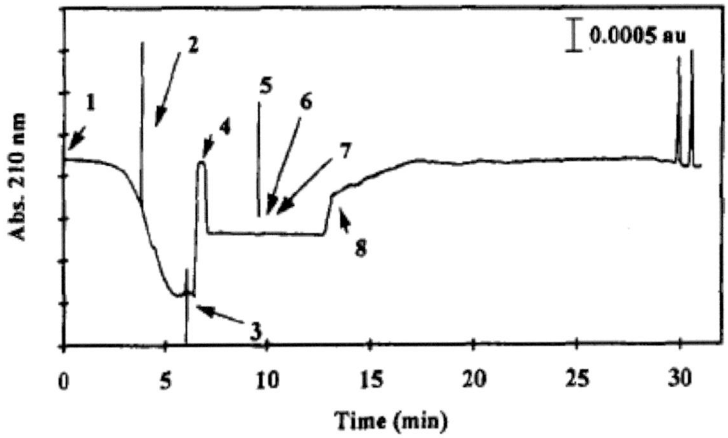

Figure 3.40. Electropherogram obtained after using the double stacking procedure followed by CE enantiomer separation. 3 μL of 400 nM *rac-terbutaline* (200 nM of each enantiomer) was injected. Arrows indicate the different events. (1) Stacking step one begins; (2) stacking peak of positive species; (3) voltage off, backpressure on; (4) zone of 5 mM phosphate buffer pH 7.5; (5) back-pressure off; (6) voltage on, stacking step two at the inlet end of the capillary; (7) back-pressure on; (8) back-pressure off, final separation step begins. The plasma samples were pretreated by on-line MLC before double stacking and CE enantioseparation. Reprinted from ref. [Pálmarsdóttir & Edholm, 1995].

Chromatography + stacking. The supported liquid membrane technique coupled on-line with CE through a MLC interface and additionally combined with a double-stacking preconcentration has been applied to a sensitive enantioselective determination of bambuterol in human plasma [Pálmarsdóttir et al., 1996, 1997]. No validation data are available for this method.

Plasma samples were pretreated and the concentration sensitivity increased by on-line MLC before double stacking and CE enantioseparation of terbutaline, see the electropherogram in Figure 3.40 [Pálmarsdóttir & Edholm, 1995]. Microlitre volumes of the cleaned sample from the MLC were concentrated directly in the electrophoresis capillary without significant loss of separation performance. The whole procedure was performed with a high degree of precision. Reproducibility of the double stacking procedure at different concentrations was as follows: RSD of migration times was 0.5-1.5%, peak areas 0.7-2.4% and peak heights 1.4-3.9% for enantiomer 1, and RSD of migration times 0.6-1.0%, peak areas 0.9-3.5%, peak heights 2.8-3.3 % for enantiomer 2. RSD of resolution was in the range of 1.1-1.9%. Other enantiomers of chiral drugs, namely bambuterol, brompheniramine, propranolol, ephedrine, were also separated using the same procedure.

Flow injection. An automatized system with on-line FI derivatization coupled to chiral CE has been developed for the enantiomeric separation of carnitine [Mardones et al., 1999]. This method allowed the determination of D-carnitine in a large excess of L-carnitine (1:100, D:L) in synthetic samples, see Figure 3.41. The reproducibility of the migration time was about 2.3%.

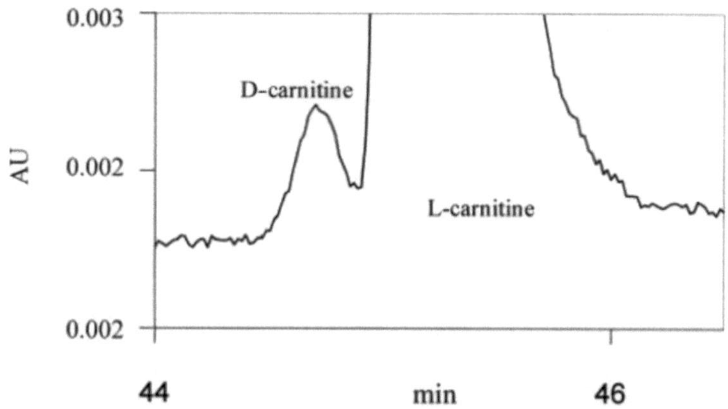

Figure 3.41. FI-CE derivatization and separation of carnitine. Electrophoretic separation of a synthetic sample containing a D-:L-carnitine ratio of 1:100, obtained with automatized FI-CE system based on FMOC derivatization and 2,6 dimethyl-β-CD as chiral selector. Reprinted from ref. [Mardones et al., 1999].

4

Advanced Combinations of Detection and Electrophoresis

4.1 Detection in electrophoresis - introduction

In the past two decades, the on-line coupling of separation techniques and appropriate (e.g., spectral, electrochemic) detection, also referred to as hyphenation, has become an important topic in analytical chemistry [Ewing et al., 1989]. In most instances hyphenation is used to obtain more information on the identity of the sample constituents, to improve analyte detectability or to enhance the speed of analysis. Therefore, in the following sections on-line detection approaches will be discussed. A list of the detection techniques hyphenated with CE and several important characteristics of these techniques are given in Table 4.1.

Detection in CE is a significant challenge as a result of the small dimensions of the capillary. Poor concentration sensitivity of CE is due to the limited sample volume that can be introduced into the capillary (typically nanolitre volumes in 25-75 μm internal diameter capillaries) and the low optical path length when the most available and used UV-VIS absorbance detection is employed. This is even worse when combining photometric absorbance detection with the MCE, resulting in a preference for other detection techniques for the microfluidic devices (e.g., fluorescence, electrochemical) [Belder, 2006]. A review of the major on-line CE detection modalities with their advantages and limitations is presented by Swinney and Bornhop [Swinney & Bornhop, 2000]. Hempel [Hempel, 2000] aimed at ascertaining strategies for how to improve the sensitivity in CE for the analysis of drugs in biological fluids, discussing sensitive detection modes such as laser-induced fluorescence detection (LIF) and mass spectrometry (MS). Hernández et al. [Hernández et al., 2008, 2010] give a general view of the different strategies used in recent years (2005-2007) to enhance the detection sensitivity in chiral analysis by CE. Molecular fluorescence, phosphorescence and chemiluminescence spectrometry as very sensitive and selective detection techniques are presented by Powe et al. [Powe et al. 2010]. Alternatively to the sensitive detection techniques (advanced detection), an advanced CE (i.e., CE with on-line sample preconcentration) or, at best, a combination of both advanced approaches, has been proposed for a significant enhancement of the sensitivity in chiral CE analyses, as comprehensively illustrated in chapters 3 and 4 of this monograph.

Analyte identification aspects in CE and CEC separation techniques are discussed by Kok et al. [Kok et al., 1998]. Attention is paid to the spectrometric techniques covering UV-VIS absorption, fluorescence line-narrowing spectroscopy, Raman spectroscopy, nuclear magnetic resonance (NMR) and MS. The most important/applied detection techniques, regarding an on-line structural identification in chiral CE analyses, are comprehensively presented in chapter 4 of this monograph.

When performing chiral analysis based on the implementation of chiral selector into the separation system, potential interferences of the chiral selector with the detection technique have to be considered and avoided, in order not to deteriorate the detection signal. Therefore, great attention must be paid to the selection of the type of chiral selector and to studying the compatibility of the chiral separation system with the linked detection technique in each particular case. Thus, chiral selectors with suppressed absorption properties must be used in absorbance detection, chiral selectors with suppressed electrochemical activity in electrochemical detection, etc. Another possibility in avoiding detection interferences caused by a chiral selector is to utilize specific electromigration effects (countercurrent migration of charged chiral selector, manipulation of the selector velocity by EOF, see chapter 2) [Iio et al., 2005; Yang L. et al., 1997; Lu W.Z. et al., 1996; Fanali et al., 1998a; Schulte et al., 1998; Lu W., 1998] or techniques (the partial filling technique, a zone of the capillary where the enantiomeric separation takes place is filled with BGE containing the chiral selector while the zone close to the detector only contains buffer without chiral selector) [Rudaz et al., 2005; Schappler et al., 2006]. These approaches are used to prevent entering the selector into the detection space. In analogy, the compatibility of chiral selectors with on-line sample preparation techniques also has to be considered in advanced CE systems (those with on-line sample preparation), as discussed in chapter 3. Therefore, the most complex situation is given when considering chiral selector (or, generally, selector) vs. on-line sample preparation vs. on-line detection. This hyphenation requires sophisticated solutions based on a deep knowledge of the particular fields, which are presented in the chapters 2-4 of this monograph.

The most important and/or the most frequently used on- and end-column detection techniques and corresponding hyphenations suitable for (advanced) CE are critically described in the following sections, also giving examples of their utilization in chiral bioanalyses of drugs (section 4.6. and Tables 2.1 and 3.1). Other, more rarely used detection techniques for CE (radioisotope detection, nuclear magnetic resonance, photothermal refraction, refractive index detection, circular dichroism, Raman-based detection, electrochemiluminescence, etc.), with their description and utilization, can be found in review papers given above. Those rare detection techniques have been mostly applied in achiral analyses, while their chiral applications available in literature are given in Table 2.1.

4.2 Photometric absorbance detection

4.2.1 Single wavelength UV-VIS absorbance detection

UV–VIS absorbance detectors working at single wavelength are the most commonly used on-column detectors for microseparations, particularly for CE, due to their interesting features, such as commercial availability, simplicity, versatility, relatively low cost, and frequently used as universal detection techniques because many organics can be detected at 195–210 nm. UV-VIS absorbance detectors produce LODs in CE corresponding to a few femtomoles of analyte (at subpicomole levels), i.e., high mass sensitivity. However, due to the need for small volumes employed in CE to avoid peak broadening that decrease the efficiency of the separation (pl to nL volumes), such sensitivity is in the micromolar range, i.e., appears modest when expressed in terms of concentration (mass detection limits are in the range of 10^{-13}-10^{-15} mol while concentration LODs ranging from 10^{-5} to 10^{-7} M depending upon the analyte being analysed). These LODs are clearly insufficient to solve many analytical problems, especially to analyse ultratrace analytes in complex matrices, being variable in qualitative and quantitative composition. Therefore, various strategies based on increasing absorbance signal (A=εdc) have been proposed to overcome the poor concentration sensitivity of UV-VIS-CE, such as (i) the selection of lower-UV wavelengths, 190–205 nm [Swinney & Bornhop, 2000], (ii) indirect absorbance detection for analytes with low values of molar absorptivity ε [Yeung, 1989], for the principle see Figure 4.1, (iii) increasing the pathlength d [Kaniansky et al., 1997; Grant & Steuer, 1990; Tsueda et al., 1990; Taylor & Yeung, 1991; Poppe, 1980; Mainka & Bachmann, 1997; Kaltenbach et al., 1997, Anaheim, CA 1997; Aiken et al., 1991] and (iv) derivatization of analytes [Mikuš & Kaniansky, 2000; Hu T. et al., 1995]. However, the strategies (i-iv) have several limitations and specific features that have to be carefully considered before being employed. These are (i) a relatively poor signal-to-noise ratio, chiral selector can also significantly absorb, (ii) use of strongly absorbing chromophores, inserted chromofores can influence complex equilibrium of analyte with chiral selector, (iii) use of capillaries with higher internal diameter, e.g., 300-800 μm (temperature dissipation and, by that, separation efficiency decrease with internal diameter), or properly designed detection window, e.g., bubble cells (see Figure 4.2a and a photo detail in Figure 4.3), Z-shaped cells (see Figure 4.2b), multireflection nanolitre scale cell (often accompanied by larger probe volumes and reduction in separation efficiency and resolution) and (iv) additional sample preparation step is needed, electrophoretic mobilities, as well as the complexing properties of derivatives, can differ from those of their native forms. Nevertheless, the detection sensitivity with UV-VIS absorbance detectors usually cannot be increased more than several tenths times, even if applying any of the presented approaches, so that sample preparation is required. On the other hand, an appropriate use of the on-line sample preparation procedures (as given in chapter 3) enables an application of UV-VIS absorbance detectors, even in ultrasensitive bioanalyses, as illustrated on several examples (in section 4.6. and Table 3.1).

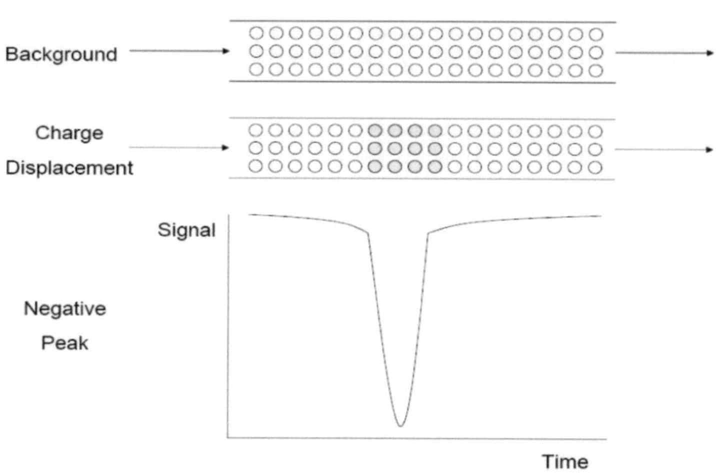

Figure 4.1. Schematic illustration of indirect absorption detection. The separation electrolyte additive provides a large background signal at the detector. Displacement occurs in the analyte zone and lower absorbance intensity is observed. White dots represent absorbing species, blue dots represent non-absorbing species. Reprinted from ref. [Yeung, 1989].

Method	Mass detection limit (moles)	Concentration detection limit (M)[b]	Advantages/ disadvantages
UV-VIS absorption	$10^{-13} - 10^{-15}$	$10^{-5} - 10^{-7}$	• Universal • Diode array offers spectral information
Fluorescence	$10^{-15} - 10^{-17}$	$10^{-7} - 10^{-9}$	• Sensitive • Usually requires sample derivatization
Laser-induced fluorescence	$10^{-18} - 10^{-20}$	$10^{-10} - 10^{-16}$	• Extremely sensitive • Usually requires sample derivatization • Expensive • Post-column LIF is 3-6 orders more sensitive than direct on-column LIF
Amperometry	$10^{-18} - 10^{-19}$	$10^{-10} - 10^{-11}$	• Sensitive • Selective but useful only for electroactive analyses • Requires special electronics and capillary modification
Conductivity	$10^{-15} - 10^{-16}$	$10^{-7} - 10^{-8}$	• Universal • Requires special electronics and capillary modification
Mass spectrometry	$10^{-16} - 10^{-17}$	$10^{-8} - 10^{-9}$	• Sensitive and offers structural information • Interface between CE and MS complicated
Indirect UV, fluorescence, amperometry	1-2 orders less than direct method	-	• Universal • Lower sensitivity than direct methods
LODs of other detection techniques [M]: Phototermal refraction (10^{-7}-10^{-8}), Potentiometric (10^{-7}-10^{-8}), Refractive index (10^{-5}-10^{-6}, capillary, 10^{-5}, chip-scale), Raman (10^{-3}-10^{-6}, preconcentration needed), Radiofrequency, NMR (10^{-3}), Radioisotope (10^{-10}), Laser-induced capillary vibration (10^{-8}, chemical derivatization, 10^{-5}, native)			

Table 4.1. Detection techniques in CE[a]

[a] adapted from refs. [Heiger, 2000; Swinney & Bornhop, 2000]

[b] assume 10 nL injection volume

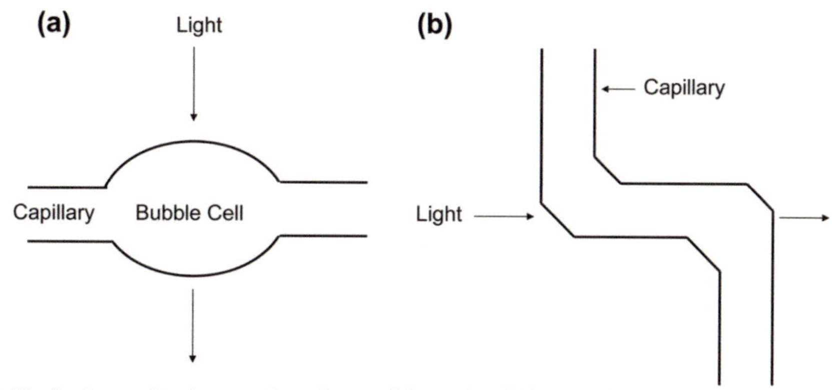

Figure 4.2. Techniques for increasing the pathlength of the capillary: (a) a bubble cell and (b) a z-cell (additional tubing). Reprinted from ref. [Skoog et al., 2007].

4.2.2 Multi-wavelength (spectral) UV-VIS absorbance detection

A diode array detector (DAD) serves as a typical multi-wavelength on-column CE detector providing UV-VIS spectra in the required interval of wavelengths [Heiger D.N. et al., 1994; Beck et al., 1993], for the instrumental scheme of the CE-DAD see Figure 4.3. Many organic compounds have characteristic spectra in the UV which can be used to help identify the substance passing through the sensor cell.

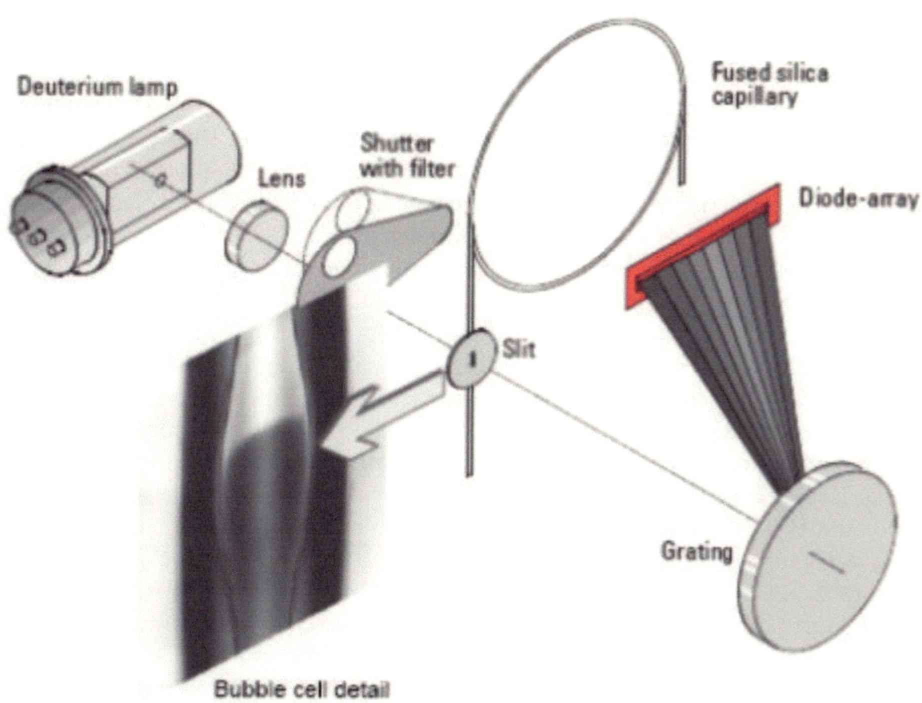

Figure 4.3. Schematic overview of the CE diode array detector (DAD) optics. Reprinted from ref. [Agilent Technologies, 2009].

a)

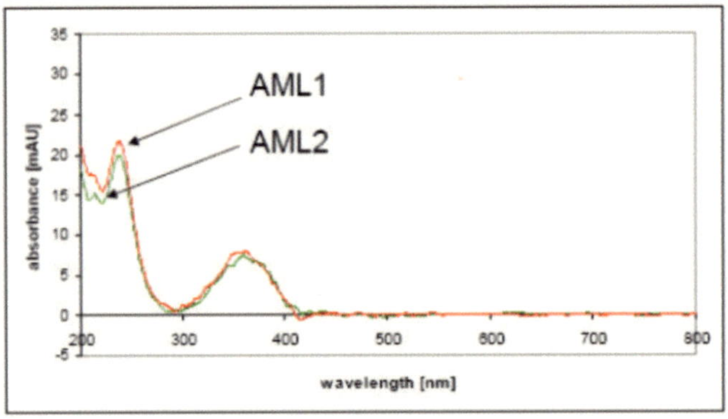

b)

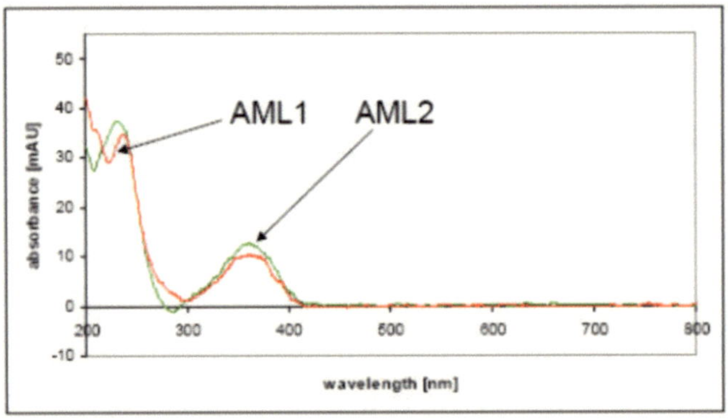

Figure 4.4. Processed UV-VIS spectra of amlodipine (AML) in different matrices. (a) AML present in demineralized water, serving as a reference spectrum, (b) AML present in 10 times diluted model urine, at a 500 ng/mL concentration level of the drug in the samples. Separating and other working conditions of the ITP-EKC-DAD method modified with (2-hydroxypropyl)-β-cyclodextrin (HP-β-CD), serving as the chiral selector, were the same for (a) and (b). AML1, AML2 - migration positions of the first migrating enantiomer of amlodipine (red spectrum), the second migrating enantiomer of amlodipine (green spectrum), respectively. Reprinted from ref. [Mikuš et al., 2008a].

Although UV-VIS spectra are not as informative as those of NMR, MS or infra-red spectrometry, they still can serve for a preliminary confirmation of peak/analyte identity and validation of peak purity [Strašík et al., 2003]. The similarity of spectral profiles can be used for the indication of structurally related compounds separated from each other while differences in spectra can indicate impurity in analyte peak. As an example, the similar profiles of the UV-VIS absorption spectra of the amlodipine enantiomers recorded in the model water and urine samples, indicating an acceptable purity of the separated electrophoretic peaks of the amlodipine enantiomers in the complex matrices (urine), are shown in Figure 4.4. With respect to spectral analysis, DAD also has significant advantages over rapid scanning detectors such as the signal-to-noise ratio of spectral data being independent of the number of wavelengths acquired, the bandwidth of individual wavelengths not being predetermined and on-line spectra being available at all times [Heiger D., 2000]. CE-DAD provides comparable sensitivity and linear detection range, and the same possibility to be combined with CE (e.g., on-line combination via optical fibres) when compared to the single wavelength UV-VIS absorbance detectors. Therefore, CE-DAD was proposed as an advantageous alternative to conventional CE-UV with the single wavelength detection and, at the same time, a pragmatic solution to the expensive CE-MS or CE-NMR, for many pharmaceutical and biomedical applications including those with the enantioselective aspects [Beck et al., 1993], see also examples in section 4.6 and Table 3.1.

4.3 Fluorescence detection

4.3.1 Conventional fluorescence detection

Fluorescence detection is a more sensitive and selective alternative to UV-VIS absorbance detection, and it is usually carried out in the on-column arrangement. For a schematic layout of on-column fluorescence detection see Figure 4.5. Mass detection limits are in the range of 10^{-15}-10^{-17} mol, while concentration LODs range from 10^{-7} to 10^{-9} M depending upon the analyte's fluorofore [Ewing et al., 1989].

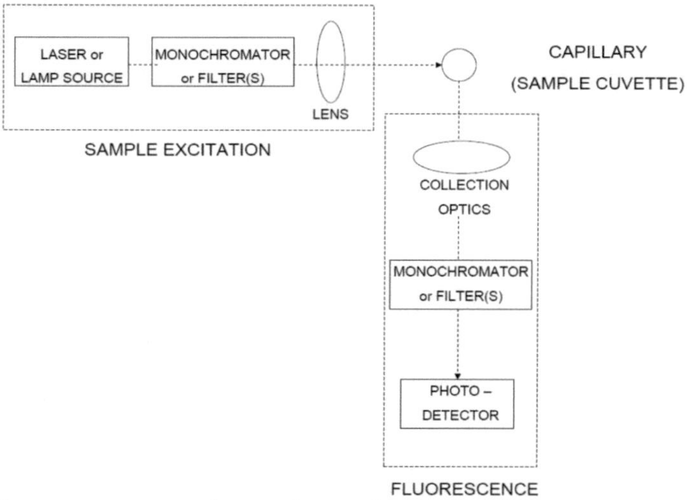

Figure 4.5. A schematic layout of on-column fluorescence detection. Adapted from ref. [Amankwa et al., 1992].

Generally, there is a considerably reduced number of compounds exhibiting natural fluorescence in comparison with UV-VIS absorbing compounds and therefore, this detection mode is very often linked with analyte derivatization. However, the complicated chemistry and time-consuming procedures associated with derivatization make fluorescence detection {conventional, as well as LIF (see below)} less attractive than universal detection methods. Another possibility to perform fluorescence detection is its indirect regime (universal). The concept of indirect fluorescence measurements is essentially the same as indirect absorbance measurements, except the background (buffer) fluoresces instead of absorbing, see Figure 4.1. Unfortunately, indirect fluorescence (likewise UV absorbance and other indirect methods) has 10-100 times less sensitivity than direct methods. Poor LODs for indirect fluorescence measurements are the result of the noisy fluorescence background. Therefore, it is not surprising that the indirect fluorescence mode has rare use in CE.

4.3.2 Laser-induced fluorescence detection

Laser-induced fluorescence (LIF), based on a fluorescence signal produced by the molecule after its illumination by a laser beam, is the most sensitive, extremely selective, small volume detection method, suitable for an on-line arrangement with the CE. It is also one of the most favoured detection techniques for microfluidic devices such as MCE. The first on-column LIF detection system was developed by Zare et al. [Gassmann et al., 1985]. For the scheme of the CE-LIF see Figure 4.5. The concentration LODs of the best CE/laser-based systems are in interval 10^{-14}-10^{-16} M with mass detection limits 10^{-18}-10^{-20} mol (individual molecules can be detected) [Ewing et al., 1989]. A variability (sensitivity, selectivity) of LIF detection is given by employing different lasers {the common argon laser (458 and 488 nm), He-Cd laser (440 nm), blue diode laser (420 nm), frequency-doubled Ar-ion laser (257 nm), frequency-doubled Kr-ion laser (284 nm)} [Hernández et al., 2008, 2010; Nie et al., 1993; Chang & Yeung, 1995; Craig D.B. et al., 1998]. To overcome problems associated with on-column detection, such as broad-band luminescence background and poor S/N ratios, Rayleigh and Raman light scattering from the capillary, several techniques based on the spatial or spectral separation of the fluorescence signal from the high background signal have been proposed (the best results have been reached with a sheath flow cuvette incorporated at the end of the capillary, performing an end-column LIF) [Cheng Y.F. & Dovichi, 1988; Chen D.Y. & Dovichi, 1996; Craig D.B. et al., 1998; Xue & Yeung, 1995]. For example, the schematic diagram of sheath-flow CE-LIF system with multichannel photomultiplier tube detection is shown in Figure 4.6.

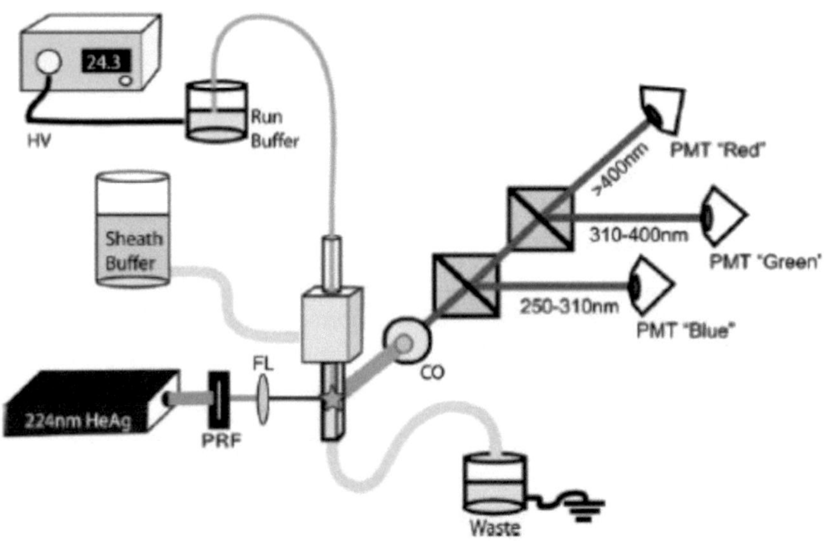

Figure 4.6. Schematic diagram of sheath-flow CE-LIF system with multichannel photomultiplier tube (PMT) detection. The beam from a HeAg laser is used for excitation of the analyte as it elutes from the capillary. Fluorescence is collected orthogonally to the excitation optics and transmitted or reflected by one or both of two custom dichroic beam-splitters. The spectrally distributed fluorescence is detected by one of three PMTs corresponding to wavelength ranges 250–310 nm (PMT "Blue"), 310–400 nm (PMT "Green"), and 400+ nm (PMT "Red"). Reprinted from ref. [Lapainis et al., 2007].

The application examples shown in section 4.6. and Tables 2.1 and 3.1 indicate that CE-LIF is a powerful tool, due to its excellent sensitivity, for the analysis of samples ranging from tissue extracts to single cells. However, one challenge for the chiral CE analysis of complex biological samples is the accurate peak identification in complex electropherograms, as often matching a migration time between an analyte and the corresponding standard may be insufficient to confirm the peak's identity. Therefore, sample preparation procedures, and, especially, their on-line modes (chapter 3), should be used to eliminate matrix interferents and, by that, simplifying the confirmation of the peak's identity, see e.g., [Cho et al., 2004] and Figure 3.33. Another interesting possibility to confirm the peak's identity reliably is based on the confirmation of analyte signal identity via a combination of single-step immunoprecipitation (specific elimination of analyte signal) and CE-LIF analysis [Miao et al., 2006], see Figure 4.7.

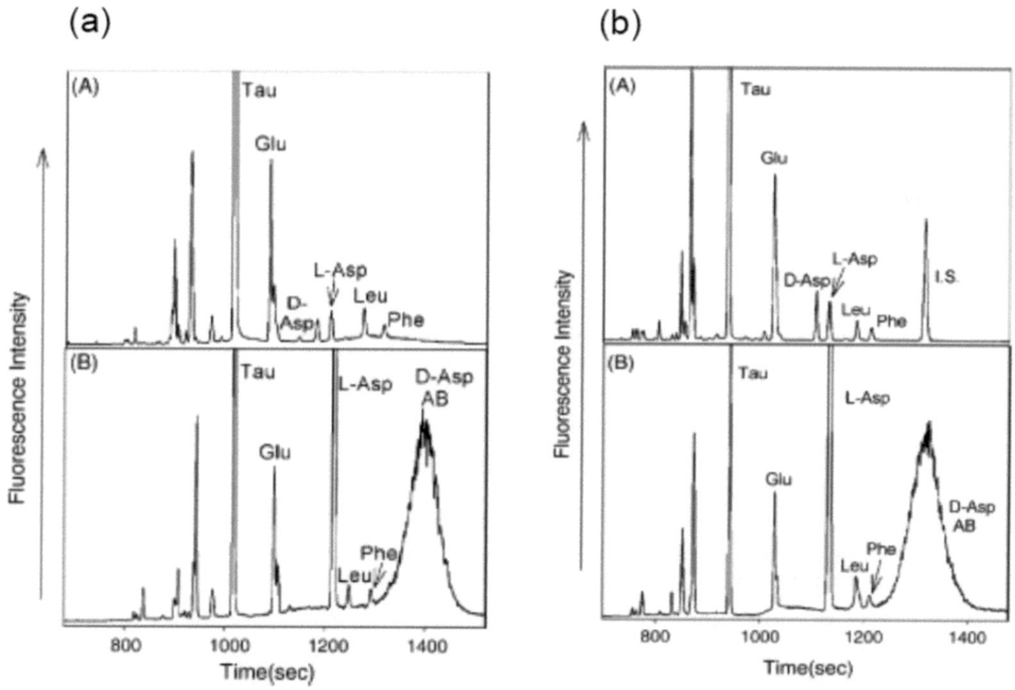

Figure 4.7. D-Asp antibody allows confirmation of analyte peak assignment in the CE-LIF analysis of complex biological samples such as nerve tissue (a) or single cell (b). Chemical information output of CE-LIF analysis is significantly enhanced by use of the antibody for signal identification. (a) Electropherograms of an anterior tentacular nerve sample before (A) and after incubation (B) with D-Asp antibody and L-Asp conjugate. (b) Electropherograms of an MCC neuron sample before (A) and after incubation (B) with D-Asp antibody and L-Asp conjugate. Increased intensity of the L-Asp signal and disappearance or decrease in the amplitude of the D-Asp peak are noticeable in (B). Internal standard (I.S.), L-cysteic acid. Adapted from ref. [Miao et al., 2006].

4.4 Electrochemical detection

Electrochemical detection for CE can be divided into three main categories: conductimetric (based on conductivity changes monitored by sensors during electrophoretic migration process) [Landers, 1997; Everaerts et al., 1979; Gebauer et al., 1997], potentiometric (based on classical ion-selective microelectrodes) [Haber et al., 1990, 1991] and amperometric (based on electrode vs. analyte redox reaction that produces a current, directly related to the analyte concentration) [Ewing et al., 1994]. Electrochemical detection provides an alternative solution for non-absorbing or non-fluorescing analytes. This detection approach offers both universal and selective modes, and provides sensitive measurements in an end-column, as well as an on-column, arrangement in the CE and MCE format [de Silva, 2003].

The most difficult problem to solve in applying electrochemical detection in CE is the need to instrumentally eliminate the effect of the strong electric field used in electrophoretic separation from the conditions of electrochemical detections. The main drawback of electrochemical detectors in their implementation with CE is that it can be extremely difficult and tedious since sensor preparation can involve complicated fabrication and handling procedures, and accurate spatial alignment of the electrodes within the capillary [Swinney & Bornhop, 2000]. Moreover, limited sensor lifetime and required recalibration, strong adsorption of the intermediate reaction products of the analyte to the electrode surface reducing its activity/response (this can be overcome by the electronic cleaning of the electrode) [Haber et al., 1991; Ewing et al., 1994] are other limiting factors that should be carefully considered when electrochemical detectors are applied. These limitations can be pronounced, especially, when complex biological samples are analysed, where sample pretreatment (especially purification) is strongly recommended for reliable and reproducible detection.

Nevertheless, recent years have provided numerous new examples of applying flow-through electrochemical detectors in chemical analysis. The review by Trojanowicz [Trojanowicz, 2009], based on about 250 original research papers cited from the current analytical literature, presents their application in flow analysis and capillary electrophoretic methods. Potentiometric detection with ion-selective electrodes predominates in flow analysis carried out mostly in a flow injection system, while amperometric and conductivity detections are most commonly employed in capillary electrophoresis and they have been applied also in the chiral field. For application examples of electrochemical detection in chiral CE, see section 4.6. and Tables 2.1 and 3.1.

4.4.1. Amperometric detection

As with other electrochemical detection methods in CE, amperometric detection is also carried out with the use of microelectrodes because of the need to adjust their size to the diameter of capillaries. There are several most commonly reported constructions of various types used for amperometric detection cells in CE, as well as various types of working electrodes resulting in interesting application possibilities and very low detection limits obtainable, as reviewed by Trojanowicz [Trojanowicz, 2009]. Schemes of the amperometric detector coupled with the hydrodynamically open (conventional) and hydrodynamically closed (unconventional) CE systems are shown in Figure 4.8 and Figure 4.9, respectively.

Amperometric detection is based on electron transfer to or from the analyte of interest at an electrode surface that is under the influence on an applied DC voltage. The result of electron transfer is a redox reaction at the electrode that produces a current that is directly related to the analyte concentration. Therefore, chiral selectors giving a redox reaction at the electrode, comparable with the redox reaction of the analyte, cannot be employed for chiral separations with this type of detection and a modified chiral system has to be used.

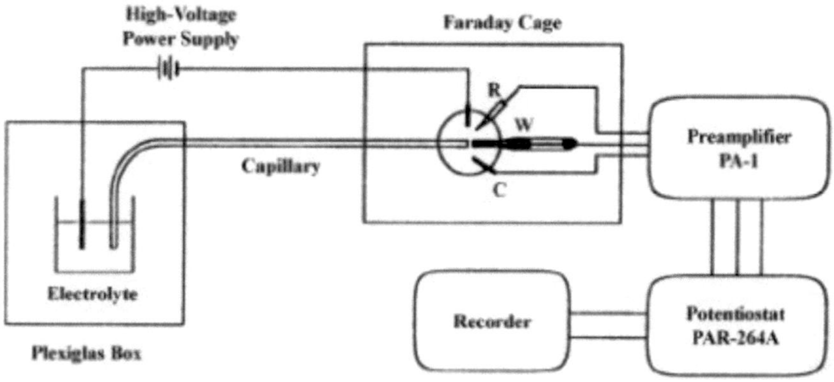

Figure 4.8. Schematic diagram of the capillary electrophoresis system with end-column amperometric detection: R, reference electrode; W, working electrode; C, counter electrode. Reprinted from ref. [His et al., 1997].

Pulsed amperometric detection (including the electrode cleaning step), an advanced detection mode, can reduce the major problem of this detection, linked with strong adsorption of the intermediate reaction products of the analyte to the electrode surface (reducing activity, i.e., electron transfer of the electrode and interfering with detection) [Ewing et al., 1994]. In this way, reproducibility of measurements, as well as sensitivity, can be considerably improved [Trojanowicz, 2009].

The conventional amperometric mode, usually used in the end-column configuration, is selective (restricted only for electroactive analytes) and can be tuned to the analyte of interest [O'Shea et al., 1993; Lu W.Z. & Cassidy, 1993]. On the other hand, the square-wave mode can be successfully applied for detection of typical nonelectroactive organic compounds, where currents associated with the non-Faradaic interfacial process due to analyte adsorption at a Pt microelectrode were used to provide the analytical signal [Gerhardt et al., 2000]. The detection limits obtained in such measurements are at least one order of magnitude lower than the ones that could be obtained by UV absorption. Moreover, such an amperometric detection mode is more universal and provides a wider application range.

Compared to the conductimetric mode, amperometric detection is much more sensitive, mass detection limits are in the range of 10^{-18}-10^{-19} mol corresponding to 10^{-10}-10^{-11} M concentration LODs [Ewing et al., 1989]. Thus, amperometric detection represents a good alternative to LIF for ultrasensitive CE determinations of another specific group of analytes. For application examples of amperometric detection in chiral CE, see section 4.6. and Tables 2.1 and 3.1.

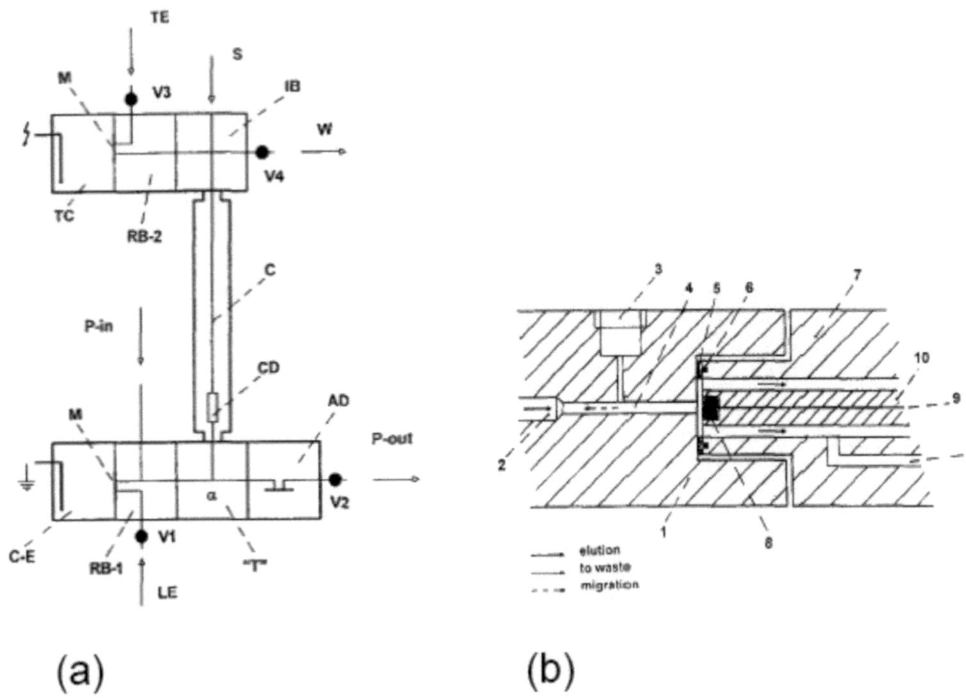

Figure 4.9. (a) Schematic diagram of the hydrodynamically closed CE separation unit with a post-column amperometric detector. IB = injection block for a microsyringe sample injection; C= capillary tube; CD =on-column conductivity detection cell; "T"=elution T-piece; α =bifurcation point; AD= amperometric detection cell; RB-1 = refilling block for the capillary tube (C); C-E=counter-electrode compartment; M = Cellophane membranes; LE = inlet for the leading electrolyte solution; P-in, P-out = inlet and outlet for the elution solution, respectively; RB-2 = refilling block for the terminating compartment (TC) and the injection block (IB); TE = inlet for the terminating electrolyte solution; W = waste; S = position for the injection of the sample; V1-V4 = valves. (b) Detail of the amperometric detection cell attached to the T-piece. l=T-piece; 2=channel to the counter electrode; 3= connection for the column; 4=elution channel (detection capillary) of 4 mm × 0.2 mm i.d.; 5=PTFE spacer (0.05 mm); 6=O-ring for a leak-proof connection; 7= amperometric cell; 8=working electrode; 9=connecting cable to the electronics of the detector; 10 = epoxy body of the electrode; 11 =connecting channel for the reference electrode. Reprinted from ref. [Kaniansky et al., 1995].

4.4.2 Conductivity detection

Conductivity detection, due to separation ions, charged particles or microorganisms in CE, has a special importance for capillary electrophoresis. The charged species are detected in the solution of electrolyte, which makes use of this detection process difficult. Nevertheless, the practical importance of this detection is justified by the fact that commercially available detectors are on the market only for this electrochemical detection for CE [Trojanowicz, 2009].

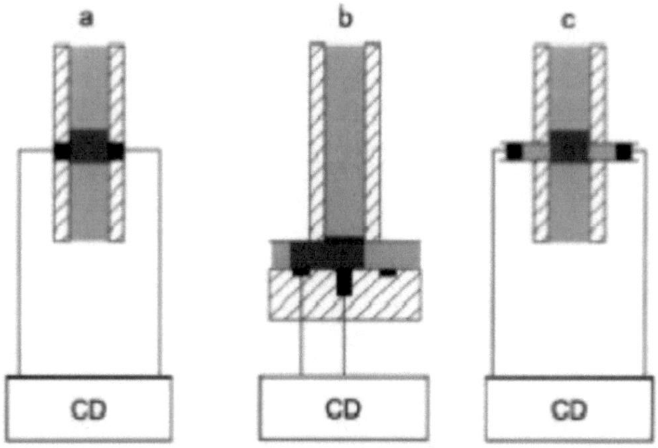

Figure 4.10. General schemes of the arrangements of the detection electrodes in contact conductivity detection cells for CZE. (a) An in-column placement of the detection electrodes exposed to direct contact with the separated constituents; (b) a post-column placement of the detection electrodes exposed to direct contact with the separated constituents; (c) an on-column placement of the detection electrodes with an electrolyte solution mediated contact with the detection compartment of the cell. CD, measuring circuitry of the detector. Reprinted from ref. [Bodor et al., 2001].

In general, conductivity detectors consist of two sensors (electrodes), in direct or indirect contact with the electrolyte solution, across which an electrical potential has been applied. General schemes of the arrangements of the detection electrodes in contact conductivity detection cells for CZE are shown in Figure 4.10. Conductimetric mode is attractive by providing universal detection in an on-line arrangement and it is the most frequently used electrochemical detection for CE. Therefore, it can be the first choice when analysing non-absorbing/fluorescing organic ions avoiding the derivatization step in the analytical protocol. However, sensitivity of the contact conductivity detection mode is moderate, mass detection limits are usually in the range of 10^{-14}-10^{-15} mol corresponding to 10^{-6}-10^{-7} M concentration LODs [Landers, 1997]. This is not sufficient for the majority of clinical and biomedical analytical problems when performed by conventional CE.

Improvement of detectability can be additionally achieved to the sub-ppb level by applying on-capillary preconcentration by electrostacking [Haber et al., 1998]. Another method of lowering the value of the detection limit in CE determinations with conductivity detection, following wide use in ion-chromatography, is to apply on-line suppressing of conductivity of BGE by the ion-exchange process [Avdalovic et al., 1993]. For example, the suppressor for determination of anions can be made of an ion-exchange sulfonated Teflon capillary tubing (1 cm long) placed between the separation capillary and the detector electrode in the wall-jet arrangement. This method can improve the detectability of about two orders of magnitude compared to indirect detection of non-UV-absorbing ions.

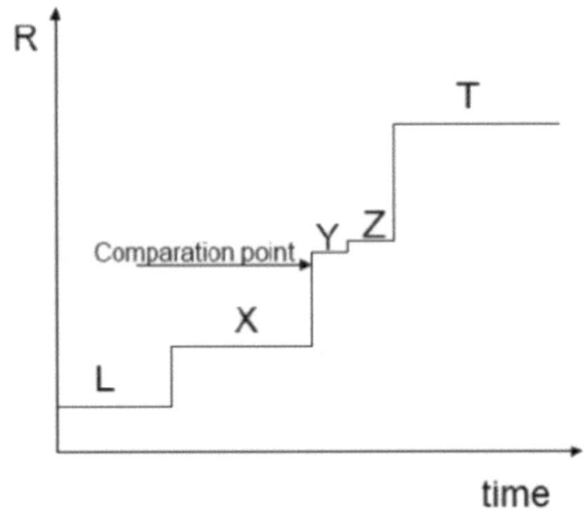

Figure 4.11. Graphical illustration of the principle of the electronic cutting of the zone of interest in the ITP stage of the ITP-CZE combination. L = leading ion, T = terminating ion, X = matrix compound(s), Y, Z = analytes, R = resistance. Reprinted from ref. [Tekel' & Mikuš, 2005].

Jumps in voltage (conductivity) between neighbouring zones result in permanently sharp boundaries between zones and are very convenient for conductivity detection. Although extremely convenient to the detection of the ITP zones (the preferred detection in this field), the conductivity detection technique has a limited applicability in the CZE separations of enantiomers. It can be caused by the measurements of small conductivity changes due to the analyte zones on a relatively high-conductivity background of the carrier electrolyte. Therefore, when monitoring the enantioseparations by the conductivity detection, mobility difference of the analyte vs. chiral selector must be carefully considered.

On the other hand, one interesting possibility of the sensitive analyses of enantiomers in multicomponent ionic samples with the aid of conductivity detection is its implementation into column-coupled CE-CE systems, see examples in ref. [Gebauer et al., 2009, 2011; Mikuš & Maráková, 2009, 2010]. Conductivity detectors in ITP produce a staircase signal, resistance (or conductivity) vs. migration time, in which the relative high of step is constant for a given analyte under given separation conditions (qualitative parameter independent on analysis time). Such an ITP profile can be beneficial in the preliminary mapping of the composition of complex (e.g., biological) samples. This also gives a good possibility of an accurately "cut" (by electronic switching) desired zone (analyte) in the preseparation stage (ITP) of ITP-EKC combination and transferring it into the analytical stage (EKC) without potential interfering compounds from the matrices, avoiding any analytical capillary overloading by the major matrix constituents [Danková et al., 1999], see Figure 4.11. In this way, chiral analytes in multicomponent matrices (e.g., biological) can be monitored and on-line preseparated/pretreated in an achiral environment before a chiral CZE (i.e., EKC) step [Mikuš et al., 2006a, 2008a, 2008b; Marák et al., 2007, 2008; Mikuš, 2010]. Anyway, the conductivity detection can be advantageously used also for the detection of enantiomers in a chiral environment as it is well documented in the literature [Mikuš et al., 2006b; Kubačák et al., 2006a, 2006b, 2007].

Chiral selectors, as well as sample matrix constituents, can influence contact conductivity detection. To reduce a decrease in detection sensitivity and reproducibility caused by a modification of the electrode surface in an ionic environment, various approaches have been proposed. A contact conductivity detection cell for CZE with an electrolyte solution mediated contact of the separated constituents with the detection electrodes (ESMC cell) was proposed to eliminate detection disturbances due to electrode reactions and adsorption of the separated constituents when these are coming into direct contact with the detection electrodes, see Figure 4.12 [Bodor et al., 2001]. Despite precautions in the construction of sensing and measuring parts of the conductivity detector, the detection in the ITP runs can be accompanied by enhanced noise of the detection signal and some detection disturbances when injecting common real samples, i.e., complex ionic samples (Figure 4.13a). Here, an electrochemical cleaning of the detection electrodes as be recommended for some conventional conductivity detection cells [Kaniansky, 1981; Kaniansky et al., 1983] provided a simple and effective solution also in microchip format [Masár et al., 2001]. Here, a pair of 100-V pulses of reversed polarities is applied between the electrodes of a particular sensor along with a stream of the leading electrolyte solution. An overall effect of this cleaning procedure is clearly illustrated by isotachopherograms in Figure 4.13a and b.

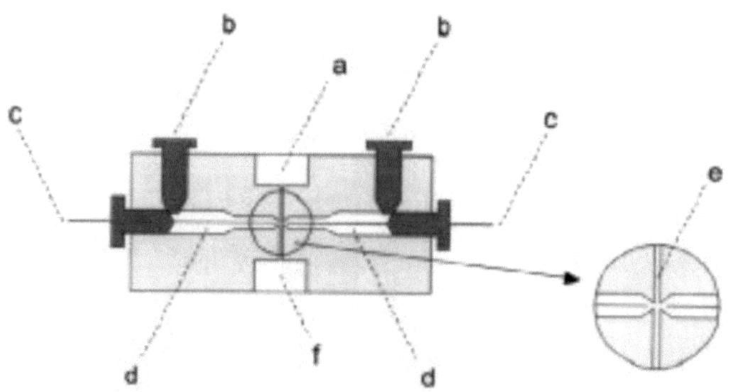

Figure 4.12. A schematic drawing of the conductivity detection cell with an electrolyte solution mediated contact of the separated constituents with the detection electrodes. (a) A connection of the cell to the separation capillary; (b) holes with screw plugs for filling the electrode channels (d) with the detection electrodes (c); (e) the detection compartment; (f) a connection of the cell to the counter-electrode compartment. A body of the cell was made of poly(methyl methacrylate). Reprinted from ref. [Bodor et al., 2001]

A contactless conductivity detector (instrumental scheme see in Figure 4.14), although a bit less sensitive than contact conductivity detector, is an advantageous alternative for the analyses of complex samples as it does not suffer from the contamination of the conductivity sensors by compounds from the electrolyte or sample (adsorption, electrochemical reactions) and, hence, the high reproducibility of detection signal can be maintained [Mikkers et al., 1979; Gebauer et al., 1997; de Silva et al., 2002; Kaniansky et al., 1999]. This detection approach was successfully applied also in ITP-EKC analyses of enantiomers in multicomponent ionic matrices, see refs. [Mikuš & Maráková, 2009, 2010] and references cited therein.

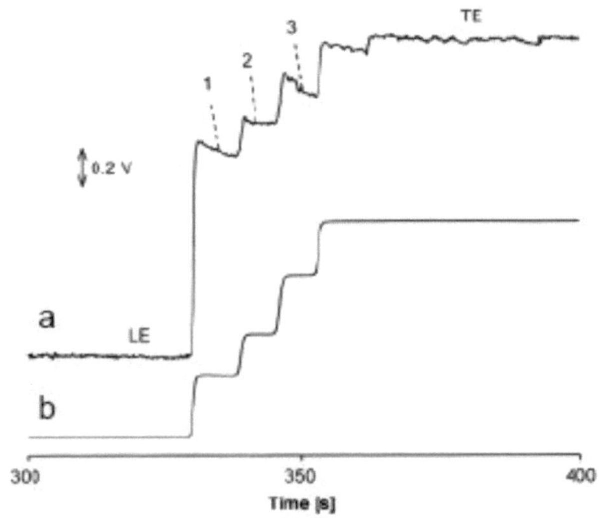

Figure 4.13. Impacts of cleaning of contaminated surfaces of the detection electrodes on the responses of the conductivity sensors in the ITP separations on the CC chips. Isotachopherograms from the separations of a three-component test mixture of anions as obtained by a particular sensor (a) before and (b) after electrochemical cleaning of its electrodes. LE=Leading anion; 1=succinate; 2=acetate; 3=benzoate; TE=terminating anion. The concentrations of the analytes in the test sample were 300 μM. The driving current was 10 μA. Reprinted from ref. [Masár et al., 2001].

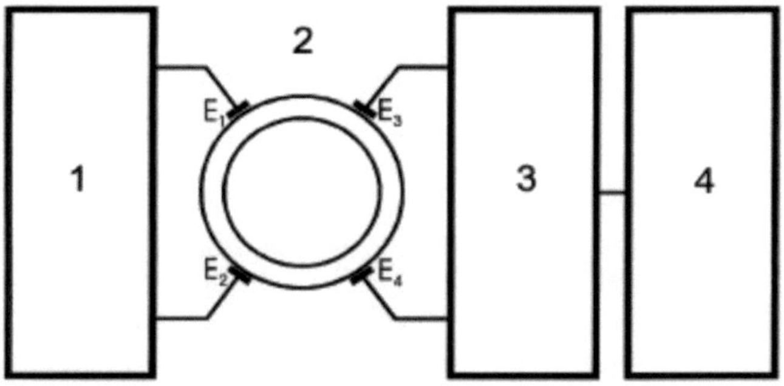

Figure 4.14. Block scheme of a high-frequency contactless conductivity detector used in this work. 1, high-frequency generator (consisting of a 4-MHz oscillator, an amplifier and inverter, phasing elements and output voltage amplifiers); 2, four-electrode (capacitive) detection cell; 3. receiver (consisting of a pre-amplifier, a narrow-band amplifier, a selective filter, a high-frequency rectifier, a d.c. amplifier and a low band-pass filter); 4, a data acquisition unit; E –E , detection electrodes. Generated from refs. [Gaš et al., 1980; Vacík et al., 1985].

4.5 Mass spectrometry

An on-line combination of CE and MS (representative scheme of CE-MS is in Figure 4.15) is a highly effective technique that separates analytes according to differences in their electrophoretic mobilities and then provides information on molecular masses and/or fragmentation of analysed substances. In this way, the on-line CE–MS technique has been established as a powerful separation and identification analytical tool. Moreover, this end-column hyphenation may enhance the sensitivity of certain compounds depending on their characteristics such as proton affinity, absorptivity, etc. In the last 10 years there have been many significant developments in CE-MS instrumentation and applications that have made CE-MS a competitive tool.

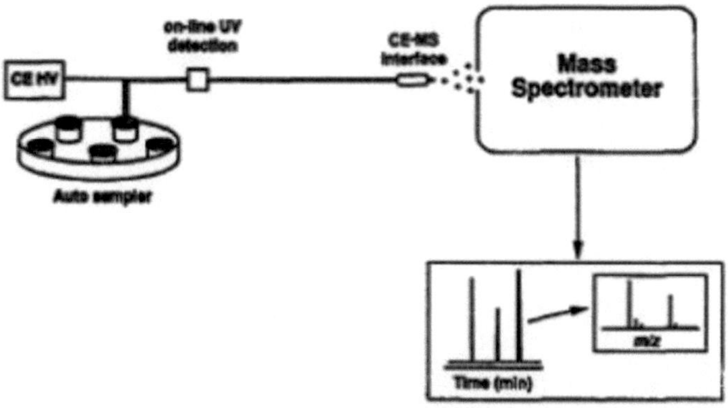

Figure 4.15. Generic illustration of a CE-MS instrumental arrangement. HV= High voltage. Reprinted from ref. [Cai & Henion, 1995].

Several recent review papers have been devoted to a combination of CE-MS, applied to the structural identification of analytes and trace analytes. Surveys on developments and applications of CE-MS in the years of 2003-2004 and 2005-2006 are given by Schmitt and Englmann [Schmitt-Kopplin & Englmann, 2005] and Gaspar et al. [Gaspar et al., 2008], respectively. The reader will rapidly find the mostly used CE-MS combinations, as well as applications classified as forensic, environmental, bioanalytical, pharmaceutical and metabolomics. Ramautar et al. [Ramautar et al., 2009] pay attention to the utilization of CE-MS in metabolomics, considering papers published between 2000 and 2008. The authors presented CE-MS to be a powerful technique for the profiling of polar metabolites in biological samples. The combination of CE with MS was chosen as a review topic also in conjunction with chiral separations in aqueous and non-aqueous media [Cai & Henion, 1995; Shamsi, 2002; Scriba, 2007]. Methodological aspects of CE–MS for quantitation were summarized and evaluated by Ohnesorge et al. [Ohnesorge et al., 2005]. Pantučková et al. [Pantučková et al., 2009] reviewed electrolyte systems for on-line CE-MS with respect to detection requirements and separation possibilities. Smyth and Rodriguez [Smyth & Rodriguez, 2007] summarized recent studies of the electro spray ionization (ESI) behaviour of selected drugs and their application in CE-MS and HPLC-MS. For application examples of chiral CE-MS, see section 4.6 and Table 3.1.

4.5.1 CE stage in CE-MS

The electrolyte systems in CE must be carefully selected regarding all the requirements of the on-line coupled MS analyser where terms such as the analyte ionization and evaporation play the key role (see section 4.5.2 CE-MS interfaces). It is obvious that both electrophoresis BGE and the solvent must support the ionization process and evaporation of droplets (i.e., volatile and low ionic strength buffers, such as acetic acid, formic acid and their ammonium salts, buffers with carbonate as a volatile anion, and alkylamines as volatile cations), otherwise, the MS signal suppression due to salt deposits on the source and decreased response due to ion-pairing with the analyte could occur (e.g., citrate, phosphate, phthalate, morpholine, Tris buffers). Operational regions in CZE recommended for use in practice for on-line CE–MS are shown in Figure 4.16. The limited choice of electrolytes that are suitable for online CE–MS brings considerable limitations not only to the CE separation itself, but also to the potential sample stacking [Pantučková et al., 2009]. For example, separation properties of typical suitable ITP systems are given in Table 4.2. Due to the high volatility and low surface tension of organic solvents like methanol or acetonitrile, the use of non-aqueous media in NACE-ESI-MS may enhance ionization, resulting in improved detection limits compared to separation in aqueous buffer systems [Servais et al., 2006].

Although numerous publications have appeared on CE-MS, this technique is still developing to be widely accepted for routine use. The major limitation of CE is the limited sample volumes that can be analysed without compromising separation efficiency. Consequently, the concentration detection limit for CE can be several orders of magnitude higher than that of chromatographic methods. Using the currently available instrumentation, CE-MS detection limits for some applications can be too high, making it unlikely to be used in routine analysis. For example, a study was conducted comparing the performance of CE-MS with that of microbore LC-MS in the determination of endogenous amounts of leucine-enkephalin and methionine-enkephalin in equine cerebrospinal fluid using identical sample clean-up and enrichment procedures [Muck & Henion, 1989]. CE-MS was found to be limited in its concentration detection capacity owing to its much smaller injection volume. Another drawback with CE-MS is that migration times tend to fluctuate with a change of temperature in the environment. Although some manufacturers have incorporated a temperature controlling system into their CE instruments, these devices cannot be effectively utilized in CE-MS applications because a large portion of the CE capillary is extended between the CE instrument and the mass spectrometer. For applications such as regulatory work or those involving unknown components in a mixture, the use of a suitable internal standard would be necessary [Pleasance et al., 1992; Henion et al., 1994]. The chemical condition of the CE capillary inner walls also plays an important role in CE separation. The reproducibility and ruggedness of CE-MS are not currently as good as those of LC-MS. Like LC-MS, the use of non-volatile buffers in CE-MS is generally avoided. Compromises are often made in choosing appropriate operational conditions for CE-MS. Sensitivity limitations, as well as ion source plugging problems, created by the use of non-volatile buffers have impeded the direct transfer of CE separation conditions to on-line CE-MS. Non-volatile additives, such as cyclodextrins, are widely used in the separation of closely related analytes including optical isomers [Ward, 1994; Novotny et al., 1994], however, the concentrations of these additives are often limited by practical restrictions [Varghese & Cole, 1993]. The MS sensitivity may deteriorate as the bulk flow of surfactant enters the mass spectrometer source region.

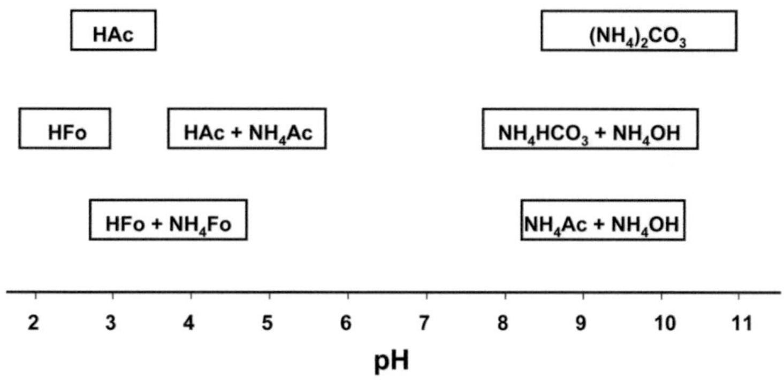

Figure 4.16. Operational regions in CZE recommended for use in practice for on-line CE-MS. The concentration of NH_4Ac usually ranges from 0.01 to 0.3M and the concentration of NH_4Fo from 0.02 to 0.9M. The pH of the buffer in the acidic range is adjusted with either HAc (0.01–1.2 M) or HFo (0.02–2 M) according to the co-ion used. Alkaline pH is usually adjusted by adding ammonia solution or alkylamine. Separation in alkaline pH is sometimes done in NH_4HCO_3 or $(NH_4)_2CO_3$ buffers in concentrations between 0.01 and 0.1 M. Reprinted from ref. [Pantučková et al., 2009].

	LE	*L*	$u_{eff,L}$ a)	pH_L	TE	*T*	$u_{eff,T}$ a)	$pH_{T,adj}$ b)
Cationic ITP								
1	10mM NH_4Ac + 5mM HAc	NH_4^+	76.2	5.06	10mM HAc	H^+	14.7	3.25
2	10mM NH_4OH + 20mM Asp	NH_4^+	56.3	8.80	10mM imidazol + 20mM Asp	$Imid^+$	7.8	7.91
Anionic ITP								
3	10mM $(NH_4)_2CO_3$	CO_3^{2-}	-47.8	9.19	10mM EACA + 20mM NH_4OH	$EACA^-$	-7.2	10.32
4	10mM NH_4Fo + 5mM HFo	Fo^-	-38.5	4.06	10mM MES + 10mM NH_4OH	MES^-	-11.2	5.92

Table 4.2. Separation properties of examples of ITP systems
a) Effective mobility (u_{eff}) of leading (*L*) or terminating (*T*) ion, in $10^{-9}m^2V^{-1}\,s^{-1}$.
b) pH adjusted.
Reprinted from ref. [Pantučková et al., 2009].

Fortunately, a CE methodology improvement for advanced CE-MS hyphenation can be performed in several ways. A number of on-line sample preparation techniques have been introduced to improve the concentration sensitivity of CE, as given in chapter 3. One of the approaches for on-line analyte concentration for CE hyphenated with MS is the chromatographic method. This concept has been incorporated into CE-ESI-MS applications [Tomlinson et al., 1994]. The pre-column was made of a small bed of HPLC packing attached to the inlet of the CE capillary. It serves as an on-line device for sample clean-up such as desalting and preconcentration for subsequent analysis by CE-ESI-MS. The capability of the ITP-CZE-ESI-MS system was demonstrated for the trace analysis of a complex matrix such as calf urine extracts. Several research groups have evaluated the ITP-CZE-ESI-MS approach [Kelly et al., 1994; Severs & Games, 1994; Moseley, 1994]. On-line ITP preconcentration has lowered the concentration detection limits of CE-MS by two orders of magnitude [Kelly et al., 1994; Moseley, 1994.]. Such an improved CE system provided much better separation efficiency than conventional LC systems. The two dimensional ITP approach based on a large volume sample injection (30 μl injection volume) and large volume ITP preseparation (800 μm i.d.) was applied for a very efficient sample preconcentration and analyte injection into a hyphenated MS stage [Tomáš et al., 2010]. The experimental arrangement of this ITP-ITP approach is illustrated in Figure 4.17. Although it has not been used for any enantiomeric separation so far, the ITP-CE approach is very promising for advanced hyphenation with the MS detection, overcoming many of the practical limitations of the CE-MS combination.

The use of small-ID capillaries was found to have improved the absolute sensitivity of CE-ESI-MS [Wahl et al., 1992, 1993]. This improvement in sensitivity is due to the high ionization efficiency associated with the very low bulk flow-rate from the small-ID capillary into the mass spectrometer. Since the ESI ion current is nearly independent of flow-rate, ESI-MS will operate as a mass-sensitive detection system when the ESI current is limited by the flow-rate of the charged species in the solution to the ESI source [Wahl et al., 1994]. For example, a 25- to 50-fold increase in absolute sensitivity can be obtained by reducing the i.d. of CE capillary from 100 to 10 μm [Wahl et al., 1993]. Another instrumental development is the use of coated capillaries. Coated capillaries are often used in the analysis of biological samples to minimize band broadening and peak tailing due to adsorption of analytes onto the capillary walls [Kohr & Engelhardt, 1993]. Moreover, the elimination of sample adsorption (mainly proteins) and EOF considerably increases reproducibility of the measurements. Several types of coated capillaries have been used in CE-MS applications such as aminopropyl silylated fused-silica capillaries [Goodlett et al., 1994; Wahl et al., 1993], capillaries coated with polyacrylamide [Thompson, T.J. et al., 1993], different hydrophilic derivatized capillaries [Cole et al., 1994] and non-covalent coated CE capillary with an overall positive charge [Thibault et al., 1991]. The use of coated capillaries to eliminate the electroosmotic flow may also be useful in minimizing the flow of non-volatile additives into the mass spectrometer [Kirby et al., 1994]. This may be of particular importance in applications such as chiral separations by CE-MS.

One solution to improving the sensitivity of CE-MS is the development of alternative types of mass spectrometers which offer the potential for greater sensitivity, as discussed in section 4.5.3.

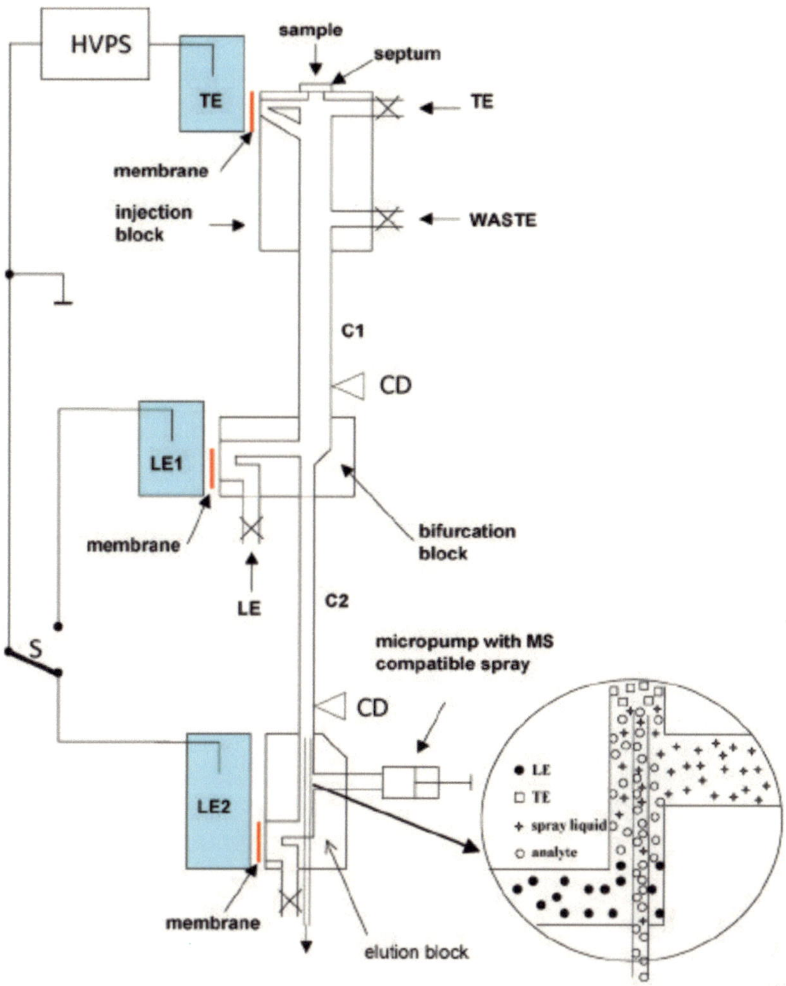

Figure 4.17. Scheme of the hydrodynamically closed isotachophoretic system. X, valves; HVPS, high voltage power supply; LE, TE, leading and terminating electrolytes and electrode reservoirs, respectively; C1, C2, preseparation and separation capillaries; CD, conductivity detectors; S, high voltage switch. Reprinted from ref. [Tomáš et al., 2010].

4.5.2 CE-MS interfaces

The transfer of analytes from the liquid phase of CE to the gas-phase for MS is facilitated via interfaces, where practically all solvent and BGE are selectively removed, and the MS inlet is reached by analytes in the gas-phase with only some rests of the BGE. Several ionization methods have been used for the hyphenation of CE with MS. These include electro spray ionization (ESI), ion spray or pneumatically assisted electro spray ionization, and continuous-flow fast atom bombardment [Cai & Henion, 1995]. These are the on-line interfaces applied for the small, as well as large, molecules. Schematic diagrams of these interfaces are illustrated and described in the next subsections. On the other hand, desorption MS interfaces are preferred for the large non-volatile molecules like proteins,

DNA etc. The coupling of CE to desorption MS can usually be off-line, although advanced (on-line) hyphenations have also recently appeared. The off-line coupling of CE with matrix-assisted laser resorption ionization and ^{252}Cf plasma desorption MS using fraction collection are reviewed by Cai and Henion [Cai & Henion, 1995]. In the recent review by Huck et al. [Huck et al., 2006] the most important techniques developed to hyphenate CE to matrix-assisted laser desorption ionisation time-of-flight mass spectrometry (MALDI-TOF-MS) are summarized. The principles of the different interfaces and ways to solve the hyphenation problem are explained and discussed in detail. Very recently, modified matrix-assisted ionization techniques have been adapted also for the analysis of low molecular weight compounds like drugs and their metabolites [Wang et al., 2011]. Therefore, this interface is principally applicable also in chiral CE-MS and a special analyte treatment is briefly mentioned here. A schematic diagram of the mechanism of MALDI is shown in Figure 4.18.

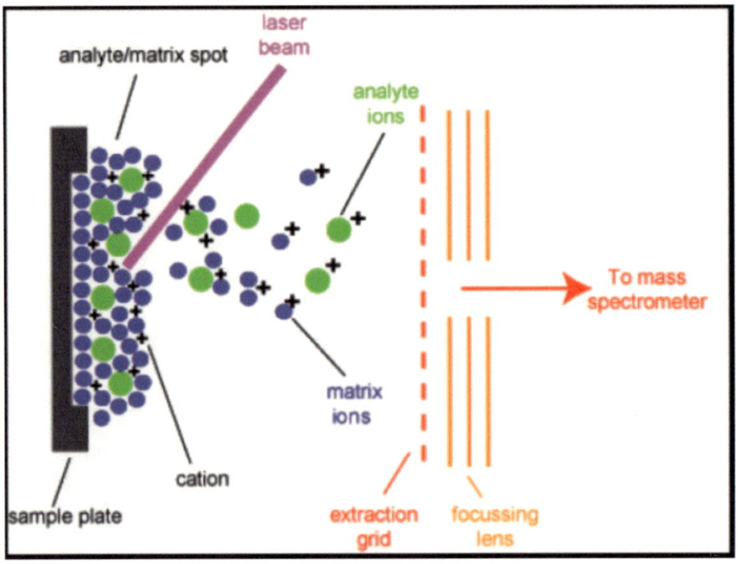

Figure 4.18. A schematic diagram of the mechanism of MALDI. The mechanism of MALDI is believed to consist of three basic steps: (i) *Formation of a 'Solid Solution'*: this is essential for the matrix to be in access thus leading to the analyte molecules being completely isolated from each other. This eases the formation of the homogenous 'solid solution' required to produce a stable desorption of the analyte. (ii) *Matrix Excitation*: the laser beam is focused onto the surface consist of the matrix-analyte solid solution. The chromaphore of the matrix couples with the laser frequency causing rapid vibrational excitation, bringing about localised disintegration of the solid solution. The clusters ejected from the surface consist of analyte molecules surrounded by matrix and salt ions. The matrix molecules evaporate away from the clusters to leave the free analyte in the gas-phase. (iii) *Analyte Ionisation*: the photo-excited matrix molecules are stabilized through proton transfer to the analyte. Cation attachment to the analyte is also encouraged during this process. In this way the characteristic $[M+X]^+$ (X= H, Na, K etc.) analyte ions are formed. These ionisation reactions take place in the desorbed matrix-analyte cloud just above the surface. The ions are then extracted into the mass spectrometer for analysis. Reprinted from ref. [http://www.chm.bris.ac.uk/ms/theory/maldi-ionisation.html].

4.5.2.1 Ion spray interface

Ion spray (ISP) is closely related to the commonly used electro spray ionization interface (ESI), the difference being the application of a nebulizing gas which permits stable electro spray operation at flow-rates up to 1 mL/min [Hopfgartner et al., 1993], whereas pure electro spray has been restricted to flow-rate below 10 μl/min [Whitehouse et al., 1985]. ISP provides a mild ionization via an ion evaporation process which results in primarily molecular mass information in the form of singly and multiply charged ions. For the schematic diagram of CE-ISP-MS interfaces see Figure 4.19.

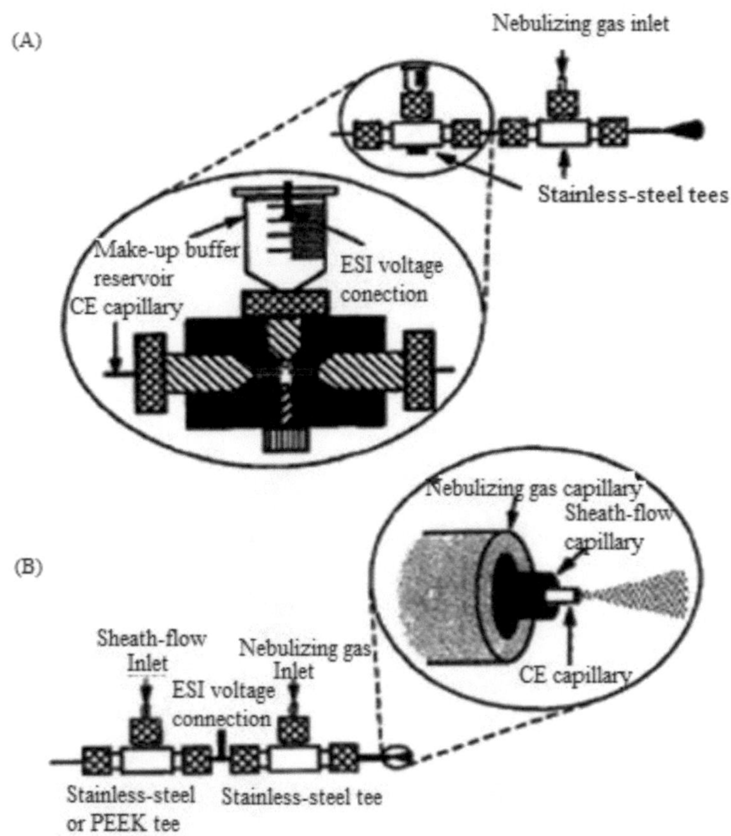

Figure 4.19. Schematic diagram of CE-ISP-MS interfaces. (A) Liquid junction and (B) coaxial sheath-flow configurations. Reprinted from ref. [Cai & Henion, 1995].

4.5.2.2 Continuous-flow fast atom bombardment interface

The continuous-flow fast atom bombardment (CF-FAB) technique can dramatically extend the capability of MS for the determination of fragile and polar compounds [Minard et al., 1988; Moseley et al., 1989a, 1989b]. For the schematic diagram of CE-CF-FAB-MS interfaces see Figure 4.20. There are several attractive features of CE-MS using the ESI interface in comparison with CF-FAB interface. Since larger-ID capillaries can be used for the ESI interface, the loading capacity should be greater than those using the coaxial sheath-flow CF-FAB interface where only small-ID capillaries (ca. 10 μm) can be used due to the pressure drop at the source region which leads to hydrodynamic flow within the CE capillary distorting the plug profile of electroosmotic flow and causing band broadening. The ESI interface also gives reduced background noise and higher sensitivity [Deterding et al., 1991; Edmonds et al., 1991].

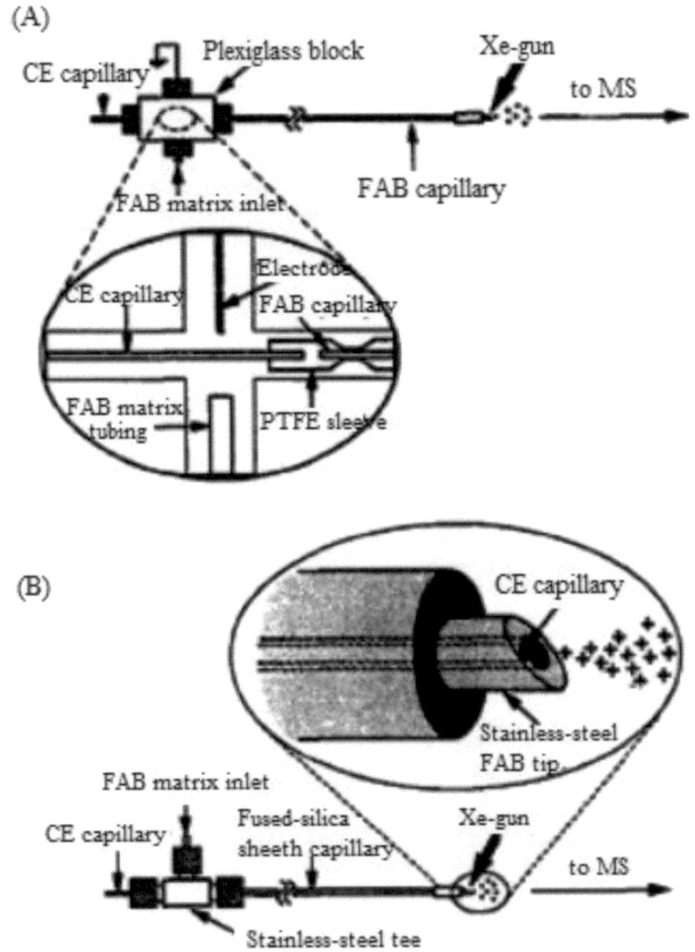

Figure 4.20. Schematic diagram of CE-CF-FAB-MS interfaces. (A) Liquid junction and (B) coaxial sheath-flow configurations. Reprinted from ref. [Cai & Henion, 1995].

4.5.2.3 Electro spray ionization interface

The ESI source is currently the preferred interface for CE-MS, as it can produce ions directly from liquids at atmospheric pressure and with high sensitivity and selectivity for a wide range of analytes. A schematic of an ESI source is in Figure 4.21. ESI is based on electrostatic effects on solution starting with the nebulization of a sample into electrically charged droplets and finishing with the formation of the gas-phase ions. A schematic of the mechanism of ion formation in ESI is in Figure 4.22.

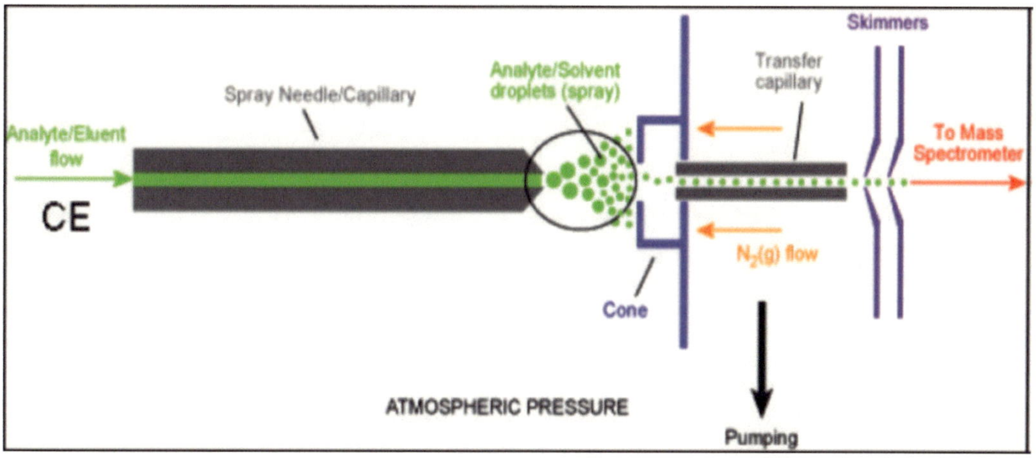

Figure 4.21. A schematic of an ESI source. The analyte is introduced to the source in solution as the eluent flow from the CE analyser. Flow-rates are typically of the order of 1μl min^{-1}. The analyte solution flow passes through the electro spray needle that has a high potential difference (with respect to the counter electrode) applied to it (typically in the range from 2.5 to 4 kV). This forces the spraying of charged droplets from the needle with a surface charge of the same polarity to the charge on the needle. The droplets are repelled from the needle towards the source sampling cone on the counter electrode (shown in blue). As the droplets traverse the space between the needle tip and the cone and solvent evaporation occurs. This is circled on the Figure 4.21 and enlarged in Figure 4.22. Reprinted from ref. [http://www.chm.bris.ac.uk/ms/theory].

Nearly all commercially available CE–MS interfaces are nowadays based upon electro spray ionization (ESI) [von Brocke et al., 2001; Schmitt-Kopplin & Frommberger, 2003]. For the schemes of ESI interfaces see Figure 4.23. Here, various configurations of ESI have been proposed in order to eliminate dead volume at the capillary terminus (Figure 4.23A) and to produce and maintain a stable electro spray signal during a CE-ESI-MS experiment (Figure 4.23B,C). Gale and Smith [Gale & Smith, 1993] compared the performance of the two ESI interfaces (i.e., sheath and sheathless) using pressure infusion. Their study showed several advantages of the sheathless version, including great sensitivity, low required flow-rates and long-term stability. In another study [Wahl et al., 1994], the performance of a gold-coated sheathless interface was compared with that of a sheath-flow interface regarding their dependence on a buffer system and concentration, as well as capillary i.d. The sheathless interface turned out to offer better analyte detectability. It was found that the sheathless configuration also eliminated the possible interferences from the sheath solvents such as charge state distribution shift [Kriger et al., 1994].

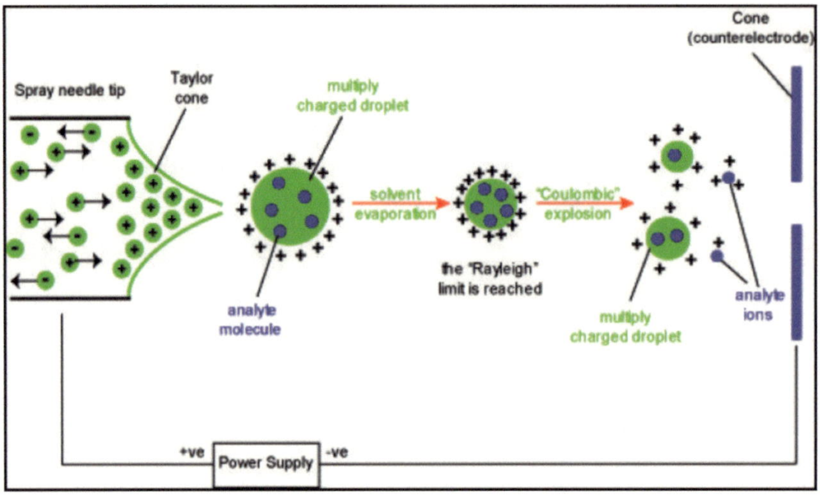

Figure 4.22. A schematic of the mechanism of ion formation in ESI. As the solvent evaporation occurs, the droplet shrinks until it reaches the point that the surface tension can no longer sustain the charge (the Rayleigh limit) at which point a "Coulombic explosion" occurs and the droplet is ripped apart. This produces smaller droplets that can repeat the process as well as naked charged analyte molecules. These charged analyte molecules (they are not strictly ions) can be singly or multiply charged. This is a very soft method of ionisation as very little residual energy is retained by the analyte upon ionisation. This is why ESI-MS is such an important technique in biological studies where the analyst often requires that non-covalent molecule-ligand (e.g., protein) interactions are representatively transferred into the gas-phase. By this technique very little (usually no) fragmentation is produced. For structural elucidation studies, this leads to the requirement for tandem mass spectrometry where the analyte molecules can be fragmented. Reprinted from ref. [http://www.chm.bris.ac.uk/ms/theory].

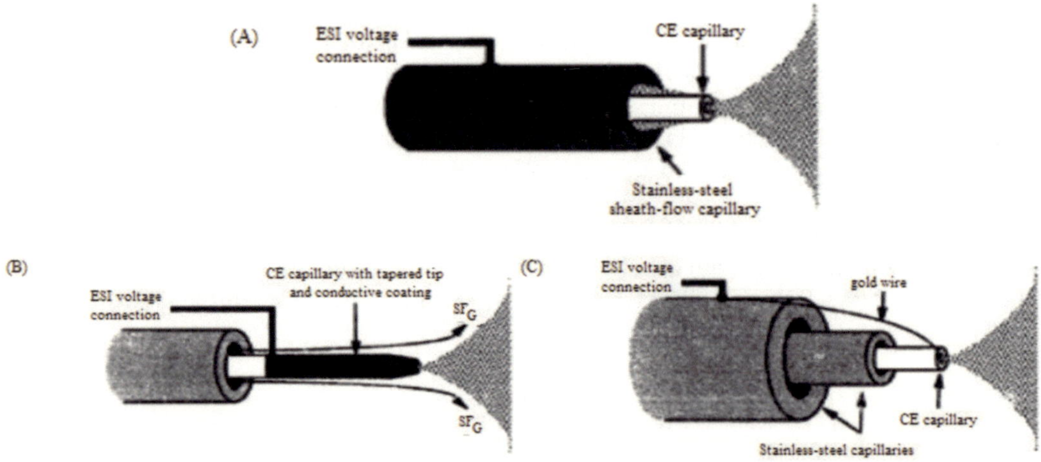

Figure 4.23. Schematic diagram of CE-ESI-MS interfaces. (A) Coaxial sheath-flow configuration, (B) sheathless interface with tapered and conductive coated CE capillary and (C) sheathless interface using a gold wire electrode. Reprinted from ref. [Cai & Henion, 1995].

4.5.3 Mass spectrometry detection approaches

So far, the triple quadrupole (TQ) and ion trap (IT) have been the most commonly used mass analysers in CE-MS for the analysis of low-molecular-weight compounds (including drugs and their metabolites) in biological samples [Soga, 2007]. A schematic of the basic set-up of a TQ mass analyser is shown in Figure 4.24 while that of IT is in Figure 4.25. These MS instruments provide (i) high sensitivity (mainly TQ) with (ii) the capability to obtain structural information on unknown compounds (mainly IT). However, a disadvantage of these mass analysers, especially with respect to fast and highly efficient CE separations, is the relatively slow scanning process, therefore, they are not able to obtain sufficient data points across a very narrow CE peak to accurately define it [Soga et al., 2003]. In addition, the mass resolution of these instruments is limited providing lower selectivity for distinguishing analysed compounds. In general, TQ and IT mass analysers are more suited for targeted metabolomic studies by CE-MS [Ramautar et al., 2006; Monton & Soga, 2007].

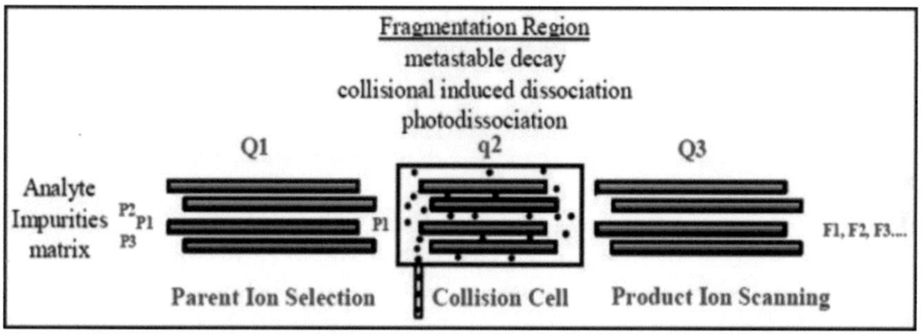

Figure 4.24. Conceptual view of tandem mass spectrometry with a tandem-in-space triple quadrupole mass analyser. The first mass analyser (Q1) selects the precursor ion of interest by allowing it only to pass while discriminating against all others. The precursor ion is then fragmented, usually by energetic collisions, in the second quadrupole (q2) that is operated in transmissive mode allowing all fragment ions to be collimated and passed into the third quadrupole (Q3). Q3 performs mass analysis on the product ions that compose the tandem mass spectra and are rationalized to a structure. Reprinted from ref. [www.noble.org/PlantBio/Sumner/metabolomics.html].

The limitations of TQ- and IT-MS can be overcome by the time-of-flight (TOF) mass analysers where ions are accelerated by an electric field [Bajad & Shulaev, 2007; Lacorte & Fernandez-Albaz, 2006]. The working principle of a linear time-of-flight mass spectrometer is illustrated in Figure 4.26. The high scan speed (e.g., 10 spectra/s), high mass accuracy and high mass resolution of TOF-MS makes this method very suitable for non-targeted metabolomics studies [Soga et al., 2003]. Despite the increased resolution of TOF analysers, potential interferences from solvent ions, adducts and compounds with the same nominal mass as the metabolites in the biological sample can still disturb the analysis. Therefore, efficient separations prior to MS analysis are of key importance. These problems could also be circumvented by using Fourier transform ion cyclotron resonance (FT-ICR) MS, which has a mass resolution of >500 000 and provides very accurate mass measurements with sub-ppm errors. However, accurate mass measurements with FT-ICR MS are relatively slow which can compromise the analysis of narrow CE peaks, and faster analysis may also lead to reduced sensitivity in FT-ICR MS [Baidoo et al., 2008].

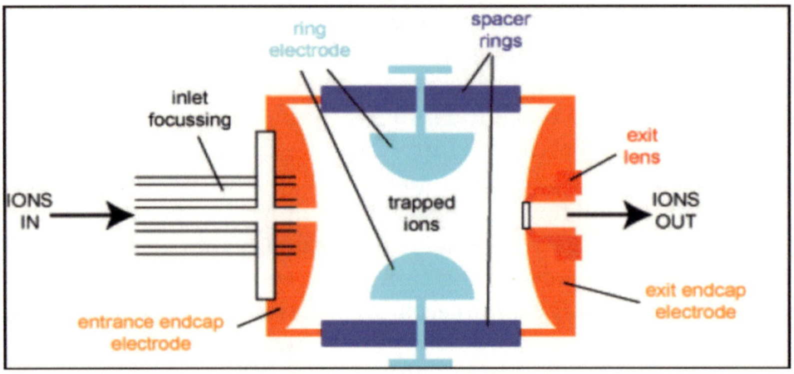

Figure 4.25. A schematic (cutaway view) of a quadrupole ion trap mass analyser. The ions, produced in the source of the instrument, enter into the trap through the inlet and are trapped through the action of the three hyperbolic electrodes: the ring electrode and the entrance and exit endcap electrodes. Various voltages are applied to these electrodes which results in the formation of a cavity in which ions are trapped. The ring electrode RF potential, an a.c. potential of constant frequency but variable amplitude, produces a 3D quadrupolar potential field within the trap. This traps the ions in a stable oscillating trajectory. The exact motion of the ions is dependent on the voltages applied and their individual mass-to-charge (*m/z*) ratios. For detection of the ions, the potentials are altered to destabilize the ion motions resulting in ejection of the ions through the exit endcap. The ions are usually ejected in order of increasing *m/z* by a gradual change in the potentials. This 'stream' of ions is focused onto the detector of the instrument to produce the mass spectrum. The very nature of trapping and ejection makes a quadrupolar ion trap especially suited to performing MS^n experiments in structural elucidation studies. It is possible to selectively isolate a particular *m/z* in the trap by ejecting all the other ions from the trap. Fragmentation of this isolated precursor ion can then be induced by collision-induced dissociation (CID) experiments. The isolation and fragmentation steps can be repeated a number of times and this is only limited by the trapping efficiency of the instrument. Reprinted from ref. [www.chm.bris.ac.uk/ms/theory/qit-massspec.html].

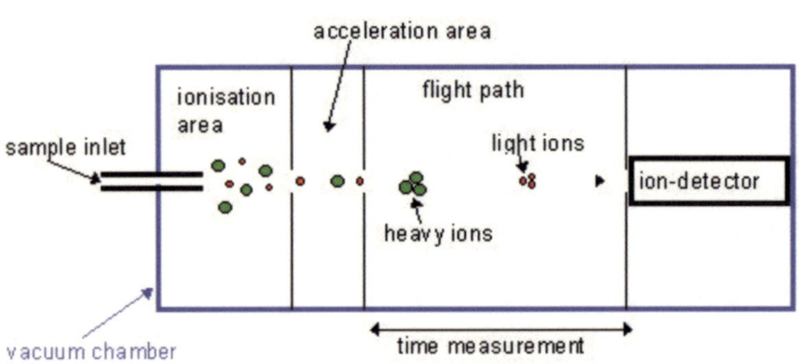

Figure 4.26. The working principle of a linear time-of-flight mass spectrometer. Time-of-flight mass spectrometers identify molecules by measuring the time that sample molecules, all starting with the same kinetic energy, require to fly a known distance. Reprinted from ref. [www.kore.co.uk/tutorial.html].

4.5.4 Chiral CE-ESI-MS

The key factor in manipulating enantioselectivity is the usage of suitable chiral selectors (see section 2.3). They are generally non-volatile molecules, whose introduction into the MS system should be avoided because they damage electro spray efficiency, and increase background noise, decreasing the sensitivity of detection [Shamsi, 2002]. It can be generalized that buffer components that interact strongly with the sample degrade the sensitivity of MS detection. For example, amphiphilic molecules give rise to intense signals in both positive and negative ion ESI, presenting a major barrier for MEKC-MS applications. The main target in such cases is to circumvent these difficulties. Therefore, an important aspect to be considered when a chiral analysis is going to be performed by CE-MS is the type of (i) chiral selector and (ii) separation mode, minimizing introduction of chiral selector into ESI-MS.

As for the selection of the proper type of chiral selector, micelles vs. micelle polymers can serve as a model example. Assuming that the enantioselective capability is comparable, micelle polymers provide several advantages over conventional micelles for MEKC-ESI-MS hyphenation (see section 2.3.8.) resulting in less background noise and higher obtainable S/N [Akbay et al., 2005; Hou et al., 2006; Rizvi et al., 2007].

As for the selection of proper separation mode minimizing the introduction of chiral selector into ESI-MS, the first possibility is immobilization of chiral selectors (CEC mode) which does not affect MS sensitivity (for CEC see section 2.2.2). The second possibility is based on the movement of the selector in the opposite direction toward the detector that can be provided by the selector's charge or by EOF in CE [Iio et al., 2005; Yang et al., 1997; Lu W. Z. et al., 1996; Fanali et al., 1998a; Schulte et al., 1998; Lu W. & Cole, 1998]. For advanced separation mechanisms see section 2.2.1.2. For example, EOF manipulation was used for micelles [Yang L. et al., 1997] and the countercurrent approach was used for antibiotics [Fanali et al., 1998a] and CD derivatives [Iio et al., 2005; Schulte et al., 1998] as chiral selectors. The partial filling of the capillary with the separation media containing the chiral selector in combination with its countercurrent migration can enhance the overall effect [Rudaz et al., 2005; Schappler et al., 2006]. Then, the concentration LODs obtainable by EKC-ESI-MS can be 10^{-8}-10^{-9} M corresponding with mass detection limits of 10^{-16}-10^{-17} mol [Ewing et al., 1989].

4.6 Applications

Absorbance detection. Mikuš et al. [Mikuš et al., 2006a] demonstrated that advanced CE systems based on (i) on-line coupled columns (ITP-EKC), enabling efficient on-line sample preparation (preconcentration of analytes, elimination of matrix constituents) and providing enhanced sample loadability (30 μl sample injection volume), and (ii) countercurrent migration of chiral selector (carboxyethyl-β-CD), allowed the use of a conventional UV detector (240 or 265 nm wavelengths were applied) for a highly efficient (~8x10^4 theoretical plates), selective (baseline enantioresolution and complete resolution from matrix compounds) and ultra-trace (LODs were in the concentration range of 1.1-4.8 ng/mL) direct determination of enantiomers of various drugs (H_1-antihistamines like pheniramine, dimethindene, dioxopromethazine) in the multicomponent ionic matrices (urine samples). The method was successfully applied for enantioselective metabolic study of pheniramine in the externally unpretreated urine samples showing its analytical potential in clinical research.

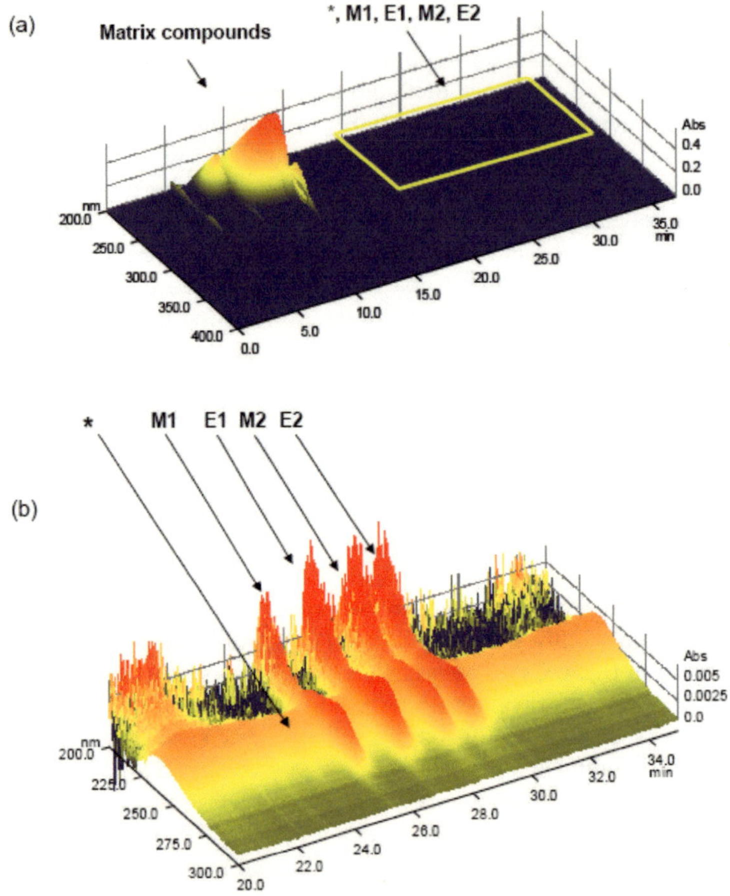

Figure 4.27. ITP-EKC-DAD method for the direct sensitive determination of enantiomers in a sample of unpretreated complex matrices with spectral characterization of electrophoretic zones. 3D traces were obtained combining electrophoretic (EKC) and spectral (DAD) data where the spectra were scanned in the interval of wavelengths 200-400 nm. (a) 3D trace illustrating the whole EKC enantioseparation of pheniramine and its metabolites in the on-line pretreated clinical urine sample (spectra of matrix constituents, well separated from the analytes, are pronounced), (b) detail on the 3D spectra showing the migration positions of pheniramine enantiomers (E1 and E2) and their structurally related metabolites (M1 and M2). The spectrum of the little unknown peak marked with the asterisk differed from the pheniramine spectrum significantly and, therefore, it was not considered as a pheniramine biodegradation product. The urine sample was taken 8.5 hours after the administration of one dose of Fervex (containing 25 mg of racemic pheniramine) to a female volunteer and it was diluted 10-fold before the injection. The separations were carried out using 10 mM sodium acetate - acetic acid, pH 4.75 as a leading electrolyte (ITP), 5 mM ε-aminocaproic acid - acetic acid, pH 4.5 as a terminating electrolyte (ITP) and 25 mM ε-aminocaproic acid - acetic acid, pH 4.5 as a carrier electrolyte (EKC). 0.1% (w/v) methyl-hydroxyethylcellulose served as an EOF suppressor in leading and carrier electrolytes. Carboxyethyl-β-CD (5 mg/mL) was used as a chiral selector in carrier electrolyte. Reprinted from ref. [Marák et al., 2007].

A very complex solution in applied biomedical analytical research was demonstrated by the hyphenation of the ITP-EKC (on-line sample preparation plus countercurrent chiral selector migration) with the spectral detector such as diode array detector (DAD). A DAD spectral characterization/identification in combination with the ITP-EKC separation was successfully applied for the enantioselective determination of drugs and their potential metabolites in unpretreated biological samples that were utilized in enantioselective pharmacokinetic and metabolic studies. Spectral monitoring of the real urine samples, taken after oral administration of 20 mg of amlodipine, carried out over a 54 hour time span, revealed the time vs. concentration profiles typical for the elimination of amlodipine enantiomers in the human body [Mikuš et al., 2008a]. These pharmacokinetic dependences clearly indicated the maxima of excluded amlodipine enantiomers and revealed the differences in elimination between the two enantiomers (enantioselective elimination). High reliability of the results was based on the fact that each point in the pharmacokinetic curves was characterized through spectra and only zones/peaks with acceptable purity (spectral homogeneity) and that matched to the reference spectra were further considered for the pharmacokinetic curve. In another work [Marák et al., 2007], ITP-EKC-DAD enabled potential pheniramine metabolites present at lower ng/mL concentration levels in real urine samples (taken after oral administration of pheniramine tablets to a female volunteer) to be distinguished, see Figure 4.27. Calculated match factors (reference vs. real spectra) gave a high statistical probability of peak identity of pheniramine enantiomers, as well as their potential metabolites. Two unknown peaks migrating close to pheniramine enantiomers peaks (Figure 4.27b) were supposed to be N-desmethyl pheniramine enantiomers, taking into account the former findings concerning the pheniramine metabolism and excretion, as well as migration times of the native and metabolized compounds. The DAD spectral analysis confirmed the high separation selectivity (i.e., producing of spectrally homogeneous analytes zones) of the ITP-EKC method with possible direct injection of unpretreated urine samples. Thus, the ITP-EKC-DAD method illustrates the benefits in (i) chiral field {countercurrent (enantio)resolution enhancement}, (ii) sample preparation (on-line preconcentration and purification) and (iii) detection (sensitivity enhancement and preliminary identification aspect) in analysis of a chiral drug and its metabolites in complex matrices.

Fluorescence detection. LIF was used for the chiral determination of many biologically active compounds [Hernández et al., 2008, 2010]. For example, CBI derivatized baclofen was determined in human plasma with LOD $5x10^{-8}$ M using the CD-EKC-LIF method (highly sulfated-β-CD as chiral selector, excitation wavelength was 442 nm, emission wavelength was 500 nm) [Kavran-Belin et al., 2005].

The main application of LIF in CE has been the analysis of amino acid enantiomers, including also biological samples [Quan et al., 2005; Zhao S.L. et al., 2005a, 2005b; Kirschner et al., 2007; Miao et al., 2005, 2006; Sheeley et al., 2005]. In all cases, the methods involved precapillary chiral derivatization of the amino acids. EKC-LIF (2-hydroxypropyl-β-CD and 2-hydroxypropyl-γ-CD as chiral selectors, excitation wavelength was 457.9 nm) was used for the chiral separation and detection of Ser, primary endogenous amino acid that binds to the Gly site of *N*-methyl-D-Asp receptor involved in a variety of physiological functions and disorders. The sensitive detection of this amino acid is essential, because it is at low concentration in biological samples. D-Ser (NBD-F or CBI derivatives) was detected in rat brain achieving LODs of about 10^{-7} M [Quan et al., 2005; Zhao S.L. et al., 2005a]. The EKC-LIF method (a highly sulfated-β-CD as chiral selector, excitation wavelength was 420 nm) for CBI-Ser was improved (and applied also for other amino acids like aspartate and Glu) by on-line preconcentration procedures. Subsequently a very high sensitivity (LODs up to 10^{-10} M) was achieved in squirrel brain samples [Kirschner et al., 2007]. Derivatized amino acids, such as CBI-Ser and NDA-Asp, were also enantioseparated and detected in invertebrate tissue (mollusc neurons) [Quan et al., 2005; Miao et al., 2005; Zhao S.L. et al., 2005b] where LODs ranged from ~10^{-7}-10^{-10} M using EKC-LIF and excitation wavelength 457.9 nm. An effectivity of the dual chiral selector system and LIF detection for the enantioseparation and identification of CBI-D/L-serine enantiomers in real biological matrices is shown in Figure 4.28 [Zhao S.L. et al., 2005b]. In this way, for the first time, peaks corresponding to L-serine and D-serine were well identified and sensitively detected (LOD was $3x10^{-8}$ M) in *Aplysia* ganglian (a sea mollusc widely used as a neuronal model) homogenates. Miao et al. [Miao et al., 2005] demonstrated an approach for the quantitative investigation of the biochemical composition of subcellular regions of single neurons. Such investigations were possible thanks to the excellent LOD ($5x10^{-10}$ M) of NDA-D-Asp and powerful separation system (CD-MEKC).

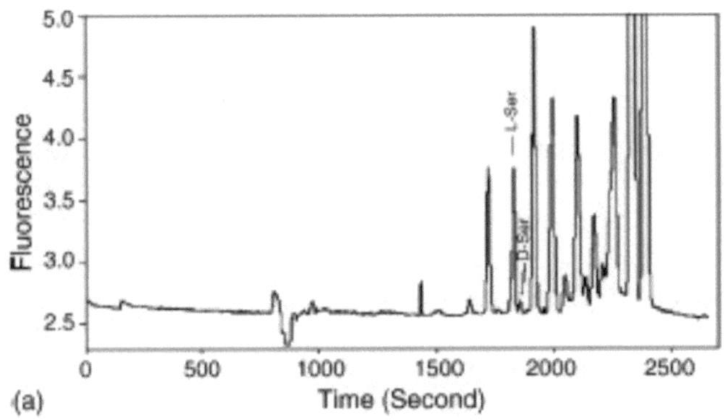

Figure 4.28. Separation and detection of CBI-Ser enantiomers in biological matrices. Separation conditions: 100mM borate (pH 9.5), 30mM β-CD and 60mM sodium deoxycholate (SDC). Electropherogram obtained from analysing an *Aplysia* pedal ganglion homogenate. Capillary was 50 μm i.d.×50 cm effective length. Voltage applied was 15 kV. Reprinted from ref. [Zhao S.L. et al., 2005b].

Electrochemical detection. Amperometric detection was introduced by Schwarz and Hauser in chiral MCE for the separation of basic drugs and biomarkers [Schwarz & Hauser, 2001, 2003]. Plate numbers of up to 20 000, chiral resolutions of 2.5 and detection limits of the order of 10^{-7} *M* were achieved. All separations were completed in less than 3 min. Detection was carried out with a two electrode amperomatric detector, eliminating the need for individual counter and reference electrodes. Because the electrochemical oxidation of catecholamines is pH-dependent, higher detection sensitivities could be obtained at higher pH values. Direct electrochemical oxidation of ephedrine and pseudoephedrine was achieved at a gold electrode at a high pH of 12.6. As the basic compounds are uncharged at this pH, a charged cyclodextrin derivative had to be used for chiral resolution. It was observed that the detection sensitivity is also affected by the type and concentration of chiral and achiral additives applied for achieving resolution. As mentioned by the authors, electrochemical detection has the advantage that derivatization can be omitted. On the other hand, the freedom of buffer choice is limited as conditions have to be arrived which satisfy the requirements for both separation and detection. Another important aspect is that electrochemical detection lacks universality.

In another paper, the detection limits using UV absorbance detector were found to be too high to determine the concentration of isoproterenol (with a speed elimination pharmacokinetics) in intravenous microdialysis samples for a sufficient time following administration to establish the pharmacokinetics. The LODs of this catecholamine were decreased three orders of magnitude (to 3 ng/mL) by using an amperometric detector. Moreover, further sensitivity enhancement (to 0.6 ng/mL) was achieved by inserting in-capillary stacking preconcentration of microdialyzed plasma samples. This provided conditions suitable for obtaining pharmacokinetic curves of isoproterenol enantiomers in plasma, see Figure 4.29 [Hadviger et al., 1996].

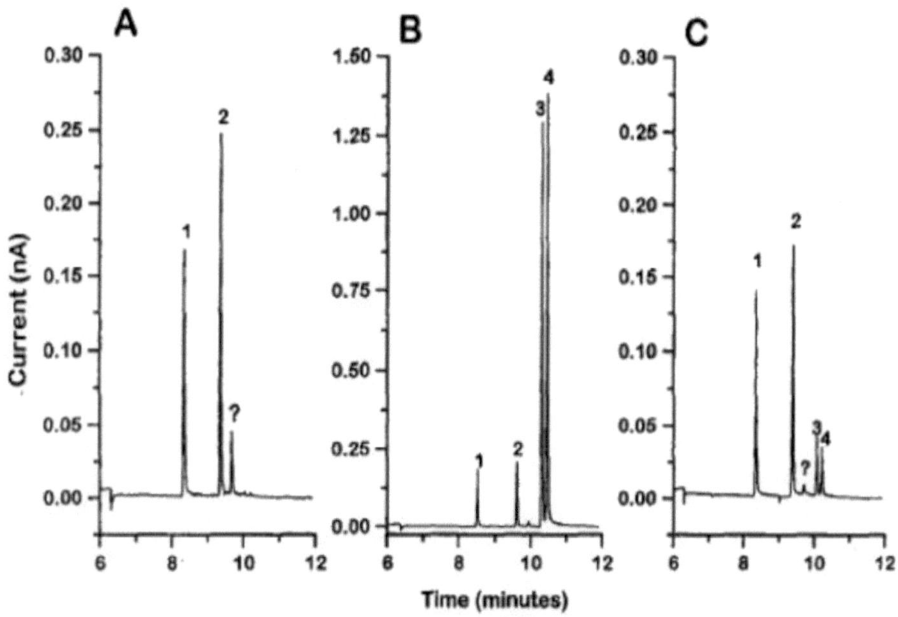

Figure 4.29. Typical CE-electrochemical detection (CE-EC) electropherograms from a pharmacokinetic experiment using on-line sample pretreatment combining dialysis and stacking. (A) Blank sample acquired prior to administering an ISP dose; (B) microdialysate acquired 6 min after dosing and (C) microdialysate acquired 54 min after dosing. Peaks: 1=3,4-Dihydroxybenzylamine(DHBA); 2=5NMHT; 3=(-)-isoproterenol (ISP); 4=(+)-ISP. Reprinted from ref. [Hadwiger et al., 1996].

While conductivity detection is regarded as rather intensive in zone electrophoresis, it can be very attractive in isotachophoresis due to the on-line focusing effect during analyses.

Mikus et al. used conductivity detection with a chiral ITP for the enantioseparation of various H1-antihistaminic drugs in dosage forms [Mikuš et al., 2006b; Kubačák et al., 2006a, 2006b, 2007]. Chiral isotachophoresis in microfluidic devices with on-column conductivity detection was successfully demonstrated by Olvecka et al. [Ölvecká et al., 2001] for the chiral separation of tryptophan enantiomers, however, only in model samples. For this purpose they used a coupled separation channel configuration. In other works, contact, as well as contactless, conductivity detection was successfully used for preliminary scanning of sample profile in the ITP stage of the ITP-EKC method when analysing various drugs present in biological samples. Thus, amlodipine, pheniramine (plus its metabolites), dioxopromethazine, and dimethindene could be easily transferred into the EKC stage for the final enantioseparation without undesired matrix constituents present in urine samples [Mikuš et al., 2006a, 2008a, 2008b; Marák et al., 2007]. The methods were applied in enantioselective metabolic [Mikuš et al., 2006a, 2008b; Marák et al., 2007] and pharmacokinetic [Mikuš et al., 2008a] studies of the drugs, see e.g., Figure 4.27.

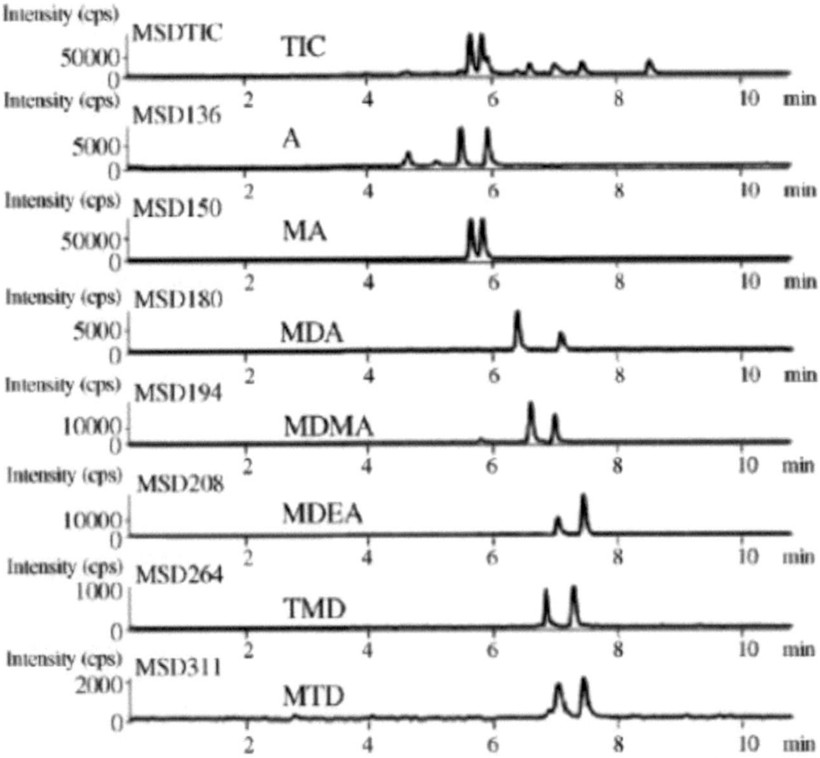

Figure 4.30. Chiral analysis of amphetamine (A), methamphetamine (MA), methylenedioxyamphetamine (MDA), methylenedioxyamphetamine (MDMA), methylenedioxyethylamphetamine (MDEA), tramadol (TMD) and methadone (MTD) amphetamine enantiomers at 0.5 ppb in plasma after LLE with EK injection. Experimental conditions: FS capillary of 75 cm and 650mm (ID); 25 kV; EK injection at 10 kV 610 s; 50% capillary filled with HS-γ-CD 0.15% in BGE 2% capillary filled with BGE post-plug; on-line CE–ESI/MS in SIM mode and extracted ion current (XIC). Reprinted from ref. [Schappler et al., 2006].

Mass spectrometry. Rudaz et al. [Rudaz et al., 2005; Schappler et al., 2006] used the EKC-MS with countercurrent migration of the negatively charged highly sulfated-γ-CD (ammonium formate electrolyte) and the partial filling technique to achieve the enantioseparation of amphetamine derivatives. The use of this strategy with a low concentration of the chiral selector allowed the rapid stereoselective separation of seven amphetamine derivatives in spiked plasma samples in analysis times of less than 6 min and concentration LODs ranging from ~$7x10^{-7}$-$3x10^{-6}$ M [Rudaz et al., 2005]. An enhancing of the detection sensitivity was accomplished with an electrokinetic injection accompanied by the introduction of an appropriate buffer plug length between the zone containing the chiral selector and the analyte injection (to overcome drawbacks linked with electrokinetic injection in the presence of a charged chiral selector) [Schappler et al., 2006], see Figure 4.30. When such complex matrices are analysed, MS signal suppression or enhancement effects are generally not reproducible and can compromise results using CE–ESI-MS. Therefore, the matrix effect was investigated with a commercially available coaxial sheath liquid ESI interface used as the post-capillary infusion system. It was found that with PP, signal suppression was observed while for LLE, no relevant matrix effect occurred in all experiments. Concentration LODs were improved by up to $4x10^{-9}$ M of each enantiomer present in plasma samples after LLE and detected by a single quadrupole MS as a detection device.

Anionic CD, heptakis(2,6-diacethyl-6-sulfato)-β-CD, migrating from the detector to the inlet of the capillary, was used for the simultaneous chiral separation of drugs [Iio et al., 2005]. This selective EKC-ESI-MS method (formic acid electrolyte) was applied to the analysis of methamphetamine, 3,4-methylenedioxyamphetamine and amphetamine in clinical human urine samples pretreated by LLE. Sufficient sensitivity was obtained when concentration LODs ranged from ~$6x10^{-8}$-10^{-7} M.

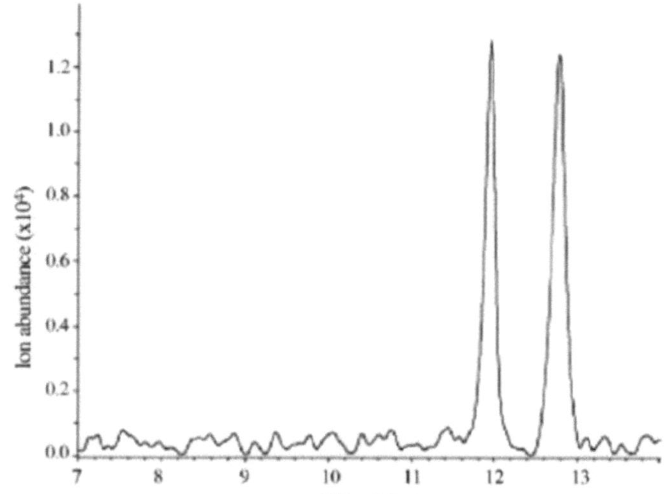

Figure 4.31. Typical electropherogram of salbutamol enantiomers at a concentration close to the LOQ obtained using SPE–NACE–ESI-MS (EIC at 240.4 *m/z*) using a BGE of 10mM ammonium formate and 15mM HDAS-β-CD in methanol acidified with 0.75M formic acid. Reprinted from ref. [Servais et al., 2006].

Micelle polymers are a promising class of chiral selectors for MS, which combine powerful chiral recognition in MEKC and high sensitivity of MS. A sensitive MEKC-MS method using poly(sodium *N*-undecenoxy carbonyl-L-leucine) sulfate (triethylamine + ammonium acetate + acetonitrile buffer) was developed for enantioselective analysis of pseudoephedrine in human urine [Rizvi et al., 2007]. The concentration LOD obtained was ~$2x10^{-6}$ M. LOD at pH 2.0 was 16 times lower than that obtained at pH 8.0, because the ionization efficiency of the MS, in the positive ionization mode, is higher when acidic solutions are used and the sulfated polymeric surfactant was effective also at low pH because of its permanent charge.

The on-line coupling of NACE and ESI-MS was used for the determination of low levels of the enantiomers of a basic chiral drug (salbutamol) in biological samples (human urine) pretreated by SPE [Servais et al., 2006]. The selected BGE (methanol acidified with formic acid containing heptakis(2,3-di-*O*-acetyl-6-*O*-sulfo)-β-CD offered good possibilities to be directly applied for MS coupling since the BGE contained volatile solvents and the non-volatile CD migrated toward the capillary inlet (countercurrent technique) away from the MS detector. After optimization of several parameters, such as sheath liquid composition and flow-rate, nebulizing gas pressure, CE counterpressure and position of the CE capillary outlet, LOQs of 18 and 20 ng/mL were obtained for the salbutamol enantiomers. The RSD at a concentration of 30 ng/mL was below 7% for both enantiomers and *R*-values were 0.9988 and 0.9966. This paper therefore proposed an easy to use and relatively sensitive NACE–ESI-MS method to determine enantiomers of a basic chiral drug in biological fluids preceded by SPE as sample clean-up. Figure 4.31 presents a typical electropherogram of the salbutamol enantiomers at a concentration close to the LOQ using SPE–NACE–ESI-MS. It is noted that, compared with the LOQ of the NACE-UV method (i.e., 375 ng/mL for an injection time of 15 s), the use of an MS detector (with an injection time of 30 s) gives rise to a significant increase in sensitivity.

5

Conclusion

This book clearly illustrates that advanced chiral CE can show real advantages over chromatographic methods in the field of chiral analysis of trace biologically active compounds present in complex matrices. Advanced chiral CE, including (i) sophisticated chiral separation mechanisms and CE formats, (ii) on-line sample preparation and (iii) hyphenation with the conventional, as well as current, top detection systems, enables automatization and miniaturization of the analytical method with the possibility of solving many real tasks based on chiral actions in biological systems.

CE offers tremendous flexibility for enantiomeric separations of new drugs, metabolites, biomarkers, etc., because of a wide variety of available chiral additives easily applicable into CE systems with the cooperation of proper electrophoretic effects (e.g., countercurrent migration of chiral selector vs. analyte). In this field the CD derivatives {especially various (selectively) sulphated CDs} dominate, but progress can also be seen in micelle systems (e.g., micelle polymers). Among a huge amount of other chiral selectors, as presented in this book, their success will be determined not only by their enantiorecognition capability, but also their compatibility with the detection system employed.

Advanced CE techniques based on effective on-line sample pretreatment (preconcentration, purification, derivatization) offer enhanced sensitivity and selectivity along with minimization of sample manipulation, simplifying the overall analytical procedure and allowing automatization and miniaturization of such systems. Although the analytical potential of the most effective and frequently used on-line sample preparation techniques based on electrophoretic principles (stacking techniques, CE-CE couplings), nonelectrophoretic principles (microextraction, microdialysis, flow injection, etc.) and their combinations is very significant, which can be demonstrated by their microscale implementations (MCE) and obtainable preconcentration factors 10^2-10^6 allowing performance of extremely fast and sensitive bioanalyses (pharmacokinetic studies, analysis of single cell contents, etc.), their utilization is still relatively rare and traditional off-line sample preparation procedures dominate. It is believed that future demands on effectivity and microscale analysis will stimulate their use.

Advanced CE methods based on hyphenated detection techniques enabling ultrasensitive quantification and/or providing structural information tend to increase their applicability in (chiral) bioanalyses. Thus, a single molecules analysis (LIF) and structural characterization of unknown biodegradation products and markers (MS) can be accomplished. However, these detection modes are still accompanied, besides their high cost, by many limitations, such as the need for analyte derivatization (LIF), restrictions in applicable buffers and chiral selectors (MS) and the need for further development. Probably, these are possible reasons for the significant domination of universal detection modes like UV-VIS absorbance photometric detection or, to a lesser extent, electrochemical detection, accompanied essentially by a sample preparation in (enantioselective) bioanalytical applications. Although the sensitivity of these later mentioned detection techniques is not sufficient for the majority of bioanalytical problems, they still have great potential to create brand new advanced methods, e.g., utilizing some of the on-line sample preparation techniques presented herein.

It is concluded that the potential, effectivity and performance parameters of CE (and also MCE and CEC) for the enantioselective drug bioanalyses can improve with an appropriate combination of progressive enantioseparation, sample preparation and detection approaches, as it was comprehensively demonstrated in this book. Indeed, new advanced combinations could lead to the development of other interesting fully automatized microscale analytical procedures suitable for reference, as well as routine, use in (chiral) biomedical research. It is apparent that their importance will continually increase with new advanced analytical tasks.

6

Acknowledgements

This work was supported by the publication fund of the Faculty of Pharmacy Comenius University, the grant from the Slovak Grant Agency for Science under the project VEGA No. 1/0664/12 and the grant from the Cultural and Educational Grant Agency of the Ministry of Education under the project KEGA No. 031UK-4/2012. Much research work by the author, included in this book, was supported by the Excellence Center of Pharmacy (ECP) at the Faculty of Pharmacy Comenius University in Bratislava. The author also would like to give his great thanks to the reviewers, excellent chemists and analysts: Prof. Dr. Ladislav Novotný, Assoc. Prof. Dr. Jozef Polonský, Prof. Dr. Emil Havránek and Prof. Dr. Milan Remko, for reviewing this scientific monograph, their valuable statements and suggestions. Last but not least, the author thanks the deputy head of Book Publishing Department and publishing process manager of InTech, Mr. Davor Vidic, for providing the editorial and stylistic revision, and his excellent assistance during the whole publication process.

7

References

[1] Adell, A. & Artigas, F. (1998). *In Vivo Neuromethods*; Boulton, A.A.; Baker, G.B.; Bateson A.N. (Eds.) Chapter 1, Humana Press: Totowa, NJ.

[2] Aebersold, R. & Morrison, H.D. (1990). Analysis of dilute peptide samples by capillary zone electrophoresis. *Journal of Chromatography A*, Vol. 516, No. 1, pp. 79-88.

[3] Afshar, M. & Thormann, W. (2006). Validated capillary electrophoresis assay for the simultaneous enantioselective determination of propafenone and its major metabolites in biological samples. *Electrophoresis*. Vol. 27, No.8, pp.1517-1525.

[4] Akbay, C.; Rizvi, S.A.A. & Shamsi, S.A. (2005). Simultaneous enantioseparation and tandem UV-MS detection of eight β-blockers in micellar electrokinetic chromatography using a chiral molecular micelle. *Analytical Chemistry*, Vol.77, No.6, pp. 1672-1683.

[5] Almeda, S.; Nozal, L.; Arce, L. & Valcárcel, M. (2007). Direct determination of chlorophenols present in liquid samples by using a supported liquid membrane coupled in-line with capillary electrophoresis equipment. *Analytica Chimica Acta*, Vol. 587, No. 1, pp. 97-103.

[6] Altria, K.D.; Mahuzier, P.-E. & Clark, B.J. (2003). Background and operating parameters in microemulsion electrokinetic chromatography. *Electrophoresis*, Vol.24, No.3, pp. 315-324.

[7] Altria, K.; Marsh, A. & Sanger-van de Griend, C. (2006). Capillary electrophoresis for the analysis of small-molecule pharmaceuticals. *Electrophoresis*, Vol.27, No.12, pp. 2263-2282.

[8] Amankwa, L.N.; Albin, M. & Kuhr, W.G. (1992). Fluorescence detection in capillary electrophoresis. *Trends in Analytical Chemistry*, Vol.11, No.3, pp. 114-120.

[9] Andersen, S.; Halvorsen, T.G.; Pedersen-Bjergaard, S.; Rasmussen, K.E.; Tanum, L. & Refsum, H. (2003). Stereospecific determination of citalopram and desmethylcitalopram by capillary electrophoresis and liquid-phase microextraction. *Journal of Pharmaceutical and Biomedical Analysis*, Vol.33, No.2, pp. 263-273.

[10] Armstrong, D.W.; Rundlett, K. & Reid III, G.L. (1994a). Use of a macrocyclic antibiotic, rifamycin B, and indirect detection for the resolution of racemic amino alcohols by CE. *Analytical Chemistry*, Vol.66, No.10, pp. 1690-1695.

[11] Armstrong, D.W.; Rundlett, K.L. & Chen, J.R. (1994b). Evaluation of the macrocyclic antibiotic vancomycin as a chiral selector for capillary electrophoresis. *Chirality*, Vol.6, No.6, pp. 496-509.

[12] Asami, T. & Imura, H. (2006). Absolute determination method for trace quantities of enantiomer of glufosinate by gamma-cyclodextrin modified capillary zone electrophoresis combined with solid-phase extraction and on-capillary concentration. *Analytical Science*, Vol. 22, No.12, pp. 1489-1493.

[13] Aturki, Z.; Scotti, V.; D'Orazio, G.; Rocco, A.; Raggi, M.A. & Fanali, S. (2007). Enantioselective separation of the novel antidepressant mirtazapine and its main metabolites by CEC. *Electrophoresis*, Vol.28, No.15, pp. 2717-2725.

[14] Avdalovic, N.; Pohl, C.A.; Rocklin, R.D. & Stillian, J.R. (1993). Determination of cations and anions by capillary electrophoresis combined with suppressed conductivity detection. *Analytical Chemistry*, Vol.65, No.10, pp. 1470-1475.

[15] Awadallah, B; Smidt, P.C & Wahl, M.A. (2003). Quantitation of the enantiomers of ofloxacin by capillary electrophoresis in the parts per billion concentration range for in vitro drug absorption studies. *Journal of Chromatography A*, Vol.988, No.1, pp. 135-143.

[16] Baidoo, E.E.K.; Benke, P.I.; Neusüss, C.; Pelzing, M.; Kruppa, G.;Leary, J.A. & Keasling, J.D. (2008). Capillary electrophoresis-fourier transforms ion cyclotron resonance mass spectrometry for the identification of cationic metabolites via a pH-mediated stacking-transient isotachophoretic method. *Analytical Chemistry*, Vol.80, No.9, pp. 3112-3122.

[17] Bajad, S. & Shulaev, V. (2007). Highly-parallel metabolomics approaches using LC-MS2 for pharmaceutical and environmental analysis. *TrAC - Trends in Analytical Chemistry*, Vol.26, No.6, pp. 625-636.

[18] Baldacci, A. & Thormann, W. (2006). Analysis of lorazepam and its 3O-glucuronide in human urine by capillary electrophoresis: Evidence for the formation of two distinct diastereoisomeric glucuronides. *Journal of Separation Science*, Vol.29, No.1, pp. 153-163.

[19] Balss, K.M.; Vreeland, W.N.; Phinney, K.W. & Ross, D. (2004). Simultaneous concentration and separation of enantiomers with chiral temperature gradient focusing. *Analytical Chemistry*, Vol.76, No.24, pp. 7243-7249.

[20] Barroso, M.B. & de Jong, A.P. (1998). A new design for large, dilute sample loading in capillary electrophoresis. *Journal of Capillary electrophoresis*, Vol.5, No. 1-2, pp. 1-7

[21] Bartos, D. & Gorog, S. (2009). Recent Advances in the Impurity Profiling of Drugs. *Current Pharmaceutical Analysis*, Vol.4, No.4, pp. 215-230.

[22] Beck, W.; Van Hoek, R. & Engelhardt, H. (1993). Application of a diode-array detector in capillary electrophoresis. *Electrophoresis*, Vol.14, No.5-6, pp. 540-546.

[23] Beckers, J.L. & Boček, P. (2000). Sample stacking in capillary zone electrophoresis: Principles, advantages and limitations. *Electrophoresis*, Vol.21, No. 14, pp. 2747-2767.

[24] Behn, F.; Michels, S.; Laer, S. & Blaschke, G. (2001). Separation of carvedilol enantiomers in very small volumes of human plasma by capillary electrophoresis with laser-induced fluorescence. *Journal of Chromatography B*, Vol.755, No.1-2, pp. 111-117.

[25] Belder, D.; Kohler, F.; Ludwig, M.; Tolba, K. & Piehl, N. (2006). Coating of powder-blasted channels for high-performance microchip electrophoresis. *Electrophoresis*, Vol.27, No.16, pp. 3277-3283

[26] Belder, D. (2006). *Chiral Analysis*, Busch, K.W.; M.A. Busch (Eds.), Chapter 9: Chiral separations in microfluidic devices, pp. 277-295, Elsevier B.V., Oxford, UK.

[27] Bertoncini, N.D. & Hennion, M.C. (2004). Immunoaffinity solid-phase extraction for pharmaceutical and biomedical trace-analysis—coupling with HPLC and CE—perspectives. *Journal of Pharmaceutical and Biomedical Analysis*, Vol.34, No.4, pp.717–736.

[28] Bjergaard, S.P. & Rasmussen, K.E. (2008). Liquid-phase microextraction with porous hollow fibers, a miniaturized and highly flexible format for liquid-liquid extraction. *Journal of Chromatography A*, Vol. 1184, No.1-2, pp. 132-142.

[29] Bjørnsdottir, I.; Hansen, S.H. & Terabe, S. (1996). Chiral separation in non-aqueous media by capillary electrophoresis using the ion-pair principle. *Journal of Chromatography A*, Vol.745, No.1-2, pp. 37-44.

[30] Blanco, M. & Valverde, I. (2003). Choice of chiral selector for enantioseparation by capillary electrophoresis. *TrAC - Trends in Analytical Chemistry,* Vol.22, No.7-8, pp. 428-439.

[31] Boček, P. (1987). *Analytical capillary isotachophoresis,* Academia, Praha, pp.133.

[32] Bodor, R.; Kaniansky, D. & Masár, M. (2001). Conductivity detection cell for capillary zone electrophoresis with a solution mediated contact of the separated constituents with the detection electrodes. *Journal of Chromatography A,* Vol. 916, No.1-2, pp. 31–40.

[33] Bonato, P.S. (2003). Recent advances in the determination of enantiomeric drugs and their metabolites in biological fluids by capillary electrophoresis-mediated microanalysis. *Electrophoresis,* Vol.24, No.22-23, pp. 4078-4094.

[34] Bonneil, E. & Waldron, K.C. (2000). On-line system for peptide mapping by capillary electrophoresis at sub-micromolar concentrations. *Talanta,* Vol. 53, No., 3, pp. 678-699.

[35] Bortocan, R. & Bonato, P.S. (2004). Enantioselective analysis of primaquine and its metabolite carboxyprimaquine by capillary electrophoresis. *Electrophoresis,* Vol.25, No.16, pp. 2848-2853.

[36] Bowser, M.T. & Kennedy, R.T. (2001). In vivo monitoring of amine neurotransmitters using microdialysis with on-line capillary electrophoresis. *Electrophoresis,* Vol.22, No.17, pp. 3668-3676.

[37] Breadmore, M.C. (2007). Recent advances in enhancing the sensitivity of electrophoresis and electrochromatography in capillaries and microchips. *Electrophoresis,* Vol.28, No.1-2, pp. 254-281.

[38] Breadmore, M.C.; Thabano, J.R.E.; Dawod, M.; Kazarian, A.A.; Quirino, J.P. & Guijt, R.M. (2009). Recent advances in enhancing the sensitivity of electrophoresis and in capillaries and microchips (2006-2008). *Electrophoresis,* Vol.30, No.1, pp. 230-248.

[39] Britz-McKibbin, P. & Chen, D.D.Y. (2000). Selective focusing of catecholamines and weakly acidic compounds by capillary electrophoresis using a dynamic pH junction. *Analytical Chemistry,* Vol.72, No. 6, pp. 1242-1252.

[40] Britz-McKibbin, P.; Otsuka, K. & Terabe, S. (2002). On-line focusing of flavin derivatives using dynamic pH junction-sweeping capillary electrophoresis with laser-induced fluorescence detection. *Analytical Chemistry,* Vol.74, No.15, pp. 3736-3743.

[41] Britz-McKibbin, P. & Terabe, S. (2003). On-line preconcentration strategies for trace analysis of metabolites by capillary electrophoresis. *Journal of Chromatography A,* Vol.1000, No.1-2, pp. 917-934.

[42] Britz-McKibbin, P.; Markuszewski, M.J.; Iyanagi, T.; Matsuda, K.; Nishioka, T. & Terabe, S. (2003). Picomolar analysis of flavins in biological samples by dynamic pH junction-sweeping capillary electrophoresis with laser-induced fluorescence detection. *Analytical Biochemistry,* Vol.313, No.1, pp. 89-96.

[43] Bushey, M.M. & Jorgenson, J.W. (1990). Automated instrumentation for comprehensive 2-dimensional high-performance liquid-chromatography capillary zone electrophoresis. *Analytical Chemistry,* Vol.62, No. 10, pp. 978-984.

[44] Cai, J. & Henion, J. (1995). Capillary electrophoresis-mass spectrometry. *Journal of Chromatography A,* Vol.703, No.1-2, pp. 667-692

[45] Camilleri, P. (1991). Biomedical applications of chiral liquid chromatography. *Biomedical Chromatography,* Vol.5, No.3, pp. 128-132.

[46] Cardoso, C.D.; Jabor, V.A.P. & Bonato, P.S. (2006). Capillary electrophoretic chiral separation of hydroxychloroquine and its metabolites in the microsomal fraction of liver homogenates. *Electrophoresis,* Vol.27, No.5-6, pp. 1248-1254.
[47] Carlavilla, D.; Moreno-Arribas, M.V.; Fanali, S. & Cifuentes, A. (2006). Chiral MEKC-LIF of amino acids in foods: Analysis of vinegars. *Electrophoresis,* Vol.27, No.13, pp. 2551-2557.
[48] Carlsson, Y.; Hedeland, M.; Bondesson, U. & Pettersson, C. (2001). Non-aqueous capillary electrophoretic separation of enantiomeric amines with (-)-2,3:4,6-di-O-isopropylidene-2-keto-L-gulonic acid as chiral counter ion. *Journal of Chromatography A,* Vol.922, No.1-2, pp. 303-311.
[49] Caslavska, J. & Thormann, W. (2011). Stereoselective determination of drugs and metabolites in body fluids, tissues and microsomal preparations by capillary electrophoresis (2000-2010). *Journal of Chromatography A,* Vol. 1218, No.4 (Sp. Iss. SI), pp. 588-601.
[50] Castro-Puyana, M.; Salgado, A.; Hazen, R.M.; Crego, A.L. & Alegre, M.L.M. (2008). The first contribution of capillary electrophoresis to the study of abiotic origins of homochirality: Investigation of the enantioselective adsorption of 3-carboxy adipic acid on minerals. *Electrophoresis,* Vol.29, No.7, pp. 1548-1555.
[51] Chang, H.T. & Yeung, E.S. (1995). Determination of catecholamines in single adrenal medullary cells by capillary electrophoresis and laser-induced native fluorescence. *Analytical Chemistry,* Vol.67, No.6, pp. 1079-1083.
[52] Chankvetadze, B.; Endresz, G. & Blaschke, G. (1994). About some aspects of the use of charged cyclodextrins for capillary electrophoresis enantioseparation. *Electrophoresis,* Vol.15, No.6, pp. 804-807.
[53] Chankvetadze, B. (1997). *Capillary Electrophoresis in Chiral Analysis.* Wiley, Chichester.
[54] Chankvetadze, B.; Burjanadze, N.; Bergenthal, D. & Blaschke, G. (1999). Potential of flow-counterbalanced capillary electrophoresis for analytical and micropreparative separations. *Electrophoresis,* Vol.20, No.13, pp. 2680-2685.
[55] Chankvetadze, B. & Blaschke, G. (2001). Enantioseparations in capillary electromigration techniques: Recent developments and future trends. *Journal of Chromatography A,* Vol.906, No.1-2, pp. 309-363.
[56] Chankvetadze, B.; Burjanadze, N. & Blaschke, G. (2001). Enantioseparation of the anticoagulant drug phenprocoumon in capillary electrophoresis with UV and laser-induced fluorescence detection and application of the method to urine samples. *Electrophoresis,* Vol.22, No.15, pp. 3281-3285.
[57] Chankvetadze, B. (2007). Enantioseparations by using capillary electrophoretic techniques. The story of 20 and a few more years. *Journal of Chromatography A,* Vol.1168, No.1-2, pp. 45-70.
[58] Chankvetadze, B. (2008). *Cyclodextrins and their Complexes.* Dodziuk, H. (Ed.), pp. 119–146, Wiley-VCH, Weinheim, Germany.
[59] Chaurasia, C.S. (1999). In vivo microdialysis sampling: theory and applications. *Biomedical Chromatography,* Vol.13, No. 5, pp. 317-332.
[60] Chen, D. & Dovichi, N.J. (1996). Single-molecule detection in capillary electrophoresis: molecular shot noise as a fundamental limit to chemical analysis. *Analytical Chemistry,* Vol.68, No.4, pp. 690-696.

[61] Chen, Y.M., Chen, C.F. & Xi, F. (1998). Chiral Dendrimers With Axial Chirality. *Chirality,* Vol.10, pp. 661–666.

[62] Chen, Y.L.; Jong, Y.J. & Wu, S.M. (2006). Capillary electrophoresis combining field-amplified sample stacking and electroosmotic flow suppressant for analysis of sulindac and its two metabolites in plasma. *Journal of Chromatography A,* Vol.1119, No.1-2, pp. 176-182.

[63] Chen, Y.; Guo, Z.; Wang, X. & Qiu, C. (2008). Sample preparation. *Journal of Chromatography A,* Vol.1184, No.1-2, pp. 191-219.

[64] Chen, J.; Du, Y.; Zhu, F. & Chen, B. (2010). Evaluation of the enantioselectivity of glycogen-based dual chiral selector systems towards basic drugs in capillary electrophoresis. *Journal of Chromatography A,* Vol.1217, No.45, pp. 7158-7163.

[65] Cheng, Y.F. & Dovichi, N.J. (1988). Subattomole amino acid analysis by capillary zone electrophoresis and laser-induced fluorescence. *Science,* Vol.242, No.4878, pp. 562-564.

[66] Cheng, J. & Kang, J. (2006). An on-column derivatization method for the determination of the enantiomeric excess of chiral primary amines via indirect enantioseparation by micellar electrokinetic chromatography. *Electrophoresis,* Vol.27, No.4, pp. 865-871.

[67] Cherkaoui, S.; Rudaz, S.; Varesio, E. & Veuthey, J.L. (2001). On-line capillary electrophoresis-electrospray mass spectrometry for the stereoselective analysis of drugs and metabolites. *Electrophoresis,* Vol.22, No.15, pp. 3308-3315.

[68] Chiang, M.T.; Chang, S.Y. & Whang, C.W. (2001). Multiple voltage-gradient gel electrophoresis system. *Electrophoresis,* Vol.22, No.1, pp. 29-32.

[69] Chien, R.L. & Burgi, D.S. (1992). On-column sample concentration using field amplification in CZE. *Analytical Chemistry,* Vol.64, No. 8, pp. 489A-496A

[70] Cho, S.I.; Shim, J.; Kim, M.S.; Kim, Y.K. & Chung, D.S. (2004). On-line sample cleanup and chiral separation of gemifloxacin in a urinary solution using chiral crown ether as a chiral selector in microchip electrophoresis. *Journal of Chromatography A,* Vol.1055, No. 1-2, pp. 241–245.

[71] Choi, K.; Kim, J.; Jang, Y.O. & Chung, D.S. (2009). Direct chiral analysis of primary amine drugs in human urine by single drop microextraction in-line coupled to CE. *Electrophoresis,* Vol.30, No.16, pp. 2905-2911.

[72] Chou, Y.W.; Huang, W.S.; Ko, C.C. & Chen, S.H. (2008). Enantioseparation of cetirizine by sulfated-β-cyclodextrin-mediated capillary electrophoresis. *Journal of Separation Science,* Vol.31, No.5, pp. 845-852.

[73] Christodoulou, E.A. (2010). An Overview of HPLC Methods for the Enantiomer Separation of Active Pharmaceutical Ingredients in Bulk and Drug Formulations, *Current Organic Chemistry,* Vol.14, No.19, pp. 2337-2347.

[74] Cole, R.B.; Varghese, J. & McCormick, R.M. (1994). Capillary Electrophoresis Electrospray Mass Spectrometry Using a Novel Hydrophilic Derivarized Capillary for Protein Analysis. *42nd ASMS Conference on Mass Spectrometry and Allied Topics, Chicago, IL, 29 May-3 June 1994.*

[75] Craig, D.B.; Arriaga, E.; Wong, J.C.Y.; Lu, H. & Dovichi, N.J. (1998). Life and Death of a Single Enzyme Molecule. *Analytical Chemistry,* Vol.70, No.1, pp. 39A-43A.

[76] Craig, S.L.; Zhong, M. & Brauman, J.I. (1998). Nonstatistical reactivity in a vibrationally excited S(N)2 intermediate [1]. *Journal of the American Chemical Society,* Vol.120, No.46, pp. 12125-12126.

[77] Cserhati, T. (2008). New applications of cyclodextrins in electrically driven chromatographic systems: a review. *Biomedical Chromatography,* Vol.22, No.6, pp. 563-571.
[78] Cucinotta, V.; Contino, A.; Giuffrida, A.; Maccarrone, G. & Messina, M. (2010). Application of charged single isomer derivatives of cyclodextrins in capillary electrophoresis for chiral analysis. *Journal of Chromatography A,* Vol.1217, No.7, pp. 953-967.
[79] Culbertson, C.T. & Jorgenson, J.W. (1994). Flow counterbalanced capillary electrophoresis. *Analytical Chemistry,* Vol.66, No.7, pp. 955-962.
[80] Culbertson, C.T. & Jorgenson, J.W. (1999). Lowering the UV absorbance detection limit and increasing the sensitivity of capillary electrophoresis using a dual linear photodiode array detector and signal averaging. *Journal of Microcolumn Separations,* Vol.11, No.9, pp. 652-662.
[81] Danger, G. & Ross, D. (2008). Development of a temperature gradient focusing method for in situ extraterrestrial biomarker analysis. *Electrophoresis* Vol.29, No.15, pp. 3107-3114.
[82] Danková, M.; Kaniansky, D.; Fanali, S. & Iványi, F. (1999). Capillary zone electrophoresis separations of enantiomers present in complex ionic matrices with on-line isotachophoretic sample pretreatment. *Journal of Chromatography A,* Vol.838, No. 1-2, pp. 31-43
[83] da Silva, J.A.F.; Guzman, N. & de Lago, C.L. (2002). Contactless conductivity detection for capillary electrophoresis: Hardware improvements and optimization of the input-signal amplitude and frequency. *Journal of Chromatography A,* Vol.942, No.1-2, pp. 249-258.
[84] da Silva, J.A.F. (2003). Detecção Eletroquímica em eletroforese capliar. *Quimica Nova,* Vol.26, No.1, pp. 56-64.
[85] de Gaitani, M.C.; Martinez, A.S. & Bonato, P.S. (2003). Study on thioridazine 5-sulfoxide epimerization and degradation by capillary electrophoresis. *Electrophoresis,* Vol.24, No.15, pp. 2723-2730.
[86] de Jong, J.; Lammertink, R.G.H. & Wessling, M. (2006). Membranes and microfluidics: a review. *Lab Chip,* Vol.6, No.9, pp. 1125-1139.
[87] de Oliveira, A.R.M.; Cardoso, C.D. & Bonato, P.S. (2007). Stereoselective determination of hydroxychloroquine and its metabolites in human urine by liquid-phase microextraction and CE. *Electrophoresis,* Vol.28, No.7, pp. 1081-1091.
[88] de Santana, F.J.M.; Lanchote, V.C. & Bonato, P.S. (2008). Capillary electrophoretic chiral determination of mirtazapine and its main metabolites in human urine after enzymatic hydrolysis. *Electrophoresis,* Vol.29, No.18, pp. 3924-3932.
[89] Denola, N.L.; Quiming, N.S.; Saito, Y. & Jinno, K. (2007). Simultaneous enantioseparation and sensitivity enhancement of basic drugs using large-volume sample stacking. *Electrophoresis,* Vol.28, No.19, pp. 3542-3552.
[90] Desiderio, C.; Polcaro, C.M.; Padiglioni, P. & Fanali, S. (1997). Enantiomeric separation of acidic herbicides by capillary electrophoresis using vancomycin as chiral selector. *Journal of Chromatography A,* Vol.781, No.1-2, pp. 503-513.
[91] Deterding, L.J.; Parker, C.E.; Perkins, J.R.; Moseley, M.A.; Jorgenson, J.W. & Tomer, K.B. (1991). Nanoscale separations. Capillary liquid chromatography-mass spectrometry and capillary zone electrophoresis-mass spectrometry for the

determination of peptides and proteins. *Journal of Chromatography*, Vol.554, No.1-2, pp. 329-338.

[92] Dhopeshwarkar, R.; Crooks, R.M.; Hlushkou, D. & Tallarek, U. (2008). Transient Effects on Microchannel Electrokinetic Filtering with an Ion-Permselective Membrane. *Analytical Chemistry*, Vol.80, pp.1039–1048.

[93] Diode-array detection in capillary electrophoresis using Agilent Extended Light Path capillaries, Agilent Technologies, 2009.

[94] Du, Y.; Taga, A.; Suzuki, S.; Liu, W. & Honda, S. (2002). Colominic acid: a novel chiral selector for capillary electrophoresis of basic drugs. *Journal of Chromatography A*, Vol.962, No.1-2, pp. 221-231.

[95] Edmonds, C.G.; Loo, J.A. & Ogorzalek Loo, R.R. (1991). Application of Electrospray Ionization Mass-Spectrometry and Tandem Mass-Spectrometry in Combination with Capillary Electrophoresis for Biochemical Investigations. *Biochemical Society Transactions*, Vol.19, No.4, pp. 943-947.

[96] El-Enany, N.; El-Sherbiny, D. & Belal, F. (2007). Spectrophotometric, spectrofluorometric and HPLC determination of desloratadine in dosage forms and human plasma. *Chemical and Pharmaceutical Bulletin*, Vol.55, No.12, pp. 1662-1670.

[97] El-Hady, D.A. & El-Maali, N.A. (2008). Determination of catechin isomers in human plasma subsequent to green tea ingestion using chiral capillary electrophoresis with a high-sensitivity cell. *Talanta*, Vol. 76, No.1, pp. 138-145.

[98] Esteban, J.; Pellín, M.D.L.C.; Gimeno, C.; Barril, J.; Mora, E.; Giménez, J. & Vilanova, E. (2004). Detection of clinical interactions between methadone and anti-retroviral compounds using an enantio selective capillary electrophoresis for methadone analysis. *Toxicology Letters*, Vol.151, No.1, pp. 243-249.

[99] Ewing, A.G.; Wallingford, R.A. & Olefirowicz, T.M. (1989). Capillary Electrophoresis. *Analytical Chemistry*, Vol.61, No.4, pp. 292A-303A.

[100] Ewing, A.G.; Mesaros, J.M. & Gavin, P.F. (1994). Electrochemical Detection in Microcolumn Separations. *Analytical Chemistry*, Vol.66, No., pp. 527A-537A.

[101] Fan, G.R.; Hong, Z.Y.; Lin, M.; Yin, X.P. & Wu, Y.T. (2004). Study of stereoselective pharmacokinetics of anisodamine enantiomers in rabbits by capillary electrophoresis. *Journal of Chromatography B*, Vol.809, No.2, pp. 265-271.

[102] Fanali, S.; Desiderio, C.; Schulte, G.; Heitmeier, S.; Strickmann, D.; Chankvetadze, B. & Blaschke, G. (1998a). Chiral capillary electrophoresis–electrospray mass spectrometry coupling using vancomycin as chiral selector. *Journal of Chromatography A*, Vol.800, No.1, pp. 69–76.

[103] Fanali, S.; Aturki, Z. & Desiderio, C. (1998b). New strategies for chiral analysis of drugs by capillary electrophoresis. *Forensic Science International*, Vol.92, No.2-3, pp. 137-155.

[104] Fanali, S.; Desiderio, C.; Ölvecká, E.; Kaniansky, D.; Vojtek, M. & Ferancová, A. (2000). Separation of enantiomers by on-line capillary isotachophoresis-capillary zone electrophoresis. *Journal of High Resolution Chromatography*, Vol.23, No.9, pp. 531-538.

[105] Fanali, S.; Catarcini, P.; Blaschke, G. & Chankvetadze, B. (2001). Enantioseparations by capillary electrochromatography. *Electrophoresis*, Vol.22, No. 15, pp. 3131-3151.

[106] Fanali, S. (2002). *Century of Separation Science*, H.J. Issaq (Ed.), pp. 579-588, Marcel Dekker, New York.

[107] Fanali, S. (2009). Chiral separations by CE employing CDs. *Electrophoresis.* Vol.30, No.SUPPL. 1, p. S203-S210.
[108] Fang, L.; Kang, J.; Yin, X.-B.; Yang, X. & Wang, E. (2006). CE coupling with end-column electrochemiluminescence detection for chiral separation of disopyramide. *Electrophoresis*, Vol.27, No.22, pp. 4516–4522.
[109] Fang, H.F.; Zeng, Z.R. & Liu, L. (2006a). Centrifuge microextraction coupled with on-line back-extraction field-amplified sample injection method for the determination of trace ephedrine derivatives in the urine and serum. *Analytical Chemistry*, Vol.78, No. 17, pp. 6043-6049.
[110] Fang, H.F.; Liu, M.M. & Zeng, Z.R. (2006b). Solid-phase microextraction coupled with capillary electrophoresis to determine ephedrine derivatives in water and urine using a sol-gel derived butyl methacrylate/silicone fiber. *Talanta*, Vol.68, No. 3, pp. 979-986.
[111] Fenyvesi, E. (1988). Cyclodextrin polymers in the pharmaceutical industry. *Journal of Inclusion Phenomena and Macrocyclic Chemistry*, Vol.6, pp. 537-545.
[112] Fillet, M.; Hubert, P. & Crommen, J. (2000). Enantiomeric separations of drugs using mixtures of charged and neutral cyclodextrins. *Journal of Chromatography A*, Vol.875, No.1-2, pp. 123-134.
[113] Frost, N.W.; Jing, M. & Bowser, M.T. (2010). Capillary Electrophoresis. *Analytical Chemistry*, Vol.82, No.12, pp. 4682-4698.
[114] Gale, D.C. & Smith, R.D. (1993). Small volume and low flow-rate electrospray ionization mass spectrometry of aqueous samples. *Rapid Communications in Mass Spectrometry*, Vol.7, No.11, pp. 1017-1021.
[115] Gaš, B.; Demjanenko, M. & Vacík, J. (1980). High frequency contactless conductivity detection in isotachophoresis. *Journal of Chromatography*, Vol.192, No. 2, pp. 253-257.
[116] Gaspar, A.; Englmann, M.; Fekete, A.; Harir, M. & Schmitt-Kopplin, P. (2008). Trends in CE-MS 2005-2006. *Electrophoresis*, Vol.29, No.1, pp. 66–79.
[117] Gassmann, E.; Kuo, J.E. & Zare, R.N. (1985). Electrokinetic separation of chiral compounds. *Science*, Vol.230, No.4727, pp. 813-814.
[118] Gatti, R. & Gioia, M.G. (2008). Liquid chromatographic fluorescence determination of amino acids in plasma and urine after derivatization with phanquinone. *Biomedical Chromatography*, Vol.22, No.2, 207-213.
[119] Gebauer, P.; Čáslavská, J.; Thormann, W. & Boček, P. (1997). Prediction of zone patterns in capillary zone electrophoresis with conductivity detection. Concept of the zone conductivity diagram. *Journal of Chromatography A*, Vol.772, No.1-2, pp. 63-71.
[120] Gebauer, P.; Malá, Z. & Boček, P. (2009). Recent progress in analytical capillary ITP. *Electrophoresis*, Vol.30, No.1, pp. 29–35.
[121] Gebauer, P.; Malá, Z. & Boček, P. (2011). Recent progress in analytical capillary isotachophoresis. *Electrophoresis*, Vol.32, No.1, pp. 83-89.
[122] Gerhardt, G.C.; Cassidy, R.M. & Baranski, A.S. (2000). Adsorption-based electrochemical detection of nonelectrochemically active analytes for capillary electrophoresis. *Analytical Chemistry*, Vol.72, No.5, pp. 908–915.
[123] Giddings, J.C. (1969). Generation of Variance, "Theoretical Plates," Resolution, and Peak Capacity in Electrophoresis and Sedimentation. *Separation Science*, Vol.4, No.3, pp. 181-189.
[124] Gilpin, R.K. & Gilpin, C.S. (2009). Pharmaceuticals and related drugs. *Analytical Chemistry*, Vol.81, No.12, pp. 4679-4694.

[125] Glowka, F.K. & Karzniewicz, M. (2004a). High performance capillary electrophoresis for determination of the enantiomers of 2-arylpropionic acid derivatives in human serum: Pharmacokinetic studies of ketoprofen enantiomers following administration of standard and sustained release tablets. *Journal of Pharmaceutical and Biomedical Analysis*, Vol.35, No.4, pp. 807-816.

[126] Glowka, F.K. & Karzniewicz, M. (2004b). Resolution of indobufen enantiomers by capillary zone electrophoresis Pharmacokinetic studies of human serum. *Journal of Chromatography A*, Vol.1032, No.1-2, pp. 219-225.

[127] Glowka, F.K. & Karazniewicz, M. (2007). Enantioselective CE method for pharmacokinetic studies on ibuprofen and its chiral metabolites with reference to genetic polymorphism. *Electrophoresis*, Vol.28, No.15, pp. 2726-2737.

[128] Goel, T.V.; Nikelly, J.G.; Simpson, R.C. & Matuszewski, B.K. (2004). Chiral separation of labetalol stereoisomers in human plasma by capillary electrophoresis. *Journal of Chromatography A*, Vol.1027, No.1-2, pp. 213-221.

[129] Gong, X.Y. & Hauser, P.C. (2006). Enantiomeric separation of underivatized small amines in conventional and on-chip capillary electrophoresis with contactless conductivity detection. *Electrophoresis*, Vol.27, No.21, pp. 4375-4382.

[130] Goodlett, D.R.; Loo, R.R.O.; Loo, J.A.; Wahl, J.H.; Udseth H.R. & Smith, R.D. (1994). A study of the thermal denaturation of ribonuclease S by electrospray ionization mass spectrometry. *Journal of American Society for Mass Spectrometry.*, Vol.5, No.7, pp. 614-622.

[131] Gotti, R.; Calleri, E.; Massolini, G.; Furlanetto, S. & Cavrini, V. (2006). Penicillin G acylase as chiral selector in CE using a pullulan-coated capillary. *Electrophoresis*, Vol.27, No.23, pp. 4746-4754.

[132] Grant, I.H. & Steuer, W. (1990). Extended path length UV absorbance detector for capillary zone electrophoresis. *Journal of Microcolumn Separations*, Vol.2, No.2, pp. 74-79.

[133] Grard, S.; Morin, P. & Ribet, J.P. (2002). Application of capillary electrophoresis with field-amplified sample injection for the detection of new adrenoreceptor antagonist enantiomers in plasma in the low ng/mL concentration range. *Electrophoresis*, Vol.23, No.15, pp. 2399-2407.

[134] Gübitz, G. & Schmid, M.G. (2000a). Recent progress in chiral separation principles in capillary electrophoresis. *Electrophoresis*, Vol.21, No., pp. 4112-4135.

[135] Gübitz, G. & Schmid, M.G. (2000b). Chiral separation by capillary electrochromatography. *Enantiomer*, Vol.5, No.1, pp. 5-11.

[136] Gübitz, G. & Schmid, M.G. (2004). Recent advances in chiral separation principles in capillary electrophoresis and capillary electrochromatography. *Electrophoresis*, Vol.25, No.23-24, pp. 3981-3996.

[137] Gübitz, G. & Schmid, M.G. (2006). Chiral separation principles in chromatographic and electromigration techniques. *Molecular Biotechnology*, Vol.32, No.2, pp. 159-179.

[138] Gübitz, G. & Schmid, M.G. (2007). Advances in chiral separation using capillary electromigration techniques. *Electrophoresis*, Vol.28, No.1-2, pp. 114-126.

[139] Gübitz, G. & Schmid, M.G. (2008). Chiral separation by capillary electromigration techniques. *Journal of Chromatography A*, Vol.1204, No.2, pp. 140-156.

[140] Guihen, E.; Hogan, A.M. & Glennon, J.D. (2009). High-Speed Microchip Electrophoresis Method for the Separation of (R,S)-Naproxen. *Chirality*, Vol.21, No.2, pp. 292-298.

[141] Ha, P.T.T.; Van Schepdael, A.; Van Vaeck, L.; Augistijns, P. & Hoogmartens, J. (2004a). Chiral capillary electrophoretic method for quantification of apomorphine. *Journal of Chromatography A,* Vol.1049, No.1-2, pp. 195-203.

[142] Ha, P.T.T.; Van Schepdael, A.; Roets, E. & Hoogmartens, J. (2004b). Investigating the potential of erythromycin and derivatives as chiral selector in capillary electrophoresis. *Journal of Pharmaceutical and Biomedical Analysis,* Vol.34, No.5, pp. 861-870.

[143] Ha, P.T.T.; Hoogmartens, J. & Van Schepdael, A. (2006). Recent advances in pharmaceutical applications of chiral capillary electrophoresis. *Journal of Pharmaceutical and Biomedical Analysis,* Vol.41, No.1, pp. 1-11.

[144] Haber, C.; Roosli, S.; Tsuda, T.; Scheidegger, D.; Müller, S. & Simon, W. (1990). The potentiometric microelectrode as a detector in fast LC and CZE. *12th Int. Symp. Capillary Chromatography, Kobe, Japan.*

[145] Haber, C.; Silvestri, I.; Roosli, S. & Simon, W. (1991). Potentiometric Detector for Capillary Zone Electrophoresis. *Chimia,* Vol.45, No.4, pp. 117-121.

[146] Haber, C.; VanSaun, R.J. & Jones, W.R. (1998). Quantitative Analysis of Anions at ppb/ppt Levels with Capillary Electrophoresis and Conductivity Detection: Enhancement of System Linearity and Precision Using an Internal Standard. *Analytical Chemistry,* Vol.70, No.11, pp. 2261–2267.

[147] Hadwiger, M.E.; Torchia, S.R.; Park, S.; Biggin, M.E. & Lunte, C.E. (1996). Optimization of the separation and detection of the enantiomers of isoproterenol in microdialysis samples by cyclodextrin-modified capillary electrophoresis using electrochemical detection. *Journal of Chromatography B,* Vol.681, No.2, pp. 241-249.

[148] Haginaka, J. (2000). Enantiomer separation of drugs by capillary electrophoresis using proteins as chiral selectors. *Journal of Chromatography A,* Vol.875, No.1-2, pp. 235-254.

[149] Hashim, N.H.; Shafie, S. & Khan, S.J. (2010). Enantiomeric fraction as an indicator of pharmaceutical biotransformation during wastewater treatment and in the environment - a review. *Environmental Technology,* Vol.31, No.12, pp. 1349-1370.

[150] Hashimoto, A.; Nishikawa, T.; Oka, T.; Takahashi, K. & Hayashi, T. (1992). Determination of free amino-acid enantiomers in rat-brain and serum by high-performance liquid-chromatography after derivatization with n-tert-butyloxycarbonyl-L-cysteine and O-phthaldialdehyde. *Journal of Chromatography A,* Vol.582, No.1-2, pp. 41-48.

[151] Hashimoto, A.; Oka, T. & Nishikawa, T. (1995). Anatomical distribution and postnatal changes in endogenous free D-aspartate and D-serine in rat-brain and periphery. *European Journal of Neuroscience,* Vol. 7, No.8, pp. 1657-1663.

[152] Hedeland, Y.; Lehtinen, J. & Pettersson, C. (2007). Ketopinic acid and diisoproylideneketogulonic acid as chiral ion-pair selectors in capillary electrophoresis - Enantiomeric impurity analysis of S-timolol and 1R,2S-ephedrine. *Journal of Chromatography A,* Vol.1141, No.2, pp. 287-294.

[153] Heiger, D.N.; Kaltenbach, P. & Sievert, H.J.P. (1994). Diode array detection in capillary electrophoresis. *Electrophoresis,* Vol.15, No.10, pp. 1234-1247.

[154] Heiger, D. (2000). *High performance capillary electrophoresis: An introduction,* Agilent Technologies, Publication No. 5968-9963E, pp. 135, Germany.

[155] Hempel, G. (2000). Strategies to improve the sensitivity in capillary electrophoresis for the analysis of drugs in biological fluids. *Electrophoresis,* Vol.21, No.4, pp. 691-698.

[156] Henion, J.; Mordehai, A. & Cai, J. (1994). Quantitative capillary electrophoresis-ion spray mass spectrometry on a benchtop ion trap for the determination of isoquinoline alkaloids. *Analytical Chemistry*, Vol.66, No.13, pp. 2103-2109.

[157] Hernández, L.S.; Crego, A.L.; Marina, M.L. & Ruiz, C.G. (2008). Sensitive chiral analysis by CE: An update. *Electrophoresis*, Vol.29, No.1, pp. 237-251.

[158] Hernández, L.S.; Ruiz, C.G.; Marina, M.L. & Crego, A.L. (2010). Recent approaches for enhancing sensitivity in enantioseparations by CE. *Electrophoresis*, Vol.31, No.1, pp. 28-43.

[159] Hödl, H.; Koidl, J.; Schmid, M.G. & Gübitz, G. (2006). Chiral resolution of tryptophan derivatives by CE using canine serum albumin and bovine serum albumin as chiral selectors. *Electrophoresis*, Vol.27, No.23, pp. 4755-4762.

[160] Hödl, H.; Krainer, A.; Holzmuller, K.; Koidl, J.; Schmid, M.G. & Gübitz, G. (2007). Chiral separation of sympathomimetics and β-blockers by ligand-exchange CE using Cu(II) complexes of L-tartaric acid and L-threonine as chiral selectors. *Electrophoresis*, Vol.28, No.15, pp. 2675-2682.

[161] Hogan, B.L.; Lunte, S.M.; Stobaugh, J.F. & Lunte, C.E. (1994). Online coupling of in-vivo microdialysis sampling with capillary electrophoresis. *Analytical Chemistry*, Vol.66, No.5, pp. 596-602.

[162] Holtzel, A. & Tallarek, U. (2007). Ionic conductance of nanopores in microscale analysis systems: Where microfluidics meets nanofluidics. *Journal of Separation Science*, Vol.30, No.10, pp. 1398-1419.

[163] Hopfgartner, G.; Wachs, T.; Bean, K. & Henion, J. (1993). High-flow ion spray liquid chromatography/mass spectrometry. *Analytical Chemistry*, Vol.65, No.4, pp. 439-446.

[164] Horáková, J.; Petr, J.; Maier, V.; Tesařová, E.; Veis, L.; Armstrong, D.W.; Gaš, B. & Ševčík, J. (2007). On-line preconcentration of weak electrolytes by electrokinetic accumulation in CE: Experiment and simulation. *Electrophoresis*, Vol.28, No.10, pp. 1540-1547.

[165] Horstkötter, C. & Blaschke, G. (2001). Stereoselective determination of ofloxacin and its metabolites in human urine by capillary electrophoresis using laser-induced fluorescence detection. *Journal of Chromatography B*, Vol.754, No.1, pp. 169-178.

[166] Hou, J.G.; He, T.X.; Mao, X.F.; Du, X.Z.; Deng, H.L. & Gao, J.Z. (2003). Enantiomeric separation using erythromycin as a new capillary zone electrophoresis chiral selector. *Analytical Letters*, Vol.36, No.7, pp. 1437-1499.

[167] Hou, J.G.; Rizvi, S.A.A.; Zheng, J. & Shamsi, S.A. (2006). Application of polymeric surfactants in micellar electrokinetic chromatography-electrospray ionization mass spectrometry of benzodiazepines and benzoxazocine chiral drugs. *Electrophoresis*, Vol.27, No.5-6, pp. 1263–1275.

[168] Hou, J.; Zheng, J. & Shamsi, S.A. (2007). Separation and determination of warfarin enantiomers in human plasma using a novel polymeric surfactant for micellar electrokinetic chromatography-mass spectrometry. *Journal of Chromatography A*, Vol.1159, No.1-2, pp. 208-216.

[169] Hsi, T.S.; Lin, J.N.; Kuo, K.Y. & Chin, J. (1997). Simultaneous Determination of Carbohydrates and Amino Acids by Capillary Zone Electrophoresis with Constant Potential Amperometric Detection at a Copper Electrode. *Journal of the Chinese Chemical Society*, Vol. 44, No.2, pp. 101–106.

[170] Hu, T.; Zuo, H.; Riley, C.M.; Stobaugh, J.F. & Lunte, S.M. (1995). Determination of α-difluoromethylornithine in blood by microdialysis sampling and capillary electrophoresis with UV detection. *Journal of Chromatography A*, Vol.716, No.1-2, pp. 381-388.

[171] Huang, Z. & Ivory, C.F. (1999). Digitally controlled electrophoretic focusing. *Analytical Chemistry*, Vol.71, No.8, pp. 1628-1632.

[172] Huang, Y.S.; Liu, J.T.; Lin, L.C. & Lin, C.H. (2003). Chiral separation of 3,4-methylenedioxymeth-amphetamine and related compounds in clandestine tablets and urine samples by capillary electrophoresis/fluorescence spectroscopy. *Electrophoresis*, Vol.24, No.6, pp. 1097-1104.

[173] Huang, L.; Lin, J.M.; Yu, L.; Xu, L. & Chen, G. (2008). Field-amplified on-line sample stacking for simultaneous enantioseparation and determination of some beta-blockers using capillary electrophoresis. *Electrophoresis*, Vol.29, No.17, pp. 3588-3594.

[174] Huang, L.; Lin, Q.; Chen, Y.T. &Chen, G. (2011). Transient isotachophoresis with field-amplified sample injection for on-line preconcentration and enantioseparation of some beta-agonists. *Analytical Methods*, Vol.3, No.2, pp. 294-298.

[175] Huck, C.W.; Bakry, R.; Huber, L.A. & Bonn, G.K. (2006). Progress in capillary electrophoresis coupled to matrix-assisted laser desorption/ionization time of flight mass spectrometry. *Electrophoresis*, Vol.27, No.11, pp. 2063–2074.

[176] Huo, Y. & Kok, W.T. (2008). Recent applications in CEC. *Electrophoresis*, Vol.29, No.1, pp. 80-93.

[177] Ibrahim, W.A.W.; Hermawan, D.; Sanagi, M.M. (2007). On-line preconcentration and chiral separation of propiconazole by cyclodextrin-modified micellar electrokinetic chromatography. *Journal of Chromatography A*, Vol.1170, No.1-2, pp. 107-113.

[178] Iio, R.; Chinaka, S.; Takayama, N. & Hayakawa, K. (2005). Simultaneous chiral analysis of methamphetamine and related compounds by capillary electrophoresis/mass spectrometry using anionic cyclodextrin. *Analytical Science*, Vol.21, No.1, pp. 15–19.

[179] Ingelse, B.; Everaerts, F.M.; Desiderio, C. & Fanali, S. (1995). Enantiomeric separation by capillary electrophoresis using a soluble neutral β-cyclodextrin polymer. *Journal of Chromatography A*, Vol.709, No.1, pp. 89-98.

[180] Ivory, C.F. (2000). A brief review of alternative electrofocusing techniques. *Separation Science and Technology*, Vol.35, No.11, pp. 1777.

[181] Jiménez, J.R. & de Castro, M.D.L. (2008). Lab-on-valve for the automatic determination of the total content and individual profiles of linear alkylbenzene sulfonates in water samples. *Electrophoresis*, Vol. 29, No. 3, pp. 590-596.

[182] Juvancz, Z.; Kendrovics, R.B.; Ivanyi, R. & Szente, L. (2008). The role of cyclodextrins in chiral capillary electrophoresis. *Electrophoresis*, Vol.29, No.8, pp. 1701-1712.

[183] Kahle, K.A. & Foley, J.P. (2006). Chiral microemulsion electrokinetic chromatography with two chiral components: Improved separations *via* synergies between a chiral surfactant and a chiral cosurfactant, *Electrophoresis*, Vol.27, No.4, pp. 896–904.

[184] Kahle, K.A. & Foley, J.P. (2007a). Review of aqueous chiral electrokinetic chromatography (EKC) with an emphasis on chiral microemulsion EKC. *Electrophoresis*, Vol.28, No.15, pp. 2503-2526.

[185] Kahle, K.A. & Foley, J.P. (2007b). Two-chiral-component microemulsion electrokinetic chromatography-chiral surfactant and chiral oil: Part 1. Dibutyl tartrate. *Electrophoresis*, Vol.28, No.11, pp., 1723–1734.

[186] Kahle, K.A. & Foley, J.P. (2007c). Two-chiral component microemulsion EKC - Chiral surfactant and chiral oil. Part 2: Diethyl tartrate. *Electrophoresis*, Vol.28, No.15, pp. 2644–2657.

[187] Kahle, K.A. & Foley, J.P. (2007d). Influence of microemulsion chirality on chromatographic figures of merit in EKC: Results with novel three-chiral-component microemulsions and comparison with one- and two-chiral-component microemulsions. *Electrophoresis*, Vol.28, No.11, pp. 3024–3040.

[188] Kaltenbach, P.; Ross, G. & Heiger, D.N. (1997). *HPCE*, Anaheim, CA.

[189] Kaniansky, D. (1981). Kapilárna izotachoforéza, kapilárna zónová elektroforéza a ich on-line spojenie. Ph.D. Thesis, Comenius University, Bratislava.

[190] Kaniansky, D.; Koval', M. & Stankoviansky, S. (1983). Simple cell for conductimetric detection in capillary isotachophoresis. *Journal of Chromatography B*, Vol.267, No.C, pp. 67-73.

[191] Kaniansky, D. & Marák, J. (1990). On-line coupling of capillary isotachophoresis with capillary zone electrophoresis. *Journal of Chromatography*, Vol.498, pp. 191-204.

[192] Kaniansky, D.; Marák, J.; Madajová, V. & Šimuničová, E. (1993). Capillary zone electrophoresis of complex ionic mixtures with on-line isotachophoretic sample pretreatment. *Journal of Chromatography*, Vol.638, No.2, pp. 137-146.

[193] Kaniansky, D.; Iványi, F. & Onuska, F.I. (1994a). Online isotachophoretic sample pretreatment in ultratrace determination of paraquat and diquat in water by capillary zone electrophoresis. *Analytical Chemistry*, Vol.66, No.11, pp. 1817-1824.

[194] Kaniansky, D.; Zelenský, I.; Hybenová, A. & Onuska, F.I. (1994b). Determination of chloride, nitrate, sulfate, nitrite, fluoride, and phosphate by on line coupled capillary isotachophoresis-capillary zone electrophoresis with conductivity detection. *Analytical Chemistry*, Vol.66, No.23, pp. 4258-4264.

[195] Kaniansky, D.; Havaši, P.; Iványi, F. & Marák, J. (1995). Galvanic decoupling of a postcolumn amperometric detector in capillary electrophoresis. *Journal of Chromatography A*, Vol.709, No.1, pp. 69-79.

[196] Kaniansky, D.; Marák, J.; Masár, M.; Iványi, F.; Madajová, V.; Šimuničová, E. & Zelenská, V. (1997). Capillary zone electrophoresis in a hydrodynamically closed separation system with enhanced sample loadability. *Journal of Chromatography A*, Vol.772, No.1-2, pp. 103-114.

[197] Kaniansky, D.; Zelenská, V.; Masár, M.; Iványi, F. & Gazdíková, Š. (1999). Contactless conductivity detection in capillary zone electrophoresis. *Journal of Chromatography A*, Vol.844, No.1-2, pp. 349–359.

[198] Kang, J.W.; Wistuba, D. & Schurig, V. (2002). Recent progress in enantiomeric separation by capillary electrochromatography. *Electrophoresis*, Vol.23, No.22-23, pp. 4005-4021.

[199] Karbaum, A. & Jira, T. (1999). Nonaqueous capillary electrophoresis: Application possibilities and suitability of various solvents for the separation of basic analytes. *Electrophoresis*, Vol.20, No.17, pp. 3396-3401.

[200] Kataoka, H. (2003). New trends in sample preparation for clinical and pharmaceutical analysis. *Trends of Analytical Chemistry*, Vol.22, No.4, pp. 232-244.

[201] Kavran-Belin, G.; Rudaz, S. & Veuthey, J.L. (2005). Enantioseparation of baclofen with highly sulfated β-cyclodextrin by capillary electrophoresis with laser-induced fluorescence detection. *Journal of Separation Science*, Vol.28, No.16, pp. 2187–2192.

[202] Kelly, J.F; Thibault, P.; Locke, S. & Ramaley, L.R. (1994). Analysis of the Oligoaccharides isolated from Glycoproteins by Capillary Elecrrophoresis-Electrospray Mass Spectrometry with Discontinuous Buffer Systems. *42nd ASMS Conference on Mass Spectrometry and Allied Topics, Chicago, IL, 29 May-3 June 1994.*

[203] Kim, J.B. & Terabe, S. (2003). On-line sample preconcentration techniques in micellar electrokinetic chromatography. *Journal of Pharmaceutical and Biomedical Analysis,* Vol.30, No.6, pp. 1625-1643.

[204] Kim, J.B.; Britz-McKibbin, P.; Hirokawa, T. & Terabe, S. (2003). Mechanistic study on analyte focusing by dynamic pH junction in capillary electrophoresis using computer simulation. *Analytical Chemistry,* Vol.75, No.16, pp. 3986-3993.

[205] Kim, M.S.; Cho, S.I.; Lee, K.N. & Kim, Y.K. (2005). Fabrication of microchip electrophoresis devices and effects of channel surface properties on separation efficiency. *Sensors and Actuators B,* Vol.107, No.2, pp. 818–824.

[206] Kirby, D.; Greve, K.F.; Foret, F.; Vouros, P.; Karger B.L. & Nashabeh, W. (1994). Capillary Electrophoresis-Electrospray Ionization-Mass Spectrometry Utilizing Background Electrolytes Containing Surfactants. *42nd ASMS Conference on Mass Spectrometry and Allied Topics, Chicago, IL, 29 May-3 June 1994.*

[207] Kirschner, D.L.; Jaramillo, M. & Green, T.K. (2007). Enantioseparation and stacking of cyanobenz[f]isoindole-amino acids by reverse polarity capillary electrophoresis and sulfated beta-cyclodextrin. *Analytical Chemistry,* Vol.79, No.2, pp. 736-743.

[208] Kitae, T.; Nakayama, T. & Kano, K. (1998). Chiral recognition of α-amino acids by charged cyclodextrins through cooperative effects of Coulomb interaction and inclusion. *Journal of Chemical Society. Perkin Transactions.,* Vol.2, No.2, pp. 207-212.

[209] Kitagawa, F.; Tsuneka, T.; Akimoto, Y.; Sueyoshi, K.; Uchiyama, K.; Hattori, A. & Otsuka, K. (2006). Toward million-fold sensitivity enhancement by sweeping in capillary electrophoresis combined with thermal lens microscopic detection using an interface chip. *Journal of Chromatography A,* Vol.1106, No.1-2., pp. 36-42.

[210] Kitagawa, F. & Otsuka, K. (2011). Recent progress in capillary electrophoretic analysis of amino acid enantiomers. *Journal of Chromatography B,* Vol.879, No.29, pp. 3078– 3095.

[211] Knudsen, C.B. & Beattie, J.H. (1997). On-line solid-phase extraction capillary electrophoresis for enhanced detection sensitivity and selectivity: application to the analysis of metallothionein isoforms in sheep fetal liver. *Journal of Chromatography A,* Vol.792, No.1-2, pp. 463-473.

[212] Kodama, S.; Yamamoto, A.; Matsunaga, A. & Hayakawa, K. (2003). Direct chiral resolution of tartaric acid by ion-pair capillary electrophoresis using an aqueous background electrolyte with (1R,2R)-(-)-1,2-diaminocyclohexane as a chiral counterion. *Electrophoresis,* Vol.24, No.15, pp. 2711-2715.

[213] Kodama, S.; Yamamoto, A.; Iio, R.; Aizawa, S.I.; Nakagomi, K., Hayakawa, K. (2005). Chiral ligand exchange micellar electrokinetic chromatography using borate anion as a central ion. *Electrophoresis,* Vol.26, No.20, pp. 3884–3889.

[214] Kodama, S.; Aizawa, S.; Taga, A.; Yamashita, T. & Yamamoto, A. (2006). Chiral resolution of monosaccharides as 1-phenyl-3-methyl-5-pyrazolone derivatives by ligand-exchange CE using borate anion as a central ion of the chiral selector. *Electrophoresis,* Vol.27, No.23, pp. 4730-4734.

[215] Koegler, W.S. & Ivory, C.F. (1996a). Field gradient focusing: A novel method for protein separation. *Biotechnology Progress,* Vol.12, No.6, pp. 822-836.

[216] Koegler, W.S. & Ivory, C.F. (1996b). Focusing proteins in an electric field gradient. *Journal of Chromatography A*, Vol.726, No.1-2, pp. 229-236.
[217] Kohr, J. & Engelhardt, H. (1993). Characterization of quartz capillaries for capillary electrophoresis. *Journal of Chromatography*, Vol. 652, No.2, pp. 309-316.
[218] Kok, S.J.; Velthorst, N.H.; Gooijer, C. & Brinkman, U.A.T. (1998). Analyte identification in capillary electrophoretic separation techniques. *Electrophoresis*, Vol.19, No.16-17, pp. 2753-2776.
[219] Konieczna, L.; Plenis, A.; Oledzka, I.; Kowalski, P. & Baczek, T. (2010). Rapid RP-LC Method with Fluorescence Detection for Analysis of Fexofenadine in Human Plasma. *Chromatographia*, Vol.71, No.11-12, pp. 1081-1086.
[220] Kraly, J.; Fazal, M.A.; Schoenherr, R.M.; Bonn, R.; Harwood, M.M.; Turner, E.; Jones, M. & Dovichi, N.J. (2006). Bioanalytical applications of capillary electrophoresis. *Analytical Chemistry*, Vol.78, No.12, pp. 4097-4110.
[221] Kriger, M.S.; Ramsey, R.S. & Cook, K.D. (1994). Evaluation of a Sheathless Capillary Electrophoresis/Electrospray Ionization Interface on an Ion Trap Mass Spectrometer. *42nd ASMS Conference on Mass Spectrometry and Allied Topics, Chicago, IL, 29 May-3 June 1994.*
[222] Kubačák, P.; Mikuš, P.; Valášková, I. & Havránek, E. (2006a). Separation of dimetinden enantiomers in drugs by means of capillary isotachophoresis. *Česká a Slovenská Farmacie*, Vol.55, No.1, pp. 32-35.
[223] Kubačák, P.; Mikuš, P.; Valášková, I. & Havránek, E. (2006b). Chiral separation of feniramine in medicaments with the use of capillary isotachophoresis. *Farmaceutický Obzor*, Vol.75, No.2-3, pp. 48-51.
[224] Kubačák, P.; Mikuš, P.; Valášková, I. & Havránek, E. (2007). Chiral separation of alkylamine antihistamines in pharmaceuticals by capillary Isotachophoresis with charged cyclodextrin. *Drug Development and Industrial Pharmacy*, Vol.33, No.11, pp. 1199-1204.
[225] Kuhn, R. (1999). Enantiomeric separation by capillary electrophoresis using a crown ether as chiral selector. *Electrophoresis*, Vol.20, No.13, pp. 2605-2613.
[226] Lacorte, S. & Fernandez-Albaz, A. R. (2006). Time of flight mass spectrometry applied to the liquid chromatographic analysis of pesticides in water and food. *Mass Spectrometry Reviews*, Vol.25, No.6, pp. 866–880.
[227] Lada, M.W. & Kennedy, R.T. (1995). Quantitative *in vivo* measurements using microdialysis on-line with capillary zone electrophoresis. *Journal of Neuroscience Methods*, Vol.63, No.1-2, pp.147-.
[228] Lada, M.W. & Kennedy, R.T. (1996). Quantitative in vivo monitoring of primary amines in rat caudate nucleus using microdialysis coupled by a flow-gated interface to capillary electrophoresis with laser-induced fluorescence detection. *Analytical Chemistry*, Vol.68, No.17, pp. 2790-2797.
[229] Lada, M.W. & Kennedy, R.T. (1997). In vivo monitoring of glutathione and cysteine in rat caudate nucleus using microdiolysis on-line with capillary zone electrophoresis-laser induced fluorescence detection. *Journal of Neuroscience Methods*, Vol. 72, No.2, pp. 153-159.
[230] Lada, M.W.; Vickroy, T.W. & Kennedy, R.T. (1997). High temporal resolution monitoring of glutamate and aspartate in vivo using microdialysis on-line with

capillary electrophoresis with laser-induced fluorescence detection. *Analytical Chemistry,* Vol.69, No.22, pp. 4560-4565.
[231] Lada, M.W.; Vickroy, T.W. & Kennedy, R.T. (1998). Evidence for neuronal origin and metabotropic receptor-mediated regulation of extracellular glutamate and aspartate in rat striatum in vivo following electrical stimulation of the prefrontal cortex. *Journal of Neurochemistry,* Vol.70, No.2, pp.617-625.
[232] Lämmerhofer, M.; Svec, F.; Frechet, J.M.J. & Lindner, W. (2000). Separation of enantiomers by capillary electrochromatography. *Trac-Trends in Analytical Chemistry,* Vol.19, No.11, pp. 676-698.
[233] Landers, J.P. (1997). *Handbook of Capillary Electrophoresis,* CRC Press, New York.
[234] Lapainis, T.; Scanlan, C.; Rubakhin, S.S. & Sweedler, J.V. (2007). A multichannel native fluorescence detection system for capillary electrophoretic analysis of neurotransmitters in single neurons. *Analytical and Bioanalytical Chemistry,* Vol.387, No.1, pp. 97-105.
[235] Lee, J.; Lee, H.K.; Rasmussen, K.E. & Bjergaard, S.P. (2008). Environmental and bioanalytical applications of hollow fiber membrane liquid-phase microextraction: A review. *Anal. Chim. Acta,* Vol.624, No.2, pp. 253-268.
[236] Li, S.F.Y. & Kricka, L.J. (2006). Clinical Analysis by Microchip Capillary Electrophoresis. *Clinical Chemistry,* Vol.52, No.1,pp. 37–45.
[237] Li, O.L.; Liu, C. & Chen, Z.G. (2008). Application of capillary electrophoresis and microfluidics in drug screening. *Chinese Journal of New Drugs,* Vol.17, No.22, pp. 1910-1914.
[238] Li, H.; Wang, P.H.; Li, C.; Wang, H. & Zhang, H.S. (2008). Steroselective determination of trihexyphenidyl using carboxylmethyl-beta-cyclodextrin by capillary electrophoresis with field-amplified sample stacking. *Microchem. J.,* Vol.89, No.1, pp. 34-41.
[239] Li, X.; Song, B.; Yuan, B.; Sun, J. & You, T. (2009). Enantioseparation of Dioxopromethazine Hydrochloride in Urine with Liquid-Liquid Extraction by CE-ECL Detection. *Chromatographia,* Vol.70, No.7-8, pp. 1291-1293.
[240] Li, Y.; Song, C.; Zhang, L.; Zhang, W. & Fu, H. (2010). Fabrication and evaluation of chiral monolithic column modified by beta-cyclodextrin derivatives. *Talanta,* Vol.80, No.3, pp. 1378-1384.
[241] Lin, C.C.; Li, Y.T. & Chen, S.H. (2003). Recent progress in pharmacokinetic applications of capillary electrophoresis. *Electrophoresis,* Vol.24, No.22-23, pp. 4106-4115.
[242] Lin, C.H. & Kaneta, T. (2004). On-line sample concentration techniques in capillary electrophoresis: Velocity gradient techniques and sample concentration techniques for biomolecules. *Electrophoresis,* Vol.25, No.23-24, pp. 4058-4073.
[243] Liu, H.C.; Yu, Y.; Wang, N.; Deng, M.; Liu, J.F. & Xue, H.Y. (2004). Pharmacokinetics of the Enantiomers of trans-Tramadol and its Active Metabolite, trans-O-Demethyltramadol, in Healthy Male and Female Chinese Volunteers. *Chirality,* Vol.16, No.2, pp. 112-118.
[244] Liu, Z. & Pawliszyn, J. (2006). Online coupling of solid-phase microextraction and capillary electrophoresis. *Journal of Chromatographic Science,* Vol.44, No.6, pp. 366–374.
[245] Lloyd, D.K. & Wätzig, H. (1995). Sodium dodecyl-sulfate solution is an effective between-run rinse for capillary electrophoresis of samples in biological matrices. *Journal of Chromatography B,* Vol.663, No.2, pp. 400-405.

[246] Long, Z.C., Liu, D.Y., Ye, N.N., Qin, J.H. & Lin, B.C. (2006). Integration of nanoporous membranes for sample filtration/preconcentration in microchip electrophoresis. *Electrophoresis*, Vol.27, No.24, pp. 4927–4934.

[247] Lord, H. & Pawliszyn, J. (2000). Evolution of solid-phase microextraction technology. *Journal of Chromatography A*, Vol.885, No.1-2, pp. 153–193.

[248] Lü, W.J.; Chen, Y.L.; Zhu, J.H. & Chen, X.G. (2009). The combination of flow injection with electrophoresis using capillaries and chips. *Electrophoresis*, Vol.30, No.1, pp.83-91.

[249] Lu, W.Z. & Cassidy, R.M. (1993). Pulsed amperometric detection of carbohydrates separated by capillary electrophoresis. *Analytical Chemistry*, Vol.65, No.20, pp. 2878-2881.

[250] Lu, W. Z.; Poon, G. K.; Carmichael, P. L &, Cole, R. B. (1996). Analysis of tamoxifen and its metabolites by on-line capillary electrophoresis electrospray ionization mass spectrometry employing nonaqueous media containing surfactants. *Analytical Chemistry*, Vol.68, No.4, pp. 668–674.

[251] Lu, W. & Cole, R. B. (1998). Determination of chiral pharmaceutical compounds, terbutaline, ketamine and propranolol, by on-line capillary electrophoresis-electrospray ionization mass spectrometry. *Journal of Chromatography B*, Vol.714, No.1, pp. 69–75.

[252] Lu, H.A. & Chen, G.N. (2011). Recent advances of enantioseparations in capillary electrophoresis and capillary electrochromatography. *Analytical Methods*, Vol.3, No.3, pp. 488-508.

[253] Lurie, I.S. (1997). Separation selectivity in chiral and achiral capillary electrophoresis with mixed cyclodextrins. *Journal of Chromatography A*, Vol.792, No.1-2, pp. 297-307.

[254] Maier, N. M.; Franco, P. & Lindner, W. (2001). Separation of enantiomers: Needs, challenges, perspectives. *Journal of Chromatography A*, Vol.906, No.1-2, pp. 3–33.

[255] Mainka, A. & Bachmann, K. (1997). UV detection of derivatized carbonyl compounds in rain samples in capillary electrophoresis using sample stacking and a Z-shaped flow cell. *Journal of Chromatography A*, Vol.767, No.1-2, pp. 241-247.

[256] Malá, Z.; Křivánková, L.; Gebauer, P. & Boček, P. (2007). Contemporary sample stacking in CE: A sophisticated tool based on simple principles. *Electrophoresis*, Vol.28, No.1-2, pp. 243-253

[257] Malá, Z.; Šlampová, A.; Gebauer, P. & Boček, P. (2009). Contemporary sample stacking in CE. *Electrophoresis*, Vol.30, No.1, pp. 215–229.

[258] Malá, Z.; Gebauer, P. & Boček, P. (2011). Contemporary sample stacking in analytical electrophoresis. *Electrophoresis*, Vol.32, No.1, pp. 116-126.

[259] Mandrioli, R.; Pucci, V.; Sabbioni, C.; Bartoletti, C.; Fanali, S. & Raggi, M.A. (2004). Enantioselective determination of the novel antidepressant mirtazapine and its active demethylated metabolite in human plasma by means of capillary electrophoresis. *Journal of Chromatography A*, Vol.1051, No.1-2, pp. 253-260.

[260] Marák, J.; Mikuš, P.; Maráková, K.; Kaniansky, D.; Valášková, I. & Havránek, E. (2007). Enantioselective analysis of pheniramine in urine by charged CD-mediated CZE provided with a fiber-based DAD and an on-line sample pretreatment by capillary ITP. *Electrophoresis*, Vol.28, No.15, pp. 2738-2747.

[261] Marák, J.; Mikuš, P.; Maráková, K.; Kaniansky, D.; Valášková, I. & Havránek, E. (2008). Potentialities of ITP-CZE method with diode array detection for enantiometric purity control of dexbrompheniramine in pharmaceuticals. *Journal of Pharmaceutical and Biomedical Analysis*, Vol.46, No.5, pp. 870-876.

[262] Mardones, C.; Ríos, A.; Valcárcel, M. & Cicciarelli, R. (1999). Enantiomeric separation of D- and L-carnitine by integrating on-line derivatization with capillary zone electrophoresis. *Journal of Chromatography A*, Vol.849, No.2, pp. 609-6166.

[263] Marsh, A.; Clark, B.; Broderick, M.; Power, J.; Donegan, S. & Altria, K. (2004). Recent advances in microemulsion electrokinetic chromatography. *Electrophoresis*, Vol.25, No.23-24, pp. 3970-3980.

[264] Martínez-Gómez, M.A.; Sagrado, S.; Villanueva-Camañas, R.M. & Medina-Hernández, M.J. (2007). Enantiomeric quality control of antihistamines in pharmaceuticals by affinity electrokinetic chromatography with human serum albumin as chiral selector. *Anal. Chim. Acta*, Vol.592, No.2, pp. 202-209.

[265] Martins, L.F.; Yegles, M. & Wennig, R. (2008). Simultaneous enantioselective quantification of methadone and of 2-ethylidene-1,5-dimethyl-3,3-diphenyl-pyrrolidine in oral fluid using capillary electrophoresis. *Journal of Chromatography B*, Vol.862, No.1-2, pp. 79-85.

[266] Masár, M.; Žúborová, M.; Bielčíková, J.; Kaniansky, D.; Jöhnck, M. & Stanislawski, B. (2001). Conductivity detection and quantitation of isotachophoretic analytes on a planar chip with on-line coupled separation channels. *Journal of Chromatography A*, Vol.916, No.1-2, pp. 101–111.

[267] McEvoy, E.; Marsh, A.; Altria, K.; Donegan, S. & Power, J. (2007). Recent advances in the development and application of microemulsion EKC. *Electrophoresis*, Vol.28, No.1-2, pp. 193-207.

[268] Mechref, Y. & El Rassi, Z. (1997). Capillary electrophoresis of herbicides .4. Evaluation of octylmaltopyranoside chiral surfactant in the enantiomeric separation of fluorescently labeled phenoxy acid herbicides and their laser-induced fluorescence detection. *Electrophoresis*, Vol.18, No.2, pp. 220-226.

[269] Miao, H.; Rubakhin, S. S. & Sweedler, J. V. (2005). Subcellular analysis of D-Aspartate. *Analytical Chemistry*, Vol.77, No.22, pp. 7190–7194.

[270] Miao, H.; Rubakhin, S. S. & Sweedler, J. V. (2006). Confirmation of peak assignments in capillary electrophoresis using immunoprecipitation: Application to D-aspartate measurements in neurons. *Journal of Chromatography A*, Vol.1106, No.1-2, pp. 56–60.

[271] Mikkers, F.E.P.; Everaerts, F.M. & Verheggen, T.P.E.M. (1979). Concentration distributions in free zone electrophoresis. *Journal of Chromatography*, Vol.169, No.C, pp. 1-10.

[272] Mikuš, P.; Kaniansky, D.; Šebesta, R. & Sališová, M. (1999). Analytical characterizations of purities of alkyl- and arylamino derivatives of β-cyclodextrin by capillary zone electrophoresis with conductivity detection. *Enantiomer*, Vol.4, No.3-4, pp. 279-287.

[273] Mikuš, P. & Kaniansky, D. (2000). Derivatization Reactions in Capillary Electrophoresis of Amino Acids [Derivatizačné reakcie v kapilárnej elektroforéze aminokyselín]. *Chemické Listy*, Vol.94, No.6, pp. 347-354.

[274] Mikuš, P.; Kaniansky, D. & Fanali, S. (2001). Separation of multicomponent mixtures of 2,4-dinitrophenyl labelled amino acids and their enantiomers by capillary zone electrophoresis. *Electrophoresis*, Vol.22, No.3, pp. 470-477.

[275] Mikuš, P.; Kaniansky, D.; Šebesta, R. & Sališová, M. (2002). Cyclodextrins and Their Complexes - Structure and Interactions. *Chemické Listy*, Vol.96, No.8, pp.696-697.

[276] Mikuš, P.; Valášková, I. & Havránek, E. (2005a). Enantioselective determination of pheniramine in pharmaceuticals by capillary electrophoresis with charged cyclodextrin. *Journal of Pharmaceutical and Biomedical Analysis*, Vol.38, No.3, pp. 442-448.

[277] Mikuš, P.; Valášková, I. & Havránek, E. (2005b). Enantioselective analysis of cetirizine in pharmaceuticals by cyclodextrin-mediated capillary electrophoresis. *Journal of Separation Science,* Vol.28, No.12, pp. 1278-1284.

[278] Mikuš, P.; Kubačák, P.; Valášková, I. & Havránek, E. (2006a). Analysis of enantiomers in biological matrices by charged cyclodextrin-mediated capillary zone electrophoresis in column-coupling arrangement with capillary isotachophoresis. *Talanta,* Vol.70, No.4, pp. 840-846.

[279] Mikuš, P.; Kubačák, P.; Valášková, I. & Havránek, E. (2006b). Comparison of capillary zone electrophoresis and isotachophoresis determination of dimethindene enantiomers in pharmaceuticals using charged carboxyethyl-beta-cyclodextrin as a chiral selector. *Methods and Findings in Experimenatal and Clinical Pharmacology,* Vol.28, No.9, pp. 595-599.

[280] Mikuš, P. & Kaniansky, D. (2007). Capillary zone electrophoresis resolutions of 2,4-dinitrophenyl labeled amino acids enantiomers by N-methylated amino-β-cyclodextrins. *Analytical Letters,* Vol.40, No.2, pp. 335-347.

[281] Mikuš, P.; Maráková, K.; Marák, J.; Nemec, I.; Valášková, I. & Havránek, E. (2008a). Direct quantitative determination of amlodipine enantiomers in urine samples for pharmacokinetic study using on-line coupled isotachophoresis-capillary zone electrophoresis separation method with diode array detection. *Journal of Chromatography B,* Vol.875, No.1, pp. 266-272.

[282] Mikuš, P.; Maráková, K.; Marák, J.; Kaniansky, D.; Valášková, I. & Havránek, E. (2008b). Possibilities of column-coupling electrophoresis provided with a fiber-based diode array detection in enantioselective analysis of drugs in pharmaceutical and clinical samples. *Journal of Chromatography A,* Vol.1179, No.1, pp. 9-16.

[283] Mikuš, P. & Maráková, K. (2009). Advanced capillary electrophoresis for chiral analysis of drugs, metabolites and biomarkers in biological samples. *Electrophoresis,* Vol.30, No.16, pp. 2773-2802.

[284] Mikuš, P. & Maráková, K. (2010). Chiral capillary electrophoresis with on-line sample preparation. *Current Pharmaceutical Analysis,* Vol.6, No.2, pp. 76-100.

[285] Mikuš, P. (2010). Chiral Capillary electrophoresis with on-line sample pretreatment and spectral detection in pharmaceutical and biomedical analysis. *Acta Facultatis Pharmaceuticae Universitatis Comenianae,* Vol.57, No.1, pp. 9-17.

[286] Mikuš, P. & Maráková, K (2011). Column Coupling Electrophoresis in Biomedical Analysis, R. Fazel-Rezai, (Ed.), in: *Biomedical Engineering - From Theory to Applications,* pp. 81-130, InTech, ISBN 978-953-307-637-0, Rijeka.

[287] Minard, R.D.; Chin-Fatt, D.; Carry, P.J. & Ewing, A.G. (1988). *36th ASMS Conference on Mass Spectrometry and Allied Topics, San Francisco, CA, 5-10 June 1988.*

[288] Mohanty, A. & Dey, J. (2006). Enantioselectivity of vesicle-forming chiral surfactants in capillary electrophoresis. Role of the surfactant headgroup structure. *Journal of Chromatography A,* Vol.1128, No.1-2, pp. 259–266.

[289] Mokhtari, B., Pourabdollah, K. & Dalali, N. (2011). Molecule and ion recognition of nano-baskets of calixarenes since 2005. *Journal of Coordination Chemistry,* Vol.64, No.5, pp. 743-794.

[290] Monton, M.R.N. & Soga, T. (2007). Metabolome analysis by capillary electrophoresis-mass spectrometry. *Journal of Chromatography A,* Vol.1168, No.1-2, pp. 237–246.

[291] Moseley, M.A.; Deterding, L.J.; Tomer, K.B. & Jorgenson, J.W. (1989a). Capillary-zone electrophoresis/fast-atom bombardment mass spectrometry: design of an on-line coaxial continuous-flow interface. *Rapid Communications in Mass Spectrometry,* Vol.3, No.3, pp. 87-93.

[292] Moseley, M.A.; Deterding, L.J.; Tomer, K.B. & Jorgenson, J.W. (1989b). Coupling of capillary zone electrophoresis and capillary liquid chromatography with coaxial continuous-flow fast atom bombardment tandem sectro mass spectrometry. *Journal of Chromatography,* Vol.480, No.C, pp. 197-209.

[293] Moseley, M.A. (1994). Preconcenrration Capillary Zone Electrophoresis Coupled with Electrospray Ionization Mass Spectrometry. *42nd ASMS Conference on Mass Spectrometry and Allied Topics, Chicago, IL, 29 May-3 June 1994.*

[294] Muck, W.M. & Henion, J.D. (1989). Determination of leucine enkephalin and methionine enkephalin in equine cerebrospinal fluid by microbore high-performance liquid chromatography and capillary zone electrophoresis coupled to tandem mass spectrometry. *Journal of Chromatography,* Vol.495, pp. 41-59.

[295] Müller, D. & Blaschke, G. (2000). Enantioselective assay of chloroquine and its main metabolite deethyl chloroquine in human plasma by capillary electrophoresis. *Journal of Chromatographic Science,* Vol.38, No.10, pp. 435-440.

[296] Natishan, T.K. (2005). Recent progress in the analysis of pharmaceuticals by capillary electrophoresis. *Journal of Liquid Chromatography and Related Technologies,* Vol.28, No.7-8, pp. 1115-1160.

[297] Nie, S.; Dadoo, R. & Zare, N. (1993). Ultrasensitive fluorescence detection of polycyclic aromatic hydrocarbons in capillary electrophoresis. *Analytical Chemistry,* Vol.65, No.24, pp. 3571-3575.

[298] Nilsson, J.; Spégel, P. & Nilsson, S. (2004) Molecularly imprinted polymer formats for capillary electrochromatography. *Journal of Chromatography B,* Vol.804, No.1, pp. 3-12

[299] Nishi, H.; Fukuyama, T. & Terabe, S. (1991). Chiral separation by cyclodextrin-modified micellar electrokinetic chromatography. *Journal of Chromatography,* Vol.553, No.1-2, pp. 503-516.

[300] Nishi, H.; Izumoto, S.; Nakamura, K.; Nakai, H. & Sato, T. (1996a). Dextran and dextrin as chiral selectors in capillary zone electrophoresis. *Chromatographia,* Vol.42, No.11-12, pp. 617-630.

[301] Nishi, H.S.; Nakamura, K.; Nakai, H. & Sato, T. (1996b). Enantiomer separation by capillary electrophoresis using DEAE-dextran and aminoglycosidic antibiotics. *Chromatographia,* Vol.43, No.7-8, pp. 426-430.

[302] Nishi, H. (1997). Enantioselectivity in chiral capillary electrophoresis with polysaccharides. *Journal of Chromatography A,* Vol.792, No.1-2, pp. 327-347.

[303] Nojavan, S. & Fakhari, A.R. (2010). Electro membrane extraction combined with capillary electrophoresis for the determination of amlodipine enantiomers in biological samples. *Journal of Separation Science,* Vol.33, No.20, pp. 3231-3238.

[304] Nojavan, S. & Fakhari, A.R. (2011). Chiral separation and quantitation of cetirizine and hydroxyzine by maltodextrin-mediated CE in human plasma: Effect of zwitterionic property of cetirizine on enantioseparation. *Electrophoresis,* Vol.32, No.6-7, pp. 764-771.

[305] Novotny, M.; Soini, H. & Stefansson, M. (1994). Chiral separation through capillary electromigration methods. *Analytical Chemistry,* Vol.66, No.11, pp. 646A-655A.

[306] Nozal, L.; Arce, L.; Simonet, B.M.; Rios, A. & Valcárcel, M. (2007). In-line liquid-phase microextraction for selective enrichment and direct electrophoretic analysis of acidic drugs. *Electrophoresis*, Vol.28, No.18, pp. 3284-3289.

[307] Nzeadibe, K. & Vigh, G. (2007). Synthesis of mono-6-deoxy-6-N,N,N',N',N'-pentamethylethylenediammonio-cyclomaltoheptaose, a single-isomer, monosubstituted, permanently dicationic β-CD and its use for enantiomer separations by CE. *Electrophoresis*, Vol.28, No.15, pp. 2589-2605.

[308] O'Brien, K.B.; Esguerra, M.; Klug, C.T.; Miller, R.F. & Bowser, M.T. (2003). A high-throughput on-line microdialysis-capillary assay for D-serine. *Electrophoresis*, Vol.24, No.7-8, pp. 1227-1235.

[309] Ohnesorge, J.; Neusüß X, Ch. & Wätzig, H. (2005). Quantitation in capillary electrophoresis-mass spectrometry. *Electrophoresis*, Vol.26, No.21, pp. 3973–3987.

[310] Ölvecká, E.; Masár, M.; Kaniansky, D.; Jöhnck, M. & Stanislawski, B. (2001). Isotachophoresis separations of enantiomers on a planar chip with coupled separation channels. *Electrophoresis*, Vol.22, No.15, pp. 3347-3353.

[311] O'Shea, T.J.; Lunte, S.M. & LaCourse, W.R. (1993). Detection of carbohydrates by capillary electrophoresis with pulsed amperometric detection. *Analytical Chemistry*, Vol.65, No.7, pp. 948-951.

[312] Ossicini, L. & Fanali, S. (1997). Enantiomeric separations by electrophoretic techniques. *Chromatographia*, Vol.45, pp. 428-432.

[313] Oswald, T.M. & Ward, T.J. (1999). Enantioseparations with the macrocyclic antibiotic ristocetin a using A countercurrent process in CE. *Chirality*, Vol.11, No.8, pp. 663-668.

[314] Otsuka, K.; Matsumura, M.; Kim, J.B. & Terabe, S. (2003). On-line preconcentration and enantio selective separation of triadimenol by electrokinetic chromatography using cyclodextrins as chiral selectors. *Journal of Pharmaceutical and Biomedical Analysis*, Vol.30, No.6, pp. 1861-1867.

[315] Ouyang, G. & Pawliszyn, J. (2006). SPME in environmental analysis. *Analytical and Bioanalytical Chemistry*, Vol.386, No.4, pp.1059–1073.

[316] Palcut, M. & Rabara, L. (2009). Host-guest Interactions of Coumarin 6 with beta-cyclodextrin in Polar Solvents. *Acta Chimica Slovenica*, Vol.56, No.4, pp. 845-851.

[317] Pálmarsdóttir, S. & Edholm, L.H. (1995). Enhancement of selectivity and concentration sensitivity in capillary zone electrophoresis by online coupling with column liquid-chromatography and utilizing a double stacking procedure allowing for microliter injections. *Journal of Chromatography A*, Vol.693, No.1, pp. 131-143.

[318] Pálmarsdóttir, S.; Mathiasson, L.; Jönsson, J.A. & Edholm, L.H. (1996). Micro-CLC as an interface between SLM extraction and CZE for enhancement of sensitivity and selectivity in bioanalysis of drugs. *Journal of Capillary Electrophoresis*, Vol.3, No.5, pp. 255-260.

[319] Pálmarsdóttir, S.; Mathiasson, L.; Jönsson, J.A. & Edholm, L.H. (1997). Determination of a basic drug, bambuterol, in human plasma by capillary electrophoresis using double stacking for large volume injection and supported liquid membranes for sample pretreatment. *Journal of Chromatography B*, Vol.688, No.1, pp. 127-134.

[320] Palmer, J.; Munro, N.J. & Landers, J.P. (1999). A universal concept for stacking neutral analytes in micellar capillary electrophoresis. *Analytical Chemistry*, Vol.71, No.9, pp. 1679-1687.

[321] Palmer, J.; Burgi, D.S. & Landers, J.P. (2001). Electrokinetic injection for stacking neutral analytes in capillary and microchip electrophoresis. *Analytical Chemistry*, Vol.73, No.4, pp. 725-731

[322] Palmer, C.P. & McCarney, J.P. (2004a). Developments in the use of soluble ionic polymers as pseudo-stationary phases for electrokinetic chromatography and stationary phases for electrochromatography. *Journal of Chromatography A*, Vol.1044, No.1-2, pp. 159-176.

[323] Palmer, C.P. & McCarney, J.P. (2004b). Recent progress in the use of soluble ionic polymers as pseudostationary phases for electrokinetic chromatography. *Electrophoresis*, Vol.25, No.23-24, pp. 4086-4094.

[324] Palmer, C.P. (2007). Recent progress in the use of ionic polymers as pseudostationary phases for EKC. *Electrophoresis*, Vol.28, No.1-2, pp. 164-173.

[325] Pantučková, P.; Gebauer, P.; Boček, P. & Křivánková, L. (2009). Electrolyte systems for on-line CE-MS: Detection requirements and separation possibilities. *Electrophoresis*, Vol.30, No.1, pp. 203–214.

[326] Park, H.; Lee, S.; Kang, S.; Jung, Y.J. & Jung, S.H. (2004). Enantioseparation using sulfated cyclosophoraoses as a novel chiral additive in capillary electrophoresis. *Electrophoresis*, Vol.25, No.16, pp. 2671-2674.

[327] Pawliszyn, J. (1997). *Solid-phase Microextraction – Theory and Practice*, Wiley-VCH: New York.

[328] Peng, X.J.; Sternberg, E. & Dolphin, D. (2002). Aberrant expression of signaling-related proteins 14-3-3 gamma and RACK1 in fetal Down Syndrome brain (trisomy 21). *Electrophoresis*, Vol.23, No.1, pp. 93-101.

[329] Petersson, M.; Wahlund, K.G. & Nilsson S. (1999). Miniaturised on-line solid-phase extraction for enhancement of concentration sensitivity in capillary electrophoresis. *Journal of Chromatography A*, Vol.841, No.2, pp. 249-261.

[330] Piehl, N.; Ludwig, M. & Belder, D. (2004). Subsecond chiral separations on a microchip. *Electrophoresis*, Vol.25, No.21-22, pp. 3848-3852.

[331] Phillips, T.M. (1998). Determination of in situ tissue neuropeptides by capillary immunoelectrophoresis. *Analytica Chimica Acta*, Vol.372, No.1-2, pp. 209-218.

[332] Pleasance, S.; Thibault, P. & Kelly, J. (1992). Comparison of liquid-junction and coaxial interfaces for capillary electrophoresis-mass spectrometry with application to compounds of concern to the aquaculture industry. *Journal of Chromatography*, Vol.591, No.1-2, pp. 325-339.

[333] Poppe, H. (1980). Characterization and design of liquid phase flow-through detector systems. *Analytica Chimica Acta*, Vol.114, No.C, pp. 59-70.

[334] Powe, A.M.; Das, S.; Lowry, M.; El-Zahab, B.; Fakayode, S.O.; Geng, M.L.; Baker, G.A.; Wang, L.; McCarroll, M.E.; Patonay, G.; Li, M.; Aljarrah, M.; Neal, S. & Warner, I.M. (2010). Molecular Fluorescence, Phosphorescence, and Chemiluminescence Spectrometry, *Analytical Chemistry*, Vol.82, No.12, pp. 4865-4894.

[335] Preinerstorfer, B.; Lubda, D.; Lindner, W. & Lämmerhofer, M. (2006). Monolithic silica-based capillary column with strong chiral cation-exchange type surface modification for enantioselective non-aqueous capillary electrochromatography. *Journal of Chromatography A*, Vol.1106, No.1-2, pp. 94–105.

[336] Preinerstorfer, B.; Lämmerhofer, M. & Lindner, W. (2009). Advances in enantioselective separations using electromigration capillary techniques. *Electrophoresis*, Vol.30, No.1, pp. 100-132.

[337] Prost, F.; Čáslavská, J. & Thormann, W. (2002). Chiral analysis of albendazole sulfoxide enantiomers in human plasma and saliva using capillary electrophoresis with on-column absorption and fluorescence detection. *Journal of Separation Science*, Vol.25, No.15-17, pp. 1043-1054.

[338] Ptolemy, A.S.; Le Bilhan, M. & Britz-McKibbin, P. (2005). On-line sample preconcentration with chemical derivatization of bacterial biomarkers by capillary electrophoresis: A dual strategy for integrating sample pretreatment with chemical analysis. *Electrophoresis*, Vol.26, No.23-24, pp. 4206-4214.

[339] Ptolemy, A.S.; Tran, L. & Britz-McKibbin, P. (2006). Single-step enantioselective amino acid flux analysis by capillary electrophoresis using on-line sample preconcentration with chemical derivatization. *Analytical Biochemistry*, Vol.354, No.2, pp. 192-204.

[340] Ptolemy, A.S. & Britz-McKibbin, P. (2006). Sample preconcentration with chemical derivatization in capillary electrophoresis - Capillary as preconcentrator, microreactor and chiral selector for high throughput metabolite screening. *Journal of Chromatography A*, Vol.1106, No.1-2, pp. 7-18.

[341] Puig, P.; Borrull, F.; Calull, M. & Aguilar, C. (2007a). Recent advances in coupling solid-phase extraction and capillary electrophoresis (SPE-CE). *Trac-Trends in Analytical Chemistry*, Vol.26, No.7, pp. 664-678.

[342] Puig, P.; Tempels, F.W.A.; Borrull, F.; Calull, M.; Aguilar, C.; Somsen, G.W & de Jong, G.J. (2007b). On-line coupling of solid-phase extraction and capillary electrophoresis for the determination of cefoperazone and ceftiofur in plasma. *Journal of Chromatography B*, Vol. 856, No.1-2, pp. 365-370.

[343] Puig, P.; Borrull, F.; Calull, M. & Aguilar, C. (2008). Sorbent preconcentration procedures coupled to capillary electrophoresis for environmental and biological applications. *Analytica Chimica Acta*, Vol.616, No.1, pp. 1-18.

[344] Quan, Z.; Song, Y.; Feng, Y.; LeBlanc, M.H. & Liu, Y.-M. (2005). Detection of D-serine in neural samples by saccharide enhanced chiral capillary electrophoresis. *Analytica Chimica Acta*, Vol.528, No.1, pp. 101–106.

[345] Quirino, J.P. & Terabe, S. (1998). Exceeding 5000-fold concentration of dilute analytes in micellar electrokinetic chromatography. *Science*, Vol.282, No.5388, pp. 465-468.

[346] Quirino, J.P. & Terabe, S. (1999). Sweeping of analyte zones in electrokinetic chromatography. *Analytical Chemistry*, Vol.71, No.8, pp. 1638-1644.

[347] Quirino, J.P. & Terabe, S. (2000). Sample stacking of cationic and anionic analytes in capillary electrophoresis. *Journal of Chromatography A*, Vol.902, No.1, pp. 119-135.

[348] Quirino, J.P.; Iwai, Y.; Otsuka, K. & Terabe, S. (2000). Determination of environmentally relevant aromatic amines in the ppt levels by cation selective exhaustive injection-sweeping-micellar electrokinetic chromatography. *Electrophoresis*, Vol.21, No.14, pp. 2899-2903.

[349] Ramautar, R.; Demirci, A. & De Jong, G. J. (2006). Capillary electrophoresis in metabolomics. *Trends in Analytical Chemistry*, Vol.25, No.5, pp. 455–466.

[350] Ramautar, R.; Somsen, G.W. & de Jong, G.J. (2009). CE-MS in metabolomics. *Electrophoresis*, Vol.30, No.1, pp. 276–291.

[351] Riekkola, M.L.; Wiedmer, S.K.; Valkó, I.E. & Sirén, H. (1997). Selectivity in capillary electrophoresis in the presence of micelles, chiral selectors and non-aqueous media. *Journal of Chromatography A*, Vol.792, No.1-2, pp. 13-35.

[352] Rizkov, D.; Mizrahi, S.; Cohen, S. & Lev, O. (2010). beta-Amino alcohol selectors for enantioselective separation of amino acids by ligand-exchange capillary zone electrophoresis in a low molecular weight organogel. *Electrophoresis,* Vol.31, No.23-24, pp. 3921-3927.

[353] Rizvi, S.A.A.; Akbay, C. & Shamsi, S.A. (2004). Polymeric alkenoxy amino acid surfactants: II. Chiral separations of β-blockers with multiple stereogenic centers. *Electrophoresis*, Vol.25, No.6, pp. 853–860.

[354] Rizvi, S.A.A. & Shamsi, S.A. (2006). Synthesis, characterization, and application of chiral ionic liquids and their polymers in micellar electrokinetic chromatography. *Analytical Chemistry*, Vol.78, No.19, pp. 7061-7069.

[355] Rizvi, S.A.A.; Zheng, J.; Apkarian, R.P.; Dublin, S.N., & Shamsi, S.A. (2007). Polymeric sulfated amino acid surfactants: A class of versatile chiral selectors for micellar electrokinetic chromatography (MEKC) and MEKC-MS. *Analytical Chemistry*, Vol.79, No.3, pp. 879–898.

[356] Rizzi, A. (2001). Fundamental aspects of chiral separations by capillary electrophoresis. *Electrophoresis*, Vol.22, No.15, pp. 3079–3106.

[357] Robinson, T.E. & Justice, J.B. (1991). *Microdialysis in the Neurosciences*, Elsevier: Amsterdam.

[358] Ross, D. & Locascio, L.E. (2002). Microfluidic temperature gradient focusing. *Analytical Chemistry*, Vol.74, No.11, pp. 2556-2564.

[359] Rudaz, S.; Cherkaoui, S.; Dayer, P.; Fanali, S. & Veuthey, J.L. (2000). Simultaneous stereoselective analysis of tramadol and its main phase I metabolites by on-line capillary zone electrophoresis-electrospray ionization mass spectrometry. *Journal of Chromatography A*, Vol.868, No.2, pp. 295-303.

[360] Rudaz, S.; Geiser, L.; Souverain, S.; Prat, J. & Veuthey, J.L. (2005). Rapid stereoselective separations of amphetamine derivatives with highly sulfated γ-cyclodextrin. *Electrophoresis*, Vol.26, No.20, pp. 3910–3920.

[361] Ruiz, C.G. & Marina, M.L. (2006). Sensitive chiral analysis by capillary electrophoresis. *Electrophoresis,* Vol.27, No.1, pp. 195-212.

[362] Rundlett, K.L. & Armstrong, D.W. (1995). Effect of micelles and mixed micelles on efficiency and selectivity of antibiotic-based capillary electrophoretic enantioseparations. *Analytical Chemistry*, Vol.67, No.13, pp. 2088-2095.

[363] Ryan, R.; Donegan, S.; Power, J.; McEvoy, E. & Altria, K. (2009). Recent advances in the methodology, optimisation and application of MEEKC. *Electrophoresis*, Vol.30, No.1, pp. 65–82.

[364] Saito, Y. & Jinno, K. (2003). Miniaturized sample preparation combined with liquid phase separations. *Journal of Chromatography A*, Vol.1000, No.1-2, pp. 53–67.

[365] Santos, B.; Simonet, B.M.; Rios, A. & Valcarcel, M. (2007). On-line coupling of solid-phase microextraction to commercial CE-MS equipment. *Electrophoresis,* Vol.28, No.9, pp. 1312–1318.

[366] Schappler, J.; Guillarme, D.; Prat, J.; Veuthey, J.L. & Rudaz, S. (2006). Enhanced method performances for conventional and chiral CE-ESI/MS analyses in plasma. *Electrophoresis*, Vol.27, No.8, pp. 1537–1546.

[367] Schappler, J.; Guillarme, D.; Prat, J.; Veuthey, J.L. & Rudaz, S. (2008). Validation of chiral capillary electrophoresis-electrospray ionization-mass spectrometry methods for ecstasy and methadone in plasma. *Electrophoresis*, Vol.29, No.10, pp. 2193-2202.

[368] Schmitt-Kopplin, P. & Frommberger, M. (2003). Capillary electrophoresis - Mass spectrometry: 15 years of developments and applications. *Electrophoresis*, Vol.24, No.22-23, pp. 3837–3867.

[369] Schmitt-Kopplin, P. & Englmann, M. (2005). Capillary electrophoresis - Mass spectrometry: Survey on developments and applications 2003-2004. *Electrophoresis*, Vol.26, No.7-8, pp. 1209-1220.

[370] Schulte, G.; Heitmeier, S.; Chankvetadze, B. & Blaschke, G. (1998). Chiral capillary electrophoresis-electrospray mass spectrometry coupling with charged cyclodextrin derivatives as chiral selectors. *Journal of Chromatography A*, Vol.800, No.1, pp. 77–82.

[371] Schwarz, M.A. & Hauser, P.C. (2001). Rapid chiral on-chip separation with simplified amperometric detection. *Journal of Chromatography A*, Vol.928, No.2, pp. 225–232.

[372] Schwarz; M.A. & Hauser, P.C. (2003). Chiral on-chip separations of neurotransmitters. *Analytical Chemistry*, Vol.75, No.17, pp. 4691-4695.

[373] Schwer, C.; Gaš, B.; Lottspeich, F. & Kenndler, E. (1993). Computer simulation and experimental evaluation of on-column sample preconcentration in capillary zone electrophoresis by discontinuous buffer systems. *Analytical Chemistry*, Vol.65, No.15, pp. 2108-2115.

[374] Scriba, G.K.E. (2002). Selected fundamental aspects of chiral electromigration techniques and their application to pharmaceutical and biomedical analysis. *Journal of Pharmaceutical and Biomedical Analysis*, Vol.27, No.3-4, pp. 373-399.

[375] Scriba, G.K.E. (2003). Pharmaceutical and biomedical applications of chiral capillary electrophoresis and capillary electrochromatography: An update. *Electrophoresis*, Vol.24, No.15, pp. 2409-2421.

[376] Scriba, G.K.E. (2007). Nonaqueous capillary electrophoresis-mass spectrometry. *Journal of Chromatography A*, Vol.1159, No.1-2, pp. 28–41.

[377] Scriba, G.K.E. (2008). Cyclodextrins in capillary electrophoresis enantioseparations - Recent developments and applications. *Journal of Separation Science*, Vol. 31, No.11, pp. 1991-2011.

[378] Scriba, G.K.E. (2011). Fundamental aspects of chiral electromigration techniques and application in pharmaceutical and biomedical analysis. *Journal of Pharmaceutical and Biomedical Analysis*, Vol.55, No.4, pp. 688-701.

[379] Ševčík, J.; Stránský, Z.; Ingelse, B. & Lemr, K. (1996). Capillary electrophoretic enantioseparation of selegiline, methamphetamine and ephedrine using a neutral β-cyclodextrin epichlorhydrin polymer. *Journal of Pharmaceutical and Biomedical Analysis*, Vol.14, No.8-10, pp. 1089-1094.

[380] Servais, A.C.; Chiap, P.; Hubert, P.; Crommen, J. & Fillet, M. (2004). Determination of salbutamol enantiomers in human urine using heptakis(2,3-di-O-acetyl-6-O-sulfo)-β-cyclodextrin in nonaqueous capillary electrophoresis. *Electrophoresis*, Vol.25, No.10-11, pp. 1632-1640.

[381] Servais, A.C.; Fillet, M.; Mol, R.; Somsen, G.W.; Chiap, P.; Jong, G.J.D. & Crommen, J. (2006). On-line coupling of cyclodextrin mediated nonaqueous capillary electrophoresis to mass spectrometry for the determination of salbutamol enantiomers in urine. *Journal of Pharmaceutical and Biomedical Analysis*, Vol.40, No.3, pp. 752–757.

[382] Severs, J.C. & Games, D.E. (1994). CZE and Transient CTTP-ES-MS Using H_20 and D_20 Based Electrolyte Systems. *42nd ASMS Conference on Mass Spectrometry and Allied Topics, Chicago, IL, 29 May-3 June 1994.*

[383] Shackman, J.G. & Ross, D. (2007). Counter-flow gradient electrofocusing. *Electrophoresis*, Vol.28, No.4, pp. 556-571.

[384] Shamsi, S.A. (2002). Chiral capillary electrophoresis-mass spectrometry: Modes and applications. *Electrophoresis*, Vol.23, No.22-23, pp. 4036–4051.

[385] Sheeley, S.A.; Miao, H.; Ewing, M.A.; Rubakhin, S.S. & Sweedler, J.V. (2005). Measuring D-amino acid-containing neuropeptides with capillary electrophoresis. *Analyst*, Vol.130, No.8, pp. 1198–1203.

[386] Shihabi, Z.K. (2002). Transient pseudo-isotachophoresis for sample concentration in capillary electrophoresis. *Electrophoresis*, Vol.23, No.11, pp. 1612-1617.

[387] Shou, C.Q., Kang, J.F. & Song, N.J. (2008). Preparation and evaluation of capillary electrophoresis column bonded by carbosilane dendrimer. *Chinese Journal of Analytical Chemistry*, Vol.36, No.3, pp. 297-300.

[388] Silva, M. (2009). Micellar electrokinetic chromatography: Methodological and instrumental advances focused on practical aspects. *Electrophoresis*, Vol.30, No.1, pp. 50–64.

[389] Simpson, S.L.; Quirino, J.P. & Terabe, S. (2008). On-line preconcentration in capillary electrophoresis Fundamentals and applications. *Journal of Chromatography A*, Vol.1184, No.1-2, pp. 504 - 541.

[390] Skoog, D.A.; Holler, F.J. & Crouch, S.R (2007). *Principles of Instrumental Analysis* 6th ed. Thomson Brooks/Cole Publishing: Belmont, CA.

[391] Smyth, W.F. & Rodriguez, V. (2007). Recent studies of the electrospray ionisation behaviour of selected drugs and their application in capillary electrophoresis-mass spectrometry and liquid chromatography-mass spectrometry. *Journal of Chromatography A*, Vol.1159, No.1-2, pp. 159–174.

[392] Soetebeer, U.B.; Schierenberg, M.O.; Schulz, H.; Andresen, P. & Blaschke, G. (2001). Direct chiral assay of tramadol and detection of the phase II metabolite O-demethyl-tramadol glucuronide in human urine using capillary electrophoresis with laser-induced native fluorescence detection. *Journal of Chromatography B*, Vol.765, No.1,pp. 3-13.

[393] Soga, T.; Ohashi, Y.; Ueno, Y.; Naraoka, H.; Tomita, M. & Nishioka, T. (2003). Quantitative Metabolome Analysis Using Capillary Electrophoresis Mass Spectrometry. *Journal of Proteome Research*, Vol.2, No.5, pp. 488–494.

[394] Soga, T. (2007). Capillary electrophoresis-mass spectrometry for metabolomics. *Methods in Molecular Biology*, Vol.358, pp. 129–137.

[395] Strašík, S.; Danková, M.; Molnárová, M.; Ölvecká, E. & Kaniansky, D. (2003). Capillary zone electrophoresis in wide bore capillary tubes with fiber-coupled diode array detection. *Journal of Chromatography A*, Vol.990, No.1-2, pp. 23-33.

[396] Suntornsuk, L. (2010). Recent advances of capillary electrophoresis in pharmaceutical analysis. *Analytical and Bioanalytical Chemistry*, Vol.398, No.1, pp. 29-52.

[397] Swinney, K. & Bornhop, D.J. (2000). Detection in capillary electrophoresis. *Electrophoresis*, Vol.21, no. 7, p. 1239-1250.

[398] Szökö, E.; Tábi, T.; Halasz, A.S.; Palfi, M.; Kalasz, M. & Magyar, K. (2004). Chiral characterization and quantification of deprenyl-N-oxide and other deprenyl metabolites in rat urine by capillary electrophoresis. *Chromatographia*, Vol.60, No.SUPPL, pp. S245-S251.

[399] Tagliaro, F.; Manetto, G.; Bellini, S.; Scarcella, D.; Smith, F.P. & Marigo, M. (1998). Simultaneous chiral separation of 3,4-methylenedioxymethamphetamine (MDMA), 3-4-methylenedioxyamphetamine (MDA), 3,4-methylenedioxyethylamphetamine (MDE),

ephedrine, amphetamine and methamphetamine by capillary electrophoresis in uncoated and coated capillaries with native beta-cyclodextrin as the chiral selector: Preliminary application to the analysis of urine and hair. *Electrophoresis*, Vol.19, No.1, pp. 42-50.

[400] Tan, L.; Wang, Y.; Liu, X.; Ju, H. & Li, J. (2005). Simultaneous determination of L- and D-lactic acid in plasma by capillary electrophoresis. *Journal of Chromatography B*, Vol.814, No.2, pp. 393-398.

[401] Tanaka, Y. & Terabe, S. (1995). Partial separation zone technique for the separation of enantiomers by affinity electrokinetic chromatography with proteins as chiral pseudo-stationary phases. *Journal of Chromatography A*, Vol.694, No.1, pp. 277-284.

[402] Taylor, J.A. & Yeung, E.S. (1991). Axial-beam absorbance detection for capillary electrophoresis. *Journal of Chromatography*, Vol.550, No.1-2, pp. 831-837.

[403] Tekeľ, J. & Mikuš, P. (2005). *Analysis of Substances in Biological Systems*; Jahnátková; A. (Ed.), pp. 135-171, Comenius University, Bratislava.

[404] Tempels, F.W.A.; Wiese, G.; Underberg, W.J.M; Somsen, G.W. & de Jong, G.J. (2006). On-line coupling of size exclusion chromatography and capillary electrophoresis via solid-phase extraction and a Tee-split interface. *Journal of Chromatography B*, Vol. 839, No.1-2, pp. 30-35.

[405] Tempels, F.W.A.; Underberg, W.J.M.; Somsen, G.W. & de Jong, G.J. (2007). On-line coupling of SPE and CE-MS for peptide analysis. *Electrophoresis*, Vol.28, No.9, pp.1319–1326.

[406] Terabe, S.; Otsuka, K.; Ichikawa, K.; Tsuchiya, A. & Ando, T. (1984). Electrokinetic separations with micellar solutions and open-tubular capillaries [2]. *Analytical Chemistry*, Vol.56, No.1, pp. 111-113

[407] Terabe, S. (1992). *Micellar Electrokinetic Chromatography*, Beckman., California

[408] Theurillat, R.; Knobloch, M.; Levionnois, O.; Larenza, P.; Mevissen, M. & Thormann, W. (2005). Characterization of the stereoselective biotransformation of ketamine to norketamine via determination of their enantiomers in equine plasma by capillary electrophoresis. *Electrophoresis*, Vol.26, No.20, pp. 3942-3951.

[409] Theurillat, R.; Knobloch, M.; Schmitz, A.; Lassahn, P.G.; Mevissen, M. & Thormann, W. (2007). Enantioselective analysis of ketamine and its metabolites in equine plasma and urine by CE with multiple isomer sulfated β-CD. *Electrophoresis*, Vol.28, No.15, pp. 2748-2757.

[410] Theurillat, R. & Thormann, W. (2008). Capillary electrophoresis evidence of the stereoselective ketoreduction of mebendazole and aminomebendazole in echinococcosis patients. *Journal of Separation Science.*, Vol.31, No.1, pp. 188-194.

[411] Thiele, C.; Auerbach, D.; Jung, G. & Wenz, G. (2011). Inclusion of chemotherapeutic agents in substituted beta-cyclodextrin derivatives, Conference Information: 1st European Cyclodextrin Conference, OCT 11-13, 2009 Aalborg, DENMARK, *Journal of Inclusion Phenomena and Macrocyclic Chemistry*, Vol.69, No.3-4 (Sp. Iss.), pp. SI 303-307.

[412] Thibault, P.; Paris, C. & Pleasance, S. (1991). Analysis of peptides and proteins by capillary electrophoresis/mass spectrometry using acidic buffers and coated capillaries. *Rapid Communications in Mass Spectrometry*, Vol.5, No.10, pp. 484-490.

[413] Thompson, T.J.; Foret, F.; Vouros, E. & Karger, B.L. (1993). Capillary electrophoresis/electrospray ionization mass spectrometry: Improvement of protein detection limits using on-column transient isotachophoretic sample preconcentration. *Analytical Chemistry*, Vol.65, No.7, pp. 900-906.

[414] Thompson, J.E.; Vickroy, T.W. & Kennedy, R.T. (1999). Rapid determination of aspartate enantiomers in tissue samples by microdialysis coupled on-line with capillary electrophoresis. *Analytical Chemistry,* Vol.71, No.13, pp.2379-2384.
[415] Tomáš, R.; Koval, M. & Foret, F. (2010). Coupling of hydronynamically closed large bore capillary isotachophoresis with electrospray mass spectrometry. *Journal of Chromatography A,* Vol.1217, No.25, pp. 4144-4149.
[416] Tomlinson, A.J.; Nevala, W.K.; Braddock, W.D.; Strausbauch, M.A.; Wettstein, P.J. & Naylor, S. (1994). Drug Metabolism Studies by On-Line CE-ESI-MS/MS. *42nd ASMS Conference on Mass Spectrometry and Allied Topics, Chicago, IL, 29 May-3 June 1994.*
[417] Toussaint, B.; Hubert, P.; Tjaden, U.R.; Van Der Greef, J. & Crommen, J. (2000). Enantiomeric separation of clenbuterol by transient isotachophoresis-capillary zone electrophoresis-UV detection - New optimization technique for transient isotachophoresis *Journal of Chromatography A,* Vol.871, No.1-2, pp. 173-180.
[418] Toussaint, B.; Palmer, M. & Chiap, P. (2001). On-line coupling of partial filling-capillary zone electrophoresis with mass spectrometry for the separation of clenbuterol enantiomers. *Electrophoresis,* Vol.22, No.7, pp. 1363-1372.
[419] Trojanowicz, M. (2009). Recent developments in electrochemical flow detections—A review, Part I. Flow analysis and capillary electrophoresis. *Analytica Chimica Acta,* Vol.653, No.1, pp. 36–58.
[420] Tsimachidis, D.; Česla, P.; Hájek, T.; Theodoridis, G. & Jandera, P. (2008). Capillary electrophoretic chiral separation of Cinchona alkaloids using a cyclodextrin selector. *Journal of Separation Science,* Vol.31, No.6-7, pp. 1130-1136.
[421] Tsuda, T.; Sweedler, J.V. & Zare, R.N. (1990). Rectangular capillaries for capillary zone electrophoresis. *Analytical Chemistry,* Vol.62, No.19, pp. 2149-2152.
[422] Turiel, E. & Martin-Esteban, A. (2004). Molecularly imprinted polymers: towards highly selective stationary phases in liquid chromatography and capillary electrophoresis. *Analytical and Bioanalytical Chemistry,* Vol.378, No.8, pp. 1876-1886
[423] Tzanavaras, P.D. (2010). Recent Advances in the Analysis of Organic Impurities of Active Pharmaceutical Ingredients and Formulations: A Review. *Current Organic Chemistry,* Vol.14, No.19, pp. 2348-2634.
[424] Urbánek, M.; Křivánková, L. & Boček, P. (2003). Stacking phenomena in electromigration: From basic principles to practical procedures. *Electrophoresis,* Vol.24, No.3, pp. 466.
[425] Vacík, J.; Zuska, J. & Muselasová, I. (1985). Improvement of the performance of a high-frequency contactless conductivity detector for isotachophoresis. *Journal of Chromatography,* Vol.320, No.1, pp. 233-240.
[426] Valkó, I.E.; Sirén, H. & Riekkola, M.L. (1996). Chiral separation of dansyl amino acids by capillary electrophoresis: Comparison of formamide and N-methylformamide as background electrolytes. *Chromatographia,* Vol.43, No.5-6, pp. 242-246.
[427] Van Eeckhaut, A. & Michotte, Y. (2006). Chiral separations by capillary electrophoresis: Recent developments and applications. *Electrophoresis,* Vol.27, No.14, pp. 2880-2895.
[428] Varghese, J.V. & Cole, R.B. (1993). Cetyltrimethylammonium chloride as a surfactant buffer additive for reversed polarity capillary electrophoresis-electrospray mass spectrometry. *Journal of Chromatography A,* Vol.652, No.2, pp. 369-372

[429] Vespalec, R. & Boček, P. (1999). Chiral separations in capillary electrophoresis. *Electrophoresis*, Vol.20, No.13, pp. 2579-2591.

[430] Vespalec, R. & Boček, P. (2000). Chiral separations in capillary electrophoresis. *Chemical Reviews*, Vol.100, No.10, pp. 3715-3753.

[431] von Brocke, A.; Nicholson, G. & Bayer, E. (2001). Recent advances in capillary electrophoresis/electrospray-mass spectrometry. *Electrophoresis*, Vol.22, No.7, pp. 1251–1266

[432] www.chm.bris.ac.uk/ms/theory/maldi-ionisation.html

[433] www.chm.bris.ac.uk/ms/theory

[434] www.chm.bris.ac.uk/ms/theory/qit-massspec.html

[435] www.csi.chemie.tu-darmstadt.de

[436] www.kore.co.uk/tutorial.htm

[437] www.ks.uiuc.edu

[438] www.noble.org/PlantBio/Sumner/metabolomics.html

[439] www.rsc.org

[440] www.sigmaaldrich.com

[441] Wahl, J.H.; Goodlett, D.R.; Udseth, H.R. & Smith, R.D. (1992). Attomole level capillary electrophoresis-mass spectrometric protein analysis using 5-μm-i.d. capillaries. *Analytical Chemistry*, Vol.64, No.24, pp. 3194-3196.

[442] Wahl, J.H.; Goodlett, D.R. & Udseth, H.R. (1993). Use of small-diameter capillaries for increasing peptide and protein detection sensitivity in capillary electrophoresis-mass spectrometry. *Electrophoresis*, Vol.14, No.5-6, pp. 448-457.

[443] Wahl, J.H.; Gale, D.C. & Smith, R.D. (1994). Sheathless capillary electrophoresis-electrospray ionization mass spectrometry using 10 μm I.D. capillaries: Analyses of tryptic digests of cytochrome c. *Journal of Chromatography* A, Vol.659, No.1, pp. 217-222.

[444] Wang, T.; Aiken, J.H.; Huie, C.W. & Hartwick, R.A. (1991). Nanoliter-scale multireflection cell for absorption detection in capillary electrophoresis. *Analytical Chemistry*, Vol.63, No.14, pp. 1372-1376.

[445] Wang, F. & Khaledi, M.G. (1996). Chiral Separations by Nonaquaous Capillary Electrophoresis. *Analytical Chemistry*, Vol.68, No.19, pp. 3460-3467.

[446] Wang, C.Y.; Shang, Z.C.; Mei, J.H. & Yu, Q.S. (2003). Synthesis of a new chiral receptor containing 1,7-diaza-12-crown-4 and its application in chiral separation. *Synthetic Communications*, Vol.33, No.19, pp. 3381-3386.

[447] Wang, Z.; Wang, J.; Hu, Z. & Kang, J. (2007). Enantioseparation by CE with vacomycin as chiral selector: Improving the separation performance by dynamic coating of the capillary with poly(dimethylacrylamide). *Electrophoresis*, Vol.28, No.6, pp. 938-943.

[448] Wang, R.; Jia, Z.P.; Fan, J.J.; Chen, L.R.; Xie, H.; Ma, J.; G, X. & Wang, J. (2007). CE, with hydroxypropyl-β-cyclodextrin as chiral selector, for separation and determination of the enantiomers of amlodipine in the serum of hypertension patients. *Chromatographia*, Vol.65, No.9-10, pp. 575-579.

[449] Wang, L.J.; Hu, S.Q.; Guo, Q.L., Yang, G.L. & Chen, X.G. (2011). Di-n-amyl L-tartrate-boric acid complex chiral selector in situ synthesis and its application in chiral nonaqueous capillary electrophoresis. *Journal of Chromatography A*, Vol.1218, No.9, pp. 1300-1309.

[450] Wang, H.Y.; Chu, X.; Zhao, Z.X.; He, X.S. & Guo, Y.L. (2011). Analysis of low molecular weight compounds by MALDI-FTICR-MS. *Journal of Chromatography* B, Vol.879, No.17-18, pp. 1166–1179.

[451] Wang, Z.Y.; Liu, C. & Kang, J.W. (2011). A highly sensitive method for enantioseparation of fenoprofen and amino acid derivatives by capillary electrophoresis with on-line sample preconcentration. *Journal of Chromatography A,* Vol.1218, No.13, pp. 1775-1779.

[452] Ward, T.J. (1994). For capillary electrophoresis. *Analytical Chemistry*, Vol.66, No.11, pp. 633A-640A.

[453] Ward, T.J.; Baker, B.A. (2008). Chiral separations. *Analytical Chemistry*, Vol.80, No.12, pp. 4363-4372.

[454] Ward, T.J. & Ward, K.D. (2010). Chiral Separations: Fundamental Review 2010. *Analytical Chemistry*, Vol.82, No.12, p. 4712-4722

[455] Weiss, D.J.; Saunders, K. & Lunte, C.E. (2001). Determination of nucleosides natural Cordyceps sinensis and cultured Cordyceps mycelia by capillary electrophoresis. *Electrophoresis,* Vol.22, No1. pp. 144-150.

[456] Weng, X.; Bi, H.; Liu, B. & Kong, J. (2006). On-chip chiral separation based on bovine serum albumin-conjugated carbon nanotubes as stationary phase in a microchannel. *Electrophoresis*, Vol.27, No.15, pp. 3129-3135

[457] Wenz, G.; Strassnig, C.; Thiele, C.; Engelke, A.; Morgenstern, B. & Hegetschweiler, K. (2008). Recognition of ionic guests by ionic beta-cyclodextrin derivatives. *Chemistry - A European Journal*, Vol.14, No.24, pp. 7202-7211.

[458] Wistuba, D. & Schurig, V. (2000a). Recent progress in enantiomer separation by capillary electrochromatography. *Electrophoresis,* Vol.21, No.18, pp. 4136-4158.

[459] Wistuba, D. & Schurig, V. (2000b). Enantiomer separation of chiral pharmaceuticals by capillary electrochromatography. *Journal of Chromatography A*, Vol.875, No.1-2, pp. 255-276.

[460] Wistuba, D.; Bogdanski, A.; Larsen, K.L. & Schurig, V. (2006). δ-Cyclodextrin as novel chiral probe for enantiomeric separation by electromigration methods. *Electrophoresis*, Vol.27, No.21, pp. 4359-4363.

[461] Whitehouse, C.M.; Dreyer, R.N.; Yamashita, M. & Fenn, J.B. (1985). Electrospray interface for liquid chromatographs and mass spectrometers. *Analytical Chemistry*, Vol.57, No.3, pp. 675-679.

[462] Wren, S.A.C. & Rowe, R.C. (1992). Theoretical aspects of chiral separation in capillary electrophoresis. I. Initial evaluation of a model. *Journal of Chromatography*, Vol.603, No.1-2, pp. 235-241.

[463] Wren, S.A.C. & Rowe, R.C. (1993). Theoretical aspects of chiral separation in capillary electrophoresis. III. Application to β-blockers. *Journal of Chromatography*, Vol.635, No.1-2, pp. 113-118.

[464] Wu, X.Z. (2003). New approaches to sample preparation for capillary electrophoresis. *Trends in Analytical Chemistry*, Vol.22, No.1, pp. 48-58.

[465] Xu, L.; Basheer, C. & Lee, H.K. (2007). Developments in single-drop microextraction. *Journal of Chromatography A*, Vol.1152, No.1-2, pp. 184-192.

[466] Xue, Q. & Yeung, E.S. (1995). Differences in the chemical reactivity of individual molecules of an enzyme. *Nature*, Vol.373, No.6516, pp. 681-683.

[467] Yang, L.; Harrata, K. & Lee, S. (1997). On-Line Micellar Electrokinetic Chromatography-Electrospray Ionization Mass Spectrometry Using Anodically Migrating Micelles. *Analytical Chemistry*, Vol.69, No.10, pp. 1820–1826.

[468] Yeung, E.S. (1989). Indirect detection methods: Looking for what is not there. *Acc. Chem. Res.*, Vol.22, No.4, pp. 125-130.

[469] Yu, C.J.; Chang, H.C. & Tseng, W.L. (2008). On-line concentration of proteins by SDS-CGE with LIF detection. *Electrophoresis*, Vol.29, No.2, pp. 483-490.

[470] Zandkarimi, M.; Shafaati, A.; Foroutan, S.M. & Lucy, Charles A. (2009). Rapid enantioseparation of amlodipine by highly sulfated cyclodextrins using short-end injection capillary electrophoresis. *Daru-Journal of Faculty of Pharmacy*, Vol.17, No.4, pp. 269-276.

[471] Zeng, A.G.; Wang, C.H.; Wang, L. & Fu, Q. (2010). Study on absorptive difference between S-amlodipine and RS-amlodipine in rat intestine. *Chinese Pharmaceutical Journal*, Vol.45, No.13, pp. 991-996.

[472] Zhang, L.H. & Wu, X.Z. (2007). Capillary electrophoresis with in-capillary solid-phase extraction sample cleanup. *Analytical Chemistry*, Vol.79, No.6, pp. 2562–2569.

[473] Zhao, J.; Hooker, T. & Jorgenson, J.W. (1999). Synchronous cyclic capillary electrophoresis using conventional capillaries: System design and preliminary results. *Journal of Microcolumn Separations*, Vol.11, No.6, pp. 431-437.

[474] Zhao, J. & Jorgenson, J.W. (1999). Application of synchronous cyclic capillary electrophoresis: Isotopic and chiral separations. *Journal of Microcolumn Separations*, Vol.11, No.6, pp. 439-449.

[475] Zhao, S.L.; Yuan, H.Y. & Xiao, D. (2005a). Detection of D-Serine in rat brain by capillary electrophoresis with laser induced fluorescence detection. *Journal of Chromatography B*, Vol.822, No.1-2, pp. 334–338.

[476] Zhao, S.L.; Song, Y.R. & Liu, Y.M. (2005b). A novel capillary electrophoresis method for the determination of d-serine in neural samples. *Talanta*, Vol.67, No.1, pp. 212–216.

[477] Zhao, S.; Wang, H.; Zhang, R.; Tang, L. & Liu, Y.M. (2006a). Degradingdehydroabietylisothiocyanate as a chiral derivatizing reagent for enantiomeric separations by capillary electrophoresis. *Electrophoresis*, Vol.27, No.17, pp. 3428-3433.

[478] Zhao, S.; Zhang, R.; Wang, H.; Tang, L. & Pan, Y. (2006b). Capillary electrophoresis enantioselective separation of vigabatrin enantiomers by precolumn derivatization with dehydroabietylisothiocyante and UV-vis detection. *Journal of Chromatography B*, Vol.833, No.2, pp. 186-190.

[479] Zhao, S.; Wang, H.; Pan, Y.; He, M. & Zhao, Z. (2007). 3-[(3-Dehydroabietamidopropyl)dimethylammonio]-1-propane-sulfonate as a new type of chiral surfactant for enantiomer separation in micellar electrokinetic chromatography. *Journal of Chromatography A*, Vol.1145, No.1-2, pp. 246-249.

[480] Zheng, J. & Shamsi, S. A. (2006). Simultaneous enantioseparation and sensitive detection of eight β-blockers using capillary electrochromatography-electrospray ionization-mass spectrometry. *Electrophoresis*, Vol.27, No.11, pp. 2139–2151.

[481] Zheng, J.; Norton, D. & Shamsi, S. A. (2006). Fabrication of internally tapered capillaries for capillary electrochromatography electrospray ionization mass spectrometry. *Analytical Chemistry*, Vol.78, No.4, pp. 1323–1330.

[482] Zhou, S.Y.; Zuo, H.; Stobaugh, J.F.; Lunte, C.E. & Lunte, S.M. (1995). Continuous in-vivo monitoring of amino-acid neurotransmitters by microdialysis sampling with online derivatization and capillary electrophoresis separation. *Analytical Chemistry*, Vol.67, No.3, pp. 594-599.

[483] Zhou, S.Y.; Heckert, D.M.; Zuo, H.; Lunte, C.E. & Lunte, S.M. (1999). Online coupling of in vivo microdialysis with capillary electrophoresis/electrochemistry. *Analytica Chimica Acta*, Vol.379, No.3, pp.307-317.

[484] Zhou, Z.; Li, X.; Chen, X. & Hao, X. (2010). Synthesis of ionic liquids functionalized β-cyclodextrin-bonded chiral stationary phases and their applications in high-performance liquid chromatography. *Analytica Chimica Acta*, Vol.678, No.2, pp. 208-214.

[485] Zhu, Z.; Zhang, L.; Marimuthu, A. & Yang, Z. (2003). Large-volume sample stacking combined with separation by 2-hydroxypropyl-b-cyclodextrin for analysis of isoxyzolylpenicillins by capillary electrophoresis. *Electrophoresis*, Vol.24, No.17, pp. 3089-3096.

8

Abbreviations

ACN	acetonitrile
AML	amlodipine
BGE/BGS	background electrolyte/background system
CBI	cyanobenz[*f*]isoindole
CC	column coupling
CDs	cyclodextrins
α/β/γ-CD	α/β-cyclodextrin
M–β-CD	methyl-β- cyclodextrin
CE-β-CD	carboxyethyl-β- cyclodextrin
S-β/γ-CD	sulphated-β/γ- cyclodextrin
CM-β/γ-CD	carboxymethyl-β/γ- cyclodextrin
HP-β/γ-CD	hydroxypropyl-β/γ- cyclodextrin
HTM-β-CD	hydroxytrimethyl -β- cyclodextrin
HDAS-β-CD	heptakisdiacethylsulfo-β- cyclodextrin
SBE-β-CD	sulfobuthylether-β- cyclodextrin
ODAS-γ-CD	oktakisdiacethylsulfo-γ- cyclodextrin
DM-β-CD	dimethyl-β- cyclodextrin
HDM-β-CD	hydroxydimethyl-β- cyclodextrin
HS-β/γ-CD	highly sulphated-β/γ- cyclodextrin
SB-β-CD	sulfobuthyl-β- cyclodextrin
CDEKC	cyclodextrin mediated electrokinetic chromatography
CID	collision-induced dissociation
CE	capillary electrophoresis
CEC	capillary electrochromatography
CF-FAB	continuous-flow fast atom bombardment
CFGF	counter-flow gradient focusing
CGE	capillary gel electrophoresis
CME	centrifuge microextraction
CSEI	cation-selective exhaustive injection
CSP	chiral stationary phase
CTAC	cetyltrimethylammonium chloride
CV	coefficients of variance
CWEs	crown ethers
CZE	capillary zone electrophoresis
DAD	diode array detection
DMR	*N*-desmethylmirtazapine
DNA	deoxyribonucleic acid
DNP	6-O-desmethylnaproxen

DPJ	dynamic pH junction
EC	electrochemical detection
ECL	electrochemiluminiscent detection
EFGF	electric-field gradient focusing
EH	enzymatic hydrolysis
EK	electrokinetic injection
EKC	electrokinetic chromatography
EKS	electrokinetic supercharging
EME	electro membrane extraction
EOF	electroosmotic flow
ESI	electro spray ionization
FCCE	flow counterbalanced capillary electrophoresis
FESI	field-enhanced sample injection
FESS	field-enhanced sample stacking
FI	flow injection
FIA	flow injection analysis
FITC	fluorescein isothiocyanate
FMN	flavin mononucleotide
FMOC-C1	9-fluorenylmethyl chloroformate
FT-ICR	Fourier transform ion cyclotron resonance
GABA	γ–amino-*n*butyric acid
HD	hydrodynamic injection
HPLC	high performance liquid chromatography
HS-Cys	highly sulfated cyclosophoraoses
IEF	isoelectric focusing
IT	ion trap
ITP	isotachophoresis
ISP	Ion spray
L/LE	leading/leading electrolyte
LIF	laser induced fluorescence detection
LLE	liquid-liquid extraction
LOD	limit of detection
LOQ	limit of quantification
LPME	liquid-phase microextraction
LVSEP-ASEI	large volume sample stacking with EOF as a pump plus anion-selective exhaustive injection
LVSS	large volume sample stacking
MALDI	matrix assisted laser desorption ionisation
MCE	microchip capillary electrophoresis
MDA	3-4-methylenedioxyamphetamine
MDE	3,4-methalenedioxyethylamphetamine
MDMA	3,4-ethylenedioxymethamphetamine
MEEKC	microemulsion electrokinetic chromatography
MEKC	micellar electrokinetic chromatography
MLC	microcolumn liquid chromatography
MRT	mirtazapine

MS	mass spectrometry
NA	noradrenaline
NACE	non-aqueous capillary electrophoresis
NBD-F	4-fluoro-7-nitro-2,1,3-benzoxadiazole
NDA	naphthalene-2,3-dicarboxaldehyde
NMDA	N-methyl-D-aspartate
NMR	nuclear magnetic resonance
NSM	normal stacking mode
OPA/NAC	o-phthalaldehyde/N-acetyl-L-cysteine
PHM	pheniramine
PMT	photomultiplier tube
PP	protein precipitation
PVA	poly(vinyl alcohol)
QC	quality control
RE	relative error
RSD	relative standard deviation
SCCE	synchronous cyclic capillary electrophoresis
SDC	sodium deoxycholate
SDLIL	sodium *N*-[4-*n*-dodecyloxybenzoyl]-L-isoleucinate
SDLL	sodium *N*-[4-*n*-dodecyloxybenzoyl]-L-leucinate
SDME	SDME=single drop microextraction
SDS	sodium dodecyl sulfate
SI	sulindac sulfide
SO	sulindac sulfone
SPCD	sample preconcentration with chemical derivatization
SPD	(5S)-pinandiol
SPE	solid-phase extraction
SPME	solid-phase microextraction
SRMP	stacking with reverse migrating phase
SU	sulindac
SWP	sweeping
T/TE	terminator/terminating electrolyte
t-ITP	transient isotachophoresis
TGF	temperature gradient focusing
TOF	time-of-flight
TQ	triple quadrupole
UV	ultraviolet
VIS	visible
ZE	zone electrophoresis

9

Index

A

B

C

D

E

M

R

S

U

V

W

Z